COMPUTED TOMOGRAPHY – CLINICAL APPLICATIONS

Edited by **Luca Saba**

Computed Tomography – Clinical Applications
Edited by Luca Saba

Published by InTech
Janeza Trdine 9, 51000 Rijeka, Croatia

Publishing Process Manager Masa Vidovic

Technical Editor Teodora Smiljanic

Cover Designer InTech Design Team

Additional hard copies can be obtained from orders@intechopen.com

Computed Tomography – Clinical Applications, Edited by Luca Saba
p. cm.
ISBN 978-953-307-378-1

For EU product safety concerns:
IN TECH d.o.o., Prolaz Marije Krucifikse Kozulić 3, 51000 Rijeka, Croatia,
info@intechopen.com or visit our website at intechopen.com.

Meet the editor

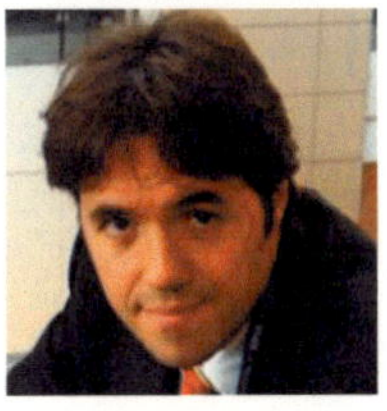

Dr. Luca Saba's research fields are focused on neuroradiology, multi-detector-row computed tomography, magnetic resonance, ultrasound, and diagnostics in vascular sciences. His work, as lead author, has been published more than 80 high impact factor, peer-reviewed journals as American Journal of Neuroradiology, European Radiology, European Journal of Radiology, Acta Radiologica, Cardiovascular and Interventional Radiology, Journal of Computer Assisted Tomography, American Journal of Roentgenology, Neuroradiology, Clinical Radiology, Journal of Cardiovascular Surgery, Cerebrovascular Diseases. Dr. Saba has written 7 book chapters and he presented more than 400 papers in national and international congresses (RSNA, ESGAR, ECR, ISR, AOCR, AINR, JRS, SIRM, AINR). He has also won 6 scientific and extracurricular awards during his career. Dr. Saba is member of the Italian Society of Radiology (SIRM), European Society of Radiology (ESR), Radiological Society of North America (RSNA), American Roentgen Ray Society (ARRS) and European Society of Neuroradiology (ESNR).

Contents

Preface

It is my pleasure to present this book entitled "Computed Tomography - Clinical Applications". Computed Tomography (CT) and in particular multi-detector-row computed tomography (MDCT), is a powerful non-invasive imaging tool with a number of advantages over the others non invasive imaging techniques.

CT has evolved into an indispensable imaging method in clinical routine. It was the first method to non-invasively acquire images of the inside of the human body that were not biased by superimposition of distinct anatomical structures.

The first generation of CT scanners developed in the 1970s and numerous innovations have improved the utility and application field of the CT, such as the introduction of helical systems that allowed the development of the "volumetric CT" concept.

A further major improvement in the CT technology is the incorporation of multiple detector row longitudinally (along the z-axis) in the gantry. In the 1998 it was proposed the first 4-detector row scanner and since then it were introduced 16-32-64-128 and 320 detector row units. A recent major improvement in the CT technology is the introduction of the dual source CT that promise exceptional potentialities in the tissue analysis and characterization. Isotropic voxels, high spatial and temporal resolution, use of fast contrast material injection rate and post-processing tools improved sensitivity and specificity of this technology in solving diagnostic medical problems.

In this book the purpose is to explore the applications of CT from medical imaging to other fields like archaeology and computer aided diagnosis. Recently interesting technical, anthropomorphic, forensic and archeological as well as paleontological applications of computed tomography have been developed. These applications further strengthen the method as a generic diagnostic tool for non-destructive material testing and three-dimensional visualization beyond its medical use.

Luca Saba, MD
Department of Science of the Images,
Policlinico Universitario,
University of Cagliari,
Italy

Part 1

Clinical Application

1

Computer-Aided Diagnosis for Acute Stroke in CT Images

Yongbum Lee, Noriyuki Takahashi and Du-Yih Tsai
Niigata University
Japan

1. Introduction

The mortality rate for cerebrovascular disease is approximately ten percents in all deaths in the world (World Health Organization [WHO], 2002). The cerebrovascular disease is a major cause of disability and is one of the three leading causes of death with heart disease and malignant neoplasm in several countries, e.g. Japan (Health and Welfare Statistics Association, 2004). Acute cerebral infarction is one of the major cerebrovascular diseases, and detection of its early signs is very important for survival and convalescence. Currently, computed tomography (CT) is still the most commonly used imaging modality in the diagnosis of acute cerebral infarction because of its wide availability and examination speed, though the advanced magnetic resonance (MR) imaging is superior to the non-enhanced CT in respect of sensitivity in the detection of cerebral ischemia within the first few hours after symptom onset (Adams et al., 2003, 2005). With the introduction of thrombolysis, much attention has been directed to identify early CT signs, which are subtle early signs of ischemic changes on CT images, over the last decade (Kummer et al., 1997; Wardlaw et al., 1999; Barber et al., 2000). Detection of early CT signs is of importance in middle cerebral artery (MCA) strokes within the first few hours of the onset of symptoms.
Computer-aided diagnosis (CAD) for detection of early CT signs must contribute to the improvement of diagnostic accuracy for acute stroke. Therefore, we developed some fundamental techniques to enhance/detect early CT signs. In this chapter, we describe two techniques to be used in CAD for acute stroke. By each technique, early CT signs are enhanced, visualized, detected and classified, respectively.

2. Enhancement of early CT signs

One of the notable early CT signs is the loss of gray-white matter interface, e.g. lenticular nuclei, due to the hypoattenuating appearance of gray matter structures (Tomura et al., 1988; Truwit et al., 1990). However, because of the subtle appearance of the loss of gray-white matter interface resulting from image noise, the radiologists may not be able to visually identify it (Schriger et al., 1998; Wardlaw & Mielke, 2005).
Recently technological innovation of CT units has dramatically advanced, so that image noise originated by the CT unit itself can be negligible. However, quantum noise due to X-ray quanta registered by the image detector cannot be prevented, even though using an ideal CT unit (Kaleder, 2000). The quantum noise degrades the visibility of low-contrast

structures such as normal gray-white matter interface on CT images. Under this condition, one can hardly recognize the normal gray-white matter interface on CT images, much less the loss of the gray-white matter interface due to cerebral ischemia. To solve this problem, it is necessary to improve the visibility of normal gray-white matter interface by removing or reducing the quantum noise with any ways. High-dose CT, for example, can reduce the quantum noise. However, this results in increasing patient radiation exposure. Hence, image processing techniques may become appropriate ways to reduce the quantum noise and consequently to improve the visibility of normal gray-white matter interface on CT images. Although various advanced digital filters for reducing image noise on CT images have been reported. However, these filters were mainly designed to deal with the reduction of radiation dose (Kalra et al., 2003; Kachelriess et al., 2001). In the present study, we focused on directly improving the visibility of normal gray-white matter interface on non-enhanced CT images by using a noise reduction filter. We believe that if noise is reduced, then the normal gray-white matter interface can be relatively enhanced. As a result, the loss of gray-white matter interface due to stroke could be more detectable. An exclusive smoothing filter is desirable to eliminate the quantum noise with almost no blurring of the edge of gray-white matter interface. To overcome this issue, an adaptive partial median filter (APMF) was proposed (Lee et al., 2007). The algorithm of APMF refers to Guis's contrast enhancement method (Guis et al., 2003) and is based on adaptive partial averaging filter (APAF) previously reported (Tsai et al., 2005; Lee et al., 2006; Takahashi et al., 2007). The distinction between APAF and APMF is simply the difference between "averaging" and "median" in a step of procedure. The APMF has a characteristic: noise can be reduced without degrading signal, i.e., edge. In the field of image processing, various image filtering techniques for noise reduction have been reported (Russ, 1995; Tukey, 1971; Davis & Rosenfeld, 1978; Wu et al., 1992; Ehrich, 1978; Lev et al., 1977; Wang et al., 1981; Nagao & Matuyama, 1978; Zamperoni, 1990; Xu et al., 2004; Kuan et al. 1985; Centeno & Haertel, 1997; Fischl & Shwarts, 1999; Westin et al., 2000; Schilham et al., 2006; Gijbels et al., 2006), and almost of them were edge-preserving smoothing techniques. The novel denoising technique, namely APMF, was compared to 14 conventional smoothing techniques by criterion-referenced performance study. Simulated CT images with gray-white matter interfaces were used for the study. Next, APMF was applied to a clinical database for application to actual clinical cases for preliminary observer performance study. Its usefulness was evaluated by receiver operator characteristic (ROC) analysis.

2.1 Adaptive partial median filter

The APMF is a specially designed filter with local median processing using a variable filter size and shape. The APMF's main steps are as follows, and illustrations corresponding to each step of APMF procedure are shown in Fig. 1.

Step 1. An averaging filter with $M \times M$ mask size is applied to the original image.

Step 2. A window image whose initial size is $W_{max} \times W_{max}$ is assigned from the original image after the averaging filter. W_{max} is a positive odd number from 3.

Step 3. A mask image is generated by assigning a binary mask value 0 if $|I(i, j)-I(i_c, j_c)|>T$, and by assigning a binary mask value 1 if $|I(i, j)-I(i_c, j_c)|\leq T$. $I(i_c, j_c)$ and $I(i, j)$ are defined as the pixel value of the center pixel and the pixel value of an arbitrary pixel in the window image, respectively.

83	82	72	65	75	73	72	62	44
82	83	79	75	66	64	67	68	43
73	67	67	53	53	34	45	44	54
62	69	83	77	56	54	52	47	53
71	62	68	59	**55**	51	49	59	32
88	43	46	48	64	62	48	62	31
90	67	64	55	53	55	46	44	45
67	66	52	50	46	48	42	48	49
68	44	48	47	42	49	71	63	81

(a)

0	0	0	1	0	0	0	1	0
0	0	0	0	0	1	0	0	0
0	0	0	1	1	0	1	0	1
1	0	0	0	1	1	1	1	1
0	1	0	1	1	1	1	1	0
0	0	1	1	1	1	1	1	0
0	0	1	1	1	1	1	0	1
0	0	1	1	1	1	0	1	1
0	0	1	1	0	1	0	1	0

(b)

0	1	1
1		1
1	1	1

P_0=12.5%

0	1	1	0	1
0				1
0				1
1				1
1	1	1	1	1

P_0=25.0%

0	0	0	0	1	0	0
0						0
0						1
1						1
0						1
0						0
0	1	1	1	1	0	1

P_0=58.3%

0	0	0	1	0	0	0	1	0
0								0
0								1
1								1
0								0
0								0
0								1
0								1
0	0	1	1	0	1	0	1	0

P_0=65.6%

(c)

83	79	75	66	64	67	68
67	67	53	53	34	45	44
69	83	77	56	54	52	47
62	68	59	**55**	51	49	59
43	46	48	64	62	48	62
67	64	55	53	55	46	44
66	52	50	46	48	42	48

(d)

Fig. 1. An example corresponding to each step of APMF procedure. (a) A window image (W_{max}=9) in Step 2. (b) Assigned mask image from (a) in case of T=10 in Step 3. (c) Calculation of the percentage of P_0 of external area at W=[3, 5, 7, 9] in Step 4. When P=60%, W=7 are determined as actual window size. (d) Median value obtained from pixel values (in dark gray pixels) corresponding with mask value 1 in the mask image (W=7) replaces the center pixel value [$I(i_c, j_c)$=55 changes to $I(i_c, j_c)$=53].

Step 4. For each window size $W \times W$ [W = 3, 5, ..., W_{max}], the percentage P_0 of 0 in the mask image is computed over the region of external area of each window image. Actual window size is determined when the percentage P_0 is not greater than P%, and is closest to P%.

Step 5. Finally, a median value is obtained from the pixel values $I(i, j)$ corresponding with mask value 1 in mask image, and the median value is used as output value at the center pixel value $I(i_c, j_c)$.

Step 6. Steps 2-5 are performed at each pixel.

Step 1 is related to differentiating between the object pixel value $I(i_c, j_c)$ and the surrounding pixel value $I(i, j)$ described in Step 3. As noise superimposed on the object pixel has to be initially reduced, otherwise the APMF will not perform well. Step 3 is based on an assumption that variation of pixel values due to noise is smaller than the difference of pixel values due to signal, and is an important process to distinguish between noise and signal components. In Step 4, actual window size will be small to enhance the quality of edge preserving if there are many pixels with pixel values larger than T in window image. In contrast, the actual window size will be large to enhance the noise reduction rate if pixel values in window image are almost uniform. As for APAF, "median" is just replaced to "averaging" in Step 5.

The performance of the APMF depends on parameters M, W_{max}, T and P. In particular, T is very important parameter because it determines rough boundary of object, e.g. lenticular nuclei on a CT image. T distinguishes object region (mask value 1) and background region (mask value 0). Then only pixel values in object region are used for computation. It means that the APMF is able to reduce local noise while preserving edge components between object and background regions. Therefore, T for application to clinical images was obtained by a simulation study described in the next section. The other parameters of M=5, W_{max}=13, and P=60 were determined using the rule of trial and error on simulated images to be described in the next section.

2.2 Objective performance test

The simulation study has two purposes. One is to determine an adequate parameter of T for application to clinical CT images. The other one is to validate the superiority of the APMF by comparing with conventional smoothing techniques. Composite images with simulated white matter (SWM) and simulated gray matter (SGM) were used for this simulation. First, in order to obtain the simulated SWM, cylindrical phantom which was Catphan CT phantom CTP486 made by The Phantom Laboratories, Inc. was scanned by CT device which was Somatom Volume Zoom made by Siemens-Asahi Medical Technologies Ltd.. Then, the SGM was put on the CT image. Concretely, 3~6HU (Hounsfield Unit) was added to the SWM by computation because the contrast of normal gray-white matter interface was approximately 6HU, and the contrast of ischemic gray-white matter interface deteriorated to approximately 3HU. Fig.2 shows a simulation image and its sketch.

The size of simulation image shown in Fig.2 is 300×300 pixels. This is a part of original image whose size is 512×512 pixels. Edge slope between SWM and SGM on the dotted line in sketch of Fig.2 has been generated as shown in Fig.3. C_x in Fig.3 corresponds to the abscissa of the dotted line in sketch of Fig.2. The *cnt* in Fig.3 corresponds to the contrast between SWM and SWM, which is 3~6HU. The CT scan specifications were Tube Voltage 120kV, Tube Current 200~400mAs, Slice Thickness 10mm, FOV (field of view) 250mm, and matrix size 512×512. The phantom was scanned ten times under the same condition, and then ten composite images were generated under the same condition to restrain variation of evaluation values that will be described in the next paragraph. The total number of simulation images was 120 which was obtained by 4 contrast levels (3~6HU, interval of 1 HU) × 3 noise levels (200~400mAs, interval of 100mAs) × 10 scans.

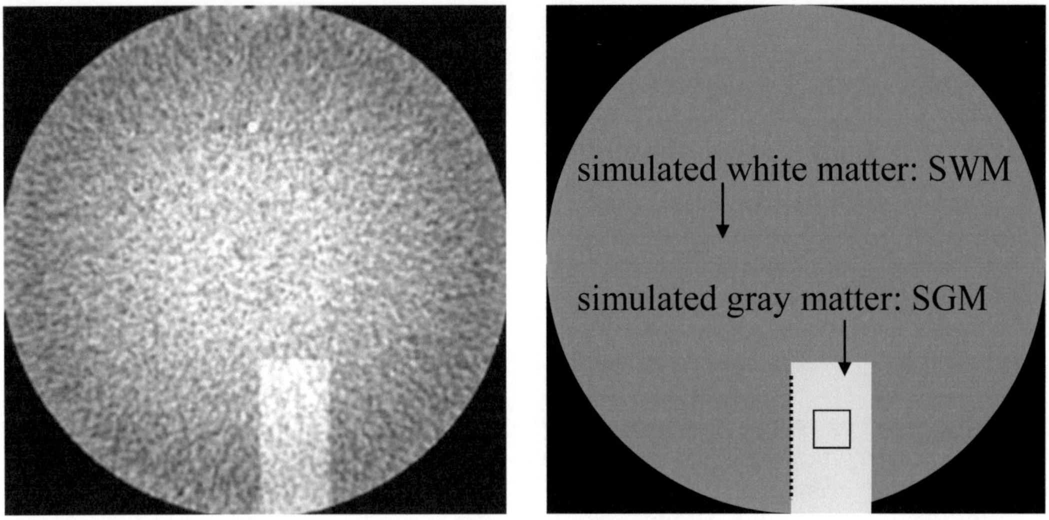

Fig. 2. A simulation image (left: 400mAs, 6HU) and its sketch (right). Dotted line in the sketch suggests a vertical edge line of 80 pixels length for ESR calculation. Its horizontal coordinate value is C_x. Square in the sketch suggests a region for SDR calculation. Its size is 20×20 pixels.

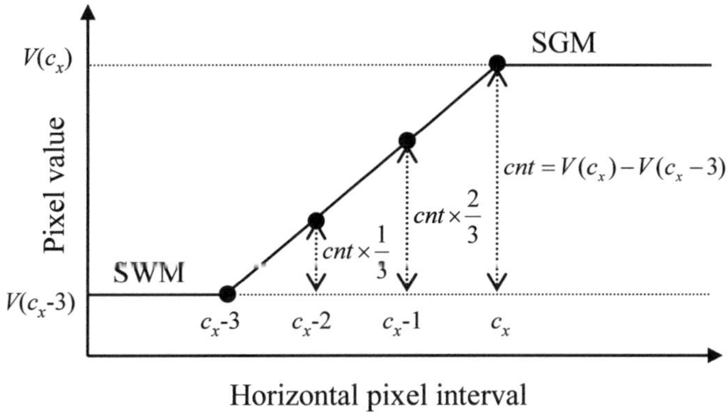

Fig. 3. Explanatory diagram with regard to edge slope of SGM-SWM interface.

The standard deviation rate (SDR) and edge slope rate (ESR) were used as two criteria for measuring the performance of the APMF and the conventional smoothing techniques. The standard deviation of the pixel values in a specified area, which was used to quantify the degree of noise reduction, was obtained from a region of 20×20 pixels on the SGM, as shown in Fig.2. To investigate the extent of edge preserving, edge slope rate was calculated from an average profile of pixel values, which was measured at the horizontal direction with respect to the edge on the dotted line shown in Fig.2. The standard deviation rate was computed by Equation (1).

$$SDR(\%) = \left(SD_{org} - SD_{prc}\right) / SD_{org} \times 100 \tag{1}$$

SD_{org} is an average standard deviation calculated from ten original composite images, and SD_{prc} is an average standard deviation calculated from ten processed images. The edge slope rate was computed by Equation (2).

$$ESR(\%) = ES_{prc} / ES_{org} \times 100 \tag{2}$$

ES_{org} is an average edge slope value calculated from ten original composite images, and ES_{prc} is an average edge slope value calculated from ten processed images. Those are defined as Equation (3) and as shown in Fig.3. High SDR means that the noise is decreased well. High ESR means that the edge is highly preserved.

$$ES = \left\{V(C_x) - V(C_x - 3)\right\} / 3 \tag{3}$$

The APMF was compared to 14 conventional smoothing filters, namely, averaging filter (AF) (Russ, 1995), median filter (MF) (Tukey, 1971), gaussian filter (GF) (Russ, 1995), k-nearest neighbor averaging (KNNA) (Davis & Rosenfeld, 1978), k-nearest neighbor median (KNNM) (Wu et al. 1992), hysteresis smoothing (HS) (Ehrich, 1978), edge and line weights smoothing (ELWS) (Lev et al., 1977), contrast sensitive weights smoothing (CSWS) (Lev et al., 1977), gradient inverse weighted smoothing (GIWS) (Wang et al., 1981), Nagao's edge preserving smoothing (EPS) (Nagao & Matuyama, 1978), adaptive rank order filter (AROF) (Zamperoni, 1990), adaptive two pass median filter (ATPMF) (Xu et al., 2004), adaptive noise smoothing filter (ANSF) (Kuan et al., 1985), and adaptive partial averaging filter (APAF) (Tsai et al., 2005, Lee et al., 2006, Takahashi et al., 2007) which was a basis of APMF. The SDR and ESR of each method were calculated from the processed composite images obtained by varying Tube Current (200, 300, 400mAs) and the contrast (3, 4, 5, 6HU) between SGM and SWM. As a sample of results, Fig.4 shows graphs of SDR and ESR in the case of 400mAs, 6HU. For those methods with variable filter size (FS), namely, AF, MF, GF, KNNA, KNNM, AROF, ATPMF and ANSF, the filter size was used as variable of the horizontal axis on the graphs. This means that SDR and ESR were calculated by varying filter size. For those methods with fixed filter size, namely, ELWS, CSWS, GIWS, and EPS, the number of iteration (NI) was used as variable of the horizontal axis on the graphs. This means that SDR and ESR were calculated by varying the number of iteration. HS has an only parameter of *Width* which is an established hysteresis cursor size, and is at least equal to the size of the largest waveform peak or valley to be removed (Ehrich, 1978). Therefore, the Width was used as variable of the horizontal axis on the graph of HS. The parameters of APAF are the same with the parameters of APMF because the difference between APAF and APMF is only whether the output value at the center pixel value $I(i_c, j_c)$ in Step 5 is the averaging value or the median value. Therefore, the parameter T was used as variable of the horizontal axis on the graph of APAF, as that of APMF. Other parameters as shown in Table 1, which were σ of GF and CSWS, a and b of ATPMF, and k of KNNA and KNNM, were determined experimentally by referring to the respective literatures.

Method	Parameters	SDR(%)	ESR(%)
Adaptive partial median filter (APMF)	M=5, Wmax=13, P=60, T=3	76.0	71.7
Adaptive partial averaging filter (APAF) [16],[17]	M=5, Wmax=13, P=60, T=3	75.6	64.0
Averaging filter (AF) [18]	FS=13	76.4	23.6
Median filter (MF) [19]	FS=15	76.1	33.1
Gaussian filter (GF) [18]	FS=55, σ=(FS-1)/4	76.1	31.2
Adaptive two pass median filter (ATPMF) [27]	FS=13, a=1, b=1	75.4	49.9
Adaptive noise smoothing filter (ANSF) [28]	FS=15	76.0	30.6
Edge and line weights smoothing (ELWS) [23]	NI=93	76.0	51.4
Contrast sensitive weights smoothing (CSWS) [23]	NI=20, σ=50	76.0	31.3
Hysteresis smoothing (HS) [22]	Width=5	35.0	69.7
k-nearest neighbor averaging (KNNA) [20]	FS=37, k=FS×FS/2	40.7	72.0
k-nearest neighbor median (KNNM) [21]	FS=31, k=FS×FS/2	47.9	71.5
Adaptive rank order filter (AROF) [26]	FS=7, k=eq.(6) in [26]	54.0	68.7
Gradient inverse weighted smoothing (GIWS) [24]	NI=352	49.5	71.7
Edge preserving smoothing (EPS) [25]	NI=10	20.1	86.7

Table 1. List of compared methods and comparison results.

Table 1 shows specific values of SDR and ESR extracted from the graphs in Fig.4. The specific values were based on SDR and ESR of APMF at T=3. We supposed that T=3 was the best value of T because ESR at T=3 was highest, and SDR at T=3 was almost highest. The details of this topic will be described in the next paragraph. In regard to AF, MF, GF, ELWS, CSWS, ATPMF, ANSF and APAF, the values of ESR were selected out when the values of SDR became closest to the SDR (76.0%) of APMF. In regard to the others that were KNNA, KNNM, HS, AROF, GIWS and ESP, the values of SDR were selected out when the values of ESR became closest to the ESR (71.7%) of APMF because the values of SDR did not become close to the SDR of APMF. In Table 1, highest ESR was 71.7% of APMF at the almost same SDR, and then in order, it was 64.0% of APAF, 51.4% of ELWS, and 49.9% of ATPMF. The ESR of the others, which were AF, MF, GF and CSWS, were less than 34.0%. In comparison in a condition of almost same ESR, highest SDR was 76.0% of APMF, and then the SDR of the others, which were KNNA, KNNM, HS, AROF, GIWS and EPS, were less than 55.0%. The processed images by each method with parameters shown in Table 1 are shown in Fig.5. These are parts of processed images around SGM-SWM interface. The image qualities are well consistent with the criterion values shown in Table 1. These comparison results clearly indicated that the APMF had the highest performance among the compared methods. The all results in conditions by varying Tube Current (200, 300, 400mAs) and the contrast (3, 4, 5, 6HU) between SGM and SWM had the same tendencies (Fig.6).

Clinical brain CT images used in this study were scanned by the ProSeed Accell made by GE Yokogawa Medical System, whose specifications were Tube Voltage 120kV, Tube Current 400mAs, Slice Thickness 10mm, FOV 250mm, and matrix size 512×512. These specifications correspond to those for sample graph of APMF shown in Fig.4. Therefore, an adequate T could be determined by referring to the simulation result of APMF as shown in Fig.4. SDR almost stop increasing from T>3, and ESR began to decrease sharply from T>3 (the peak at T=3).

Fig.7 shows the processed images obtained by varying the threshold value T [0, 1, 2, 3, 4, 5, 6] of APMF. The APMF image at T=3 looks very well with regard to edge sharpness and noise reduction. The APMF images at T=0, 1, 2 are insufficient on the degree of noise reduction, and the APMF images at T=4, 5, 6 are too blurry. Considering these data, T=3

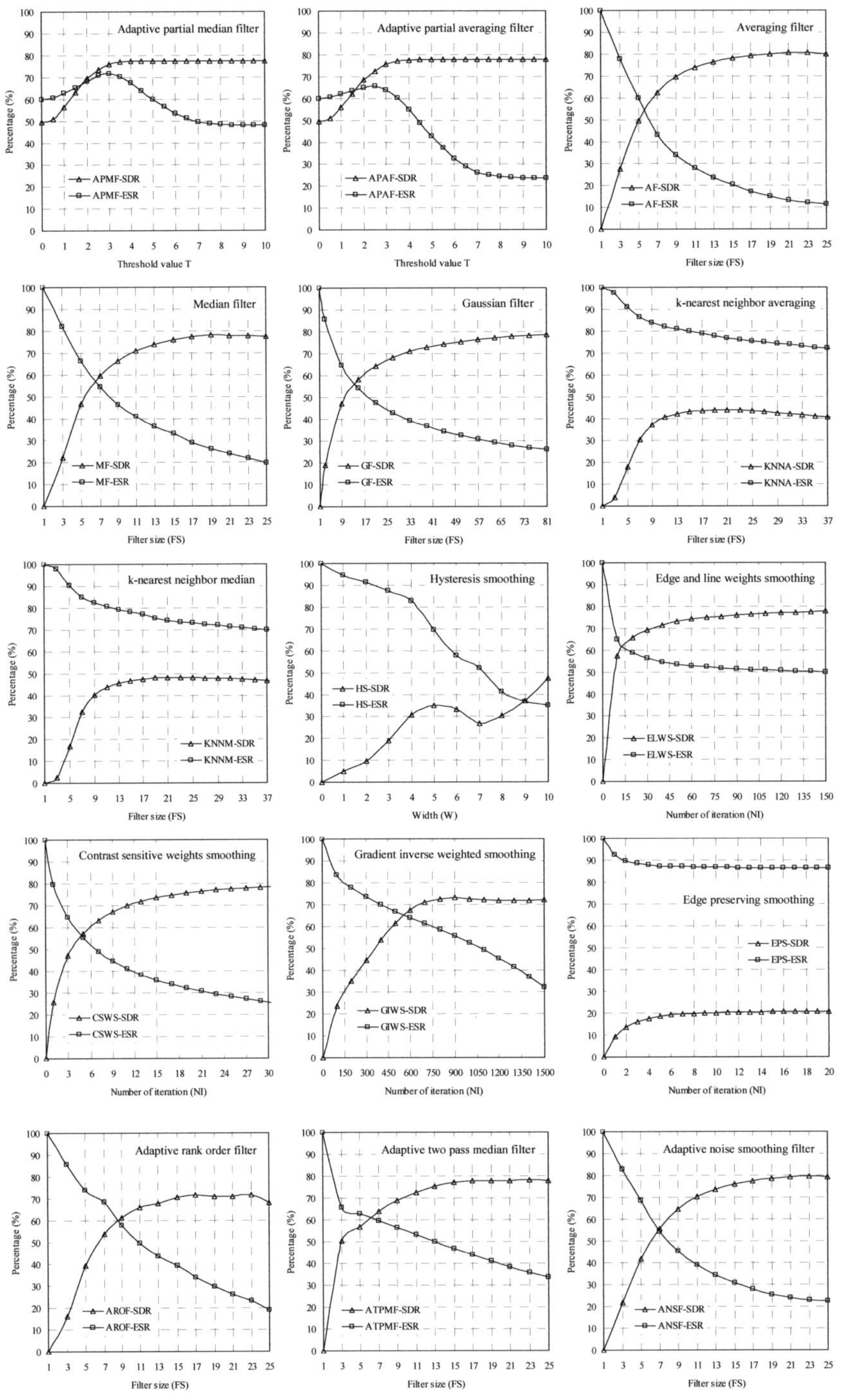

Fig. 4. Graphs of SDR and ESR obtained from simulation images in condition of 400mAs, 6HU.

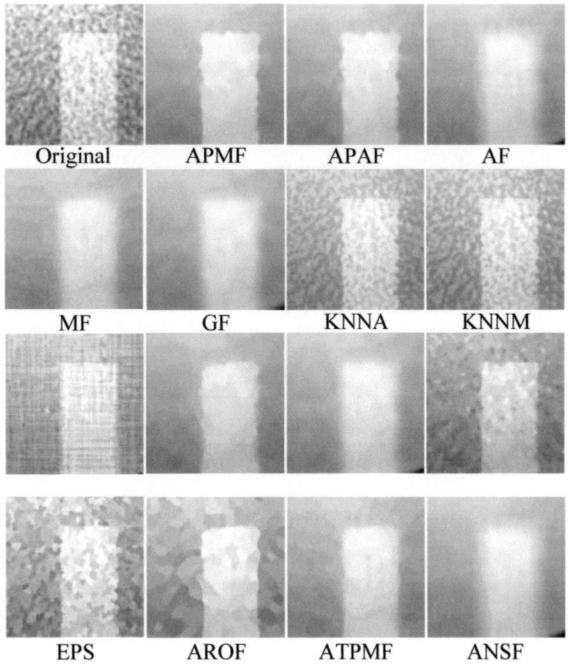

Fig. 5. Various processed images (400mAs, 6HU) with parameters in Table 1.

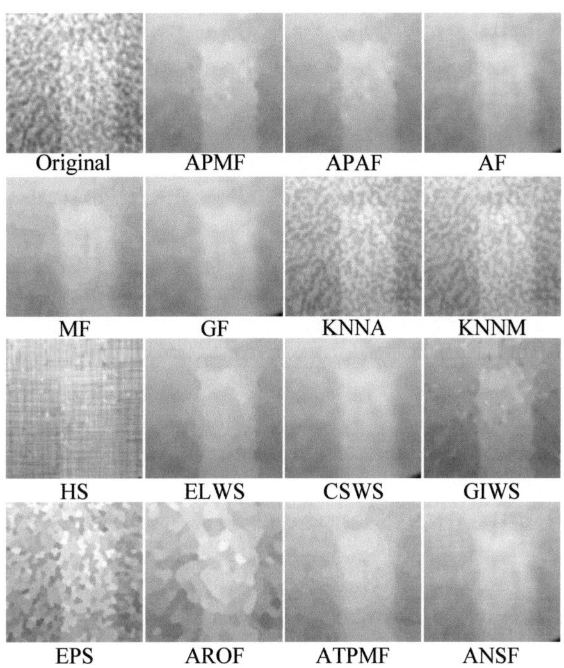

Fig. 6. Various processed images (400mAs, 3HU) corresponding to either SDR≈75% or ESR≈49%. These numerical values were obtained from APMF images.

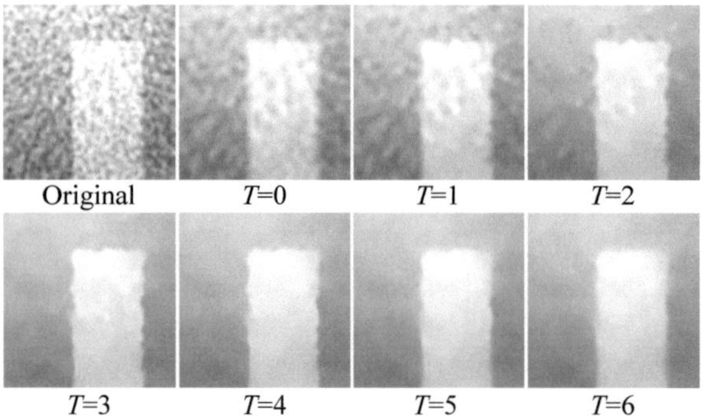

Fig. 7. APMF processed images (400mAs, 6HU) by varying T.

might be an adequate threshold value in the condition of 400mAs and on the assumption that the contrast of gray-white matter interface on clinical brain CT image was approximately 6HU. Therefore, *T*=3 was determined as an adequate parameter for applying to clinical CT images in this study.

2.3 Subjective performance test

The APMF at *T*=3 was applied to 51 non-enhanced brain CT images which consisted of 18 abnormal images and 33 normal images, and then observer study with ROC analysis was performed by 4 radiologists. The abnormal images were obtained from 18 patients (mean age, 74 years) with acute (within 5 hours) cerebral infarction, and all of them showed subtle loss of the gray-white matter interface in the cortical ribbon and/or in the lentiform nucleus. The normal images were obtained from 33 control patients (mean age, 68 years). Two samples of abnormal cases used in this study are shown in Fig.8. A sample supplies three CT images, which are original image, APMF image and follow-up image obtained several days after the onset of symptoms. The original image of case 1 illustrated on the upper left in Fig.8 was obtained in an 83-year-old-female with right hemiplegia at 2.4 hours after stroke onset. The APMF image shows that the loss of the gray-white matter interface at the left lentiform nucleus, the so-called obscured outline of the lentiform nucleus, is clearly detectable (arrows). The outline of the right normal lentiform nucleus is obviously visible compared to the corresponding contralateral one. The follow-up image demonstrates infarction in the left middle cerebral artery (MCA) and anterior cerebral artery (ACA) distributions. The original image of case 2 illustrated on the lower left in Fig.8 was obtained in an 83-year-old-male with right hemiplegia at 1.5 hours after stroke onset. The APMF image shows that the loss of the gray-white matter interface of posterior part of the left lentiform nucleus is clearly detectable. The follow-up image demonstrates infarction in the left middle cerebral artery (MCA) and posterior cerebral artery (PCA) distributions. Two samples vividly indicated that early CT signs of acute cerebral infarction were remarkably enhanced in the APMF images.

Four radiologists including two attending radiologists (years of experience, 14-18 years) and two radiology resident (years of experience, 1-3 years) independently interpreted the cases on the monitor for this observer study. First diagnostic decisions of them were determined by interpreting only original images. Window width (WW) and window level (WL) were free in their interpreting. Although there were some reports that diagnostic accuracy would be improved by using narrow WW in interpreting on the monitor (Lev et al., 1999), narrow

WW enhances not only edge such as gray-white matter interface but quantum noise in non-enhanced CT image. Therefore, default WW and WL for original images were 80 and 35HU, respectively, because it was the general condition for diagnosis in radiologist's daily work in Japan. After first interpreting, they could correct their decisions by reinterpreting both original and the APMF images. Default WW and WL for the APMF images were 20 and 35HU, respectively. Narrow WW was used for the APMF images as default condition because quantum noises were sufficiently decreased by APMF. Narrow WW after decreasing noises in the APMF images enhances only edges such as gray-white matter interface. The radiologists indicated their confidence rating regarding the presence or absence of early CT sign on each case. The scale of confidence rating ranged from 0 to 100. A computer program (LABMRMC; Charles E. Metz, University of Chicago) (Dolfman et al., 1992) was used for obtaining ROC curves and the statistical significance of the difference between the ROC curves by only original images and by original images with APMF images.

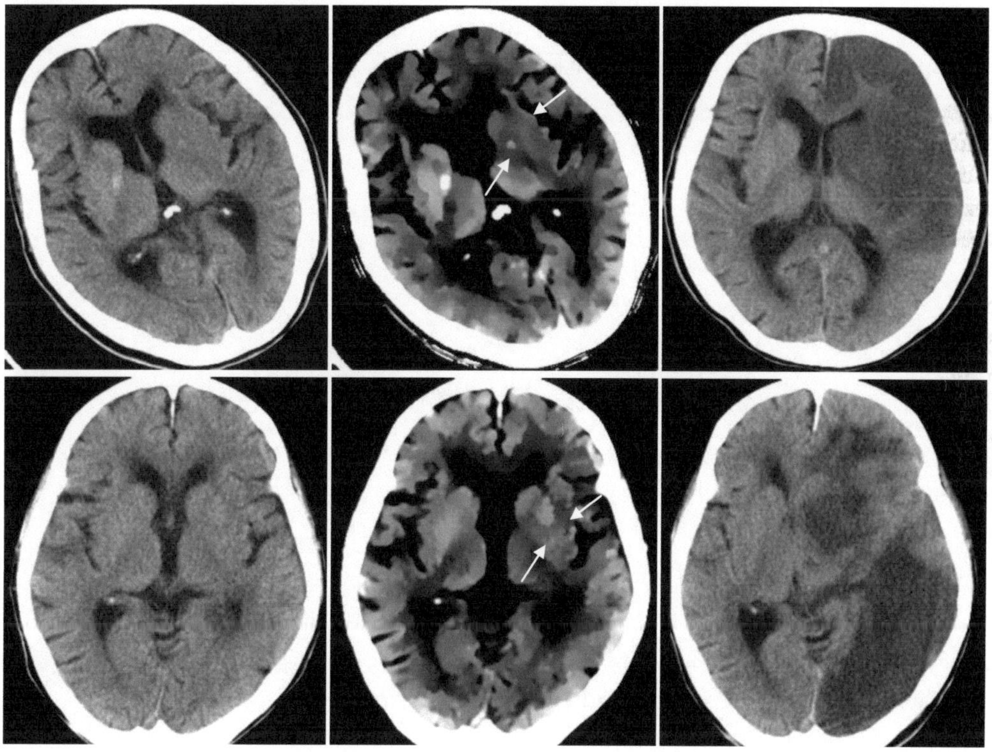

Fig. 8. Two examples of abnormal cases. Lefts are original images (WL=35, WW=80). Middles are APMF images (WL=35, WW=20). Rights are follow-up images obtained several days after the onset of symptoms (WL=35, WW=80). Arrows indicate obscuration of the lentiform nucleus.

The area under the ROC curves plotted in the unit square (A_z) was calculated for each fitted curve. The overall performance is illustrated in Table 2 and Fig.9. Table 2 shows the A_z values without the APMF images and with the APMF images for each radiologist. Figure 9 shows the average ROC curves of four radiologists without the APMF images and with the APMF images. The performance of all observers was improved when the APMF image was used. The average A_z values for all radiologists increased from 0.876 without the APMF images to 0.926 with the APMF images, and this difference was statistically significant (P=0.04). This preliminary result of observer study is suggesting that the APMF can be an useful technique for diagnosis of acute cerebral infarction in non-enhanced CT images. The observer performance study using much more cases and by more observers would be required to more clearly prove the usefulness of APMF to clinical cases in the future work. We believe that the results from two performance studies demonstrate the usefulness of APMF.

	Az value	
Observer	Only original images	Original + APMF images
A	0.912	0.952
B	0.881	0.922
C (resident)	0.842	0.914
D (resident)	0.866	0.916
Mean	0.876	0.926

Note.-The difference was statistically significant with a *P* value of 0.04.

Table 2. A_z values for each observer.

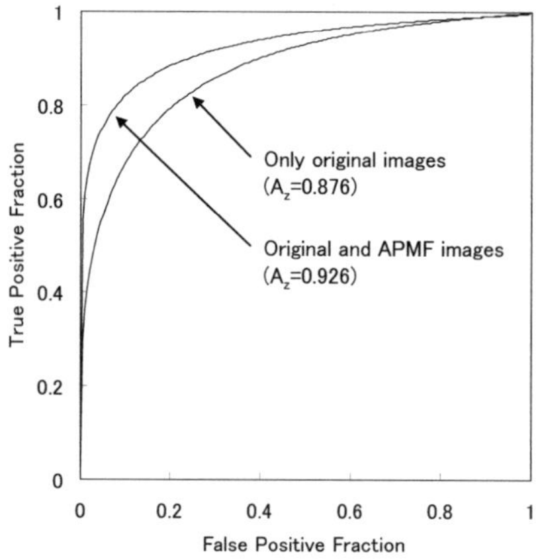

Fig. 9. Average ROC curves of four radiologists for diagnosis of acute stroke from brain CT images without the APMF images and with the APMF images.

3. Detection of hypoattenuation in CT images

Unenhanced computed tomographic (CT) imaging still plays an important role in the assessment of eligible patients for receiving thrombolytic therapy for hyperacute ischemic stroke, because of its wide accessibility and convenience, although diffusion-weighted MR imaging (DWI) in acute stroke has been supported (Adams et al., 2003, 2005). Patients showing large ischemic lesions (parenchymal hypoattenuation or brain swelling) on CT images have a high risk of fatal hemorrhagic complications after thrombolytic therapy (Kummer et al., 1997; Barber et al., 2000; Kalafut et al., 2000). Therefore, quantification of the extent of areas of ischemic lesions appeared on CT images is mandatory to avoid the risk. However, because the detection of hypoattenuation (a subtle attenuation change of ischemic brain tissue) is difficult, inter-rater homogeneity is poor in the assessment of the extent of areas of ischemic lesions (Fiebach et al. 2002). Thus, the detectability of hypoattenuation largely depends on the skill and experiences of the interpreters (Schriger et al., 1998; Wardlaw et al., 2005). To cope with this issue, a quantitative CT scoring system, the Alberta Stroke Programme Early CT Score (ASPECTS) (Barber et al., 2000), has been proposed to help interpreters in quantifying the extent of ischemic lesions in the territory of the middle cerebral artery (MCA). However, the sensitivity for the detection of acute stroke was less than 50% on unenhanced CT images, even when the ASPECTS method was used (Camargo et al., 2007).

Recently, a *z*-score mapping method on the basis of a voxel-by-voxel analysis has been developed to assist interpreters in quantifying the extent of hypoattenuation regions of hyperacute ischemic stroke on unenhanced CT images (Takahashi et al., 2010a, 2010b). The method was applied to patients with the MCA territory infarction within 3 hours of symptom onset for its performance test. The result of the test has shown that the method is effective in the visualization of hypoattenuation areas. However, observer performance study on the quantification of the extent of hypoattenuation regions of hyperacue stroke by use of the method has not yet been made.

We evaluated the usefulness of the *z*-score mapping method on neuroradiologists' performance in the quantification of the extent of hypoattenuation regions of hyperacute stroke using the ASPECTS score system. Accuracies of the quantification without and with the *z*-score maps were calculated to evaluate observers' performance in the quantification of the extent of hypoattenuation regions. Moreover, receiver operating characteristic (ROC) analysis was used to evaluate observers' performance in the detection of focal hypoattenuation.

3.1 Z-score mapping method

Z-score mapping method (Takahashi et al., 2010a, 2010b) consisted of five main steps, i.e., anatomic standardization, the construction of a normal reference database, calculation of the *z*-score, the elimination of cerebrospinal fluid (CSF) areas, and display of *z*-score maps.

First, all data sets were transformed into a standard brain atlas using Statistical Parametric Mapping 2 (SPM2) software (The Welcome Department of Cognitive Neurology, London, United Kingdom) (Friston et al., 1995; Ashbumer & Friston, 1999). The matrix size used for normalization was 79×95×69 voxels (2-mm anisotropic voxel size). Processed data sets were then smoothed with a 4-mm full width at half maximum isotropic Gaussian kernel.

Second, two normal data sets for reference were constructed by computing the averages and standard deviations (SDs) of image voxel values from the normalized CT database. The CT database was comprised of 28 normal controls.

Third, the *z*-score was calculated on a voxel-by-voxel basis as shown in Fig.10 and was defined as Equation (4).

$$Z-score_{(x,y,z)} = \left(C_{mean(x,y,z)} - Input_{(x,y,z)}\right) \Big/ N_{SD(x,y,z)} \quad (4)$$

$C_{mean}(x, y, z)$ and $N_{SD}(x, y, z)$ represent the mean and standard deviation of the normal reference data at the coordinate of (x, y, z), respectively. $Input(x, y, z)$ is the value of spatially normalized patient data set at the same coordinate system. Before the calculation of *z*-scores, an offset was used to remove variation among patients in attenuation coefficients of the normal brain parenchyma on unenhanced CT images.

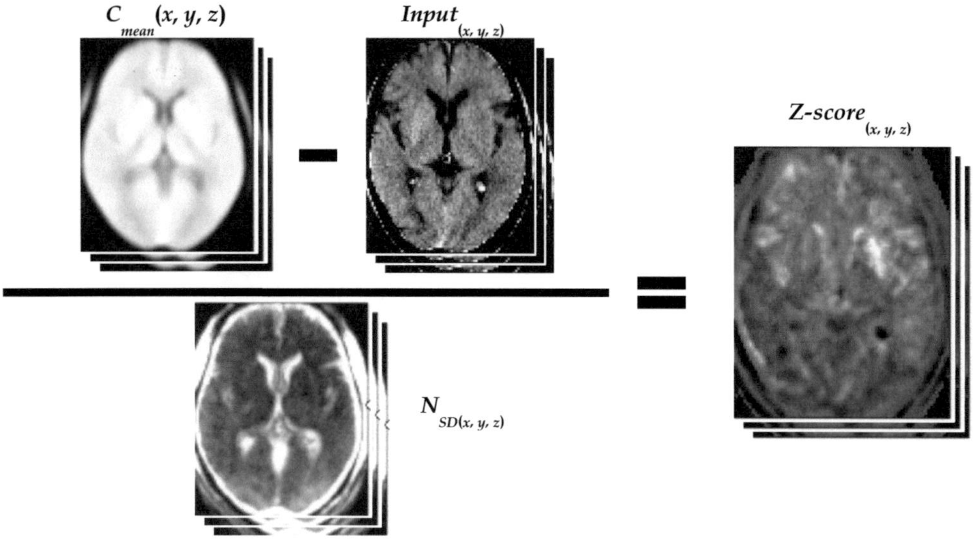

Fig. 10. Calculation of *z*-score for input CT scan

In the fourth step, CSF areas which may give rise to false-positive (FP) results, were eliminated from *z*-score data set by use of a gray-scale thresholding technique (Fig.11). Note that CT values of CSF areas may be lower than those of hypoattenuation areas. Therefore, after using adaptive thresholding, the CSF areas can be removed while maintaining hypoattenution areas. After the elimination of CSF areas, the area of the brain parenchyma except the MCA territory was also removed from the *z*-score data set.

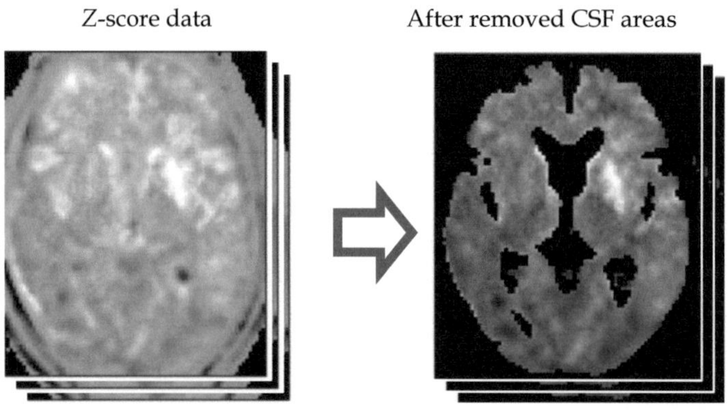

Fig. 11. Elimination of false positive areas.

Finally, the normalized input CT data set and the *z*-score map were reconstructed with a slice thickness of 4 mm. The *z*-score map was then superimposed on the normalized CT data set and was color-coded to reflect ranges of *z*-scores, as shown in Fig.12. Small clusters having 50 voxels or less were removed from the z-score map before displaying the z-score map.

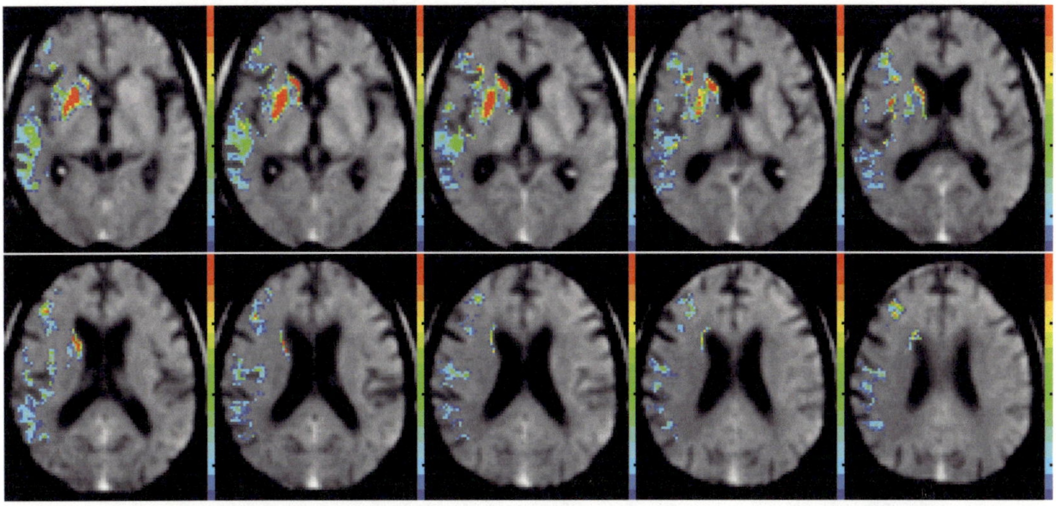

Fig. 12. Display of z-score maps.

3.2 Observer performance study

Data from 34 consecutive patients with embolic infarction in the MCA territory stroke who underwent unenhanced CT scan at Sendai City Hospital, Sendai, Japan, between April 2007 and December 2008 were collected for this study. From the 34 collected CT files, 21 patients were selected using the following inclusion criteria: (1) the first CT scan was performed within 3 hours after stroke onset, and (2) no patients had evidence of old infarctions. The 21 patients consisted of 14 men and 7 women (age range, 46-92 years; mean age, 66.5 years). The median National Institute of Health Stroke Scale score was 12 (range, 1-27) in the 21 patients. All patients underwent the first unenhanced CT scan within 3 hours (mean, 1.86 hours; range, 0.67-3 hours) after the onset of stroke ictus. All images were acquired using a 16-slice multidetector CT scanner (Emotion16; Siemens Medical Solutions, Forchheim, Germany). At our institution, CT scans are routinely obtained using a matrix size of 512×512 and a field of view of 230 mm, with 4.8-mm contiguous sections. Figure 13 shows 10 ASPECTS defined regions in the MCA territory on 2 standardized axial section images. These regions included the lentiform nucleus (L), insula (I), caudate nucleus (C), internal capsule (IC), anterior inferior frontal lobe (M1), temporal lobe (M2), inferior parietal and posterior temporal lobe (M3), anterior superior frontal lobe (M4), precentral and superior frontal lobe (M5), and superior parietal lobe (M6). To constitute a criterion standard of hypoattenuation region on unenhanced CT images for the selected 21 patients, 2 neuroradiologists (31 and 19 years of neuroimaging review experience, respectively) determined criterion standard regions on unenhanced CT images in consensus. Hypoattenuation was defined as an area of abnormally low density of brain structures relative to attenuation of the contralateral hemisphere. The neuroradiologists identified the existence of hypoattenuation in each of the 10 regions of the MCA territory on the cerebral hemisphere suspected of hyperacute ischemic stroke in each patient by referring followup CT images. Diffusion-weighted MR images were used only for help in determining the criterion standard if necessary. Three of the 21 patients presented no hypoattenuation regions on CT images but presented hyperintense lesions on diffusion-weighted MR images. The mean number of hypoattenuation regions per patient was 3.2 (range, 0Y9) in the 21 patients. Figure 14 shows the distribution of the number of hypoattenuation regions identified by the 2 neuroradiologists from the 21 patients.

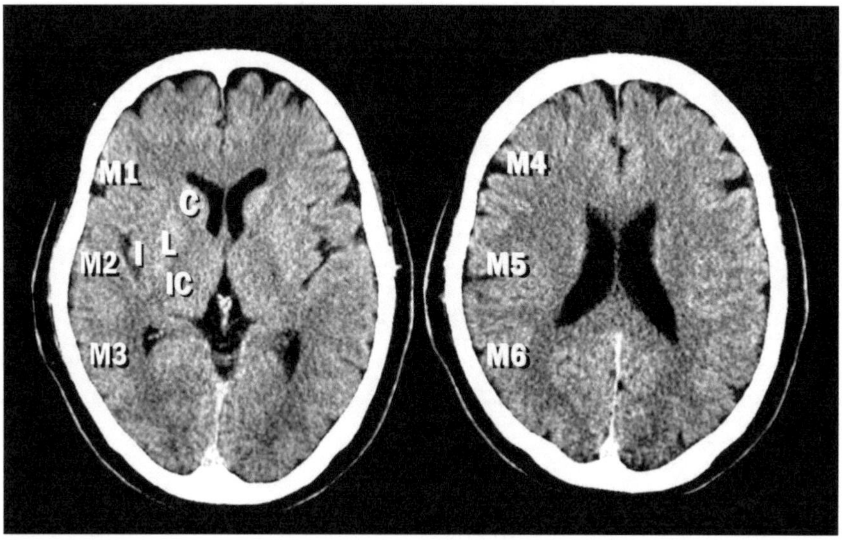

Fig. 13. Ten Alberta Stroke Programme Early CT Score (ASPECTS)-defined regions in the MCA territory for the performance evaluation on unenhanced CT images. These regions include lentiform nucleus (L), insula (I), caudate nucleus (C), internal capsule (IC), anterior inferior frontal lobe (M1), temporal lobe (M2), inferior parietal and posterior temporal lobe (M3), anterior superior frontal lobe (M4), precentral and superior frontal lobe (M5), and superior parietal lobe (M6).

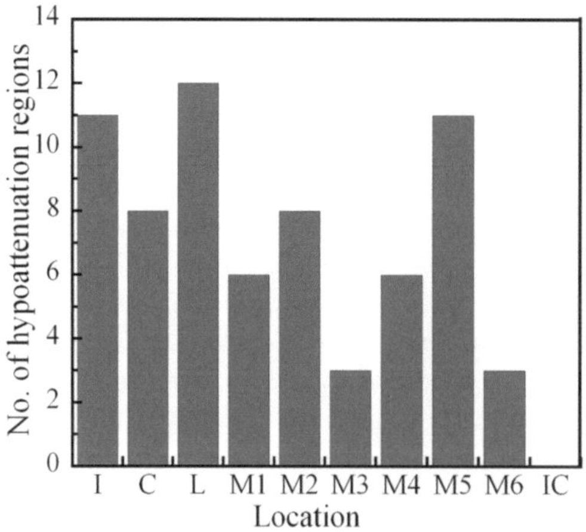

Fig. 14. Distribution of the number of hypoattenuation regions identified by two neuroradiologists from 21 patients.

Five neuroradiologists (years of experience 9-31 years) took part in the observer performance study. The two of them, who selected the patients, did not participate as an observer. All observers were blinded to all clinical and patient information, except that the information about the side of the hemisphere with stroke symptoms was provided. We used a sequential test method (Uozumi et al., 2001). Each observer first viewed CT images only for the initial rating, and then viewed both the original and the *z*-score maps for the second rating. During the rating process, the observers were asked to indicate their confidence level regarding the presence of parenchymal hypoattenuation at each of the 10 regions in the affected hemisphere of each patient by using a continuous rating scale (Metz et al., 1998). Each observer reviewed randomly the 21 patients, and rated his/her confidence level for the 210 regions of the 21 patients.

Before the observer test, each observer underwent a training session with four training cases to become familiar with the characteristics of *z*-score maps and the test procedure. The four training cases were not included in the observer performance study. The procedure that observers undertook is described as follows: (1) unenhanced CT images were displayed on a color monitor without *z*-score maps; (2) each observer rated the confidence level in the presence or absence of hypoattenuation in each of the 10 locations of every patient; (3) a series of eight *z*-score maps, including two standardized axial sections defined by the ASPECTS method were then displayed next to the original CT images; (4) The observer viewed both the original CT images and the *z*-score maps and rated them again if the ratings were different from the first ones.

When reviewing on the monitor, a continuous rating scale was displayed for each location with a 100-point scale, the left, right end, and the center of which indicates "definitely absent", "definitely present" and "ambiguous", respectively. The indicator was originally set at the point of 50 (ambiguous) before an initial rating. The observers were permitted to review the entire sequence of CT slices of each patient and were also allowed to adjust window width and center level settings as necessary. Reading time was not limited in this study.

To evaluate observers' performance in the quantification of the extent of hypoattenuation regions without and with the *z*-score maps using the ASPECTS score system, we calculated the accuracy of quantification. The accuracy was defined as the sum of true-positive and true-negative regions per 10 ASPECTS-defined regions in each patient. A positive finding and a negative finding were assumed to be a point of higher than 50 and a point of less than 50, respectively, on a 100-point confidence rating scale. The point of 50 considered as ambiguous was initially indicated on a bar. The difference between the average accuracy values obtained without and with the *z*-score maps was estimated using a paired Student *t* test.

Observers' performance in the detection of focal hypoattenuation for the 210 regions without and with the *z*-score map was evaluated using receiver operating characteristic (ROC) analysis. A computer program (ROCKIT 0.9B; C. E. Metz, University of Chicago, Ill., USA) was used for obtaining binormal ROC curves from the continuous rating data (Uozumi et al., 2001). The statistical significance of the difference in the areas under these curves (AUC) obtained without and with *z*-score maps was tested by use of the jackknife method that involves an analysis of variance approach (Dorfman et al. 1992). A computer program (LABMRMC; C. E. Metz, University of Chicago, Ill., USA) was used for the test.

In the detection of focal hypoattenuation, average sensitivities and specificities without and with the *z*-score map were calculated. The statistical significances of the difference in the sensitivities and the specificities without and with the *z*-score map were evaluated using the Wilcoxon matched-pairs signed-ranks test. Moreover, to validate the usefulness of the *z*-score mapping method, we determined the change in observers' findings without and with the *z*-score map in the detection of focal hypoattenuation. We assumed that a "clinically reverse action" in confidence levels occurred only when a finding was reversed between first and second ratings on the 100-point confidence rating scale. In hypoattenuation regions, a change from a negative finding or ambiguous to a positive finding implied that the use of the *z*-score map was beneficial. Similarly, a change from a positive finding or ambiguous to a negative finding implied that the use of the map was detrimental. In normal regions, inversely, a change from a positive finding or ambiguous to a negative finding implied that the use of the *z*-score map was beneficial. Similarly, a change from a negative finding or ambiguous to positive finding implied that the use of the map was detrimental. We calculated the number of regions in which the use of the *z*-score map led the observers to take the clinically reverse actions among the 210 regions. The differences between the median numbers of the clinically reverse actions without and with the use of the *z*-score maps for the five observers were evaluated using the Wilcoxon matched-pairs signed-ranks test. In all the analyses, a P value of less than 0.05 was considered to indicate a significant difference.

The average accuracy of the five observers for the quantification of the extent of hypoattenuation regions obtained without and with the *z*-score maps were 82.6% and 86.6%, respectively, indicating a significant difference ($P<0.0001$). Table 3 shows the accuracy values for the five observers without and with the *z*-score maps. Note that all observers improved the accuracies when viewing the *z*-score maps.

Observer	Without *Z*-Score Maps	With *Z*-Score Maps
A	77.6%	80.0%
B	77.6%	84.8%
C	85.2%	87.6%
D	88.1%	92.4%
E	84.3%	88.1%
Mean	82.6%	86.6% ($P < 0.0001$)

Table 3. Accuracy values for 5 neuroradiologists in quantification of the extent of hypoattenuation regions.

The average ROC curves for the five observers in the detection of focal hypoattenuation from the 210 regions without and with the *z*-score map are shown in Fig.15. The average AUC value was increased from 0.883 to 0.925 when the observers viewed the original CT images together with the *z*-score maps, and this difference was statistically significant ($P=0.01$). Table 4 shows the AUC values for the five observers without and with the *z*-score maps. Note that all observers improved the performance when viewing the *z*-score maps.

The average sensitivity in the detection of focal hypoattenuation was improved significantly from 80.6% (274 of 340 regions) to 88.8% (303 of 340 regions) by using the *z*-score map ($P=0.042$). The 340 regions were the product of the 68 hypoattenuation regions and five readings by the observers. The average specificity was improved from 77% (547 of 710 observations) to 80.4% (571 of 710 observations) when the observers used the *z*-score maps. The 710 observations were the product of the 142 normal regions and five readings by the observers. No significant difference in the specificities between without and with the z-score maps was found (P=0.13).

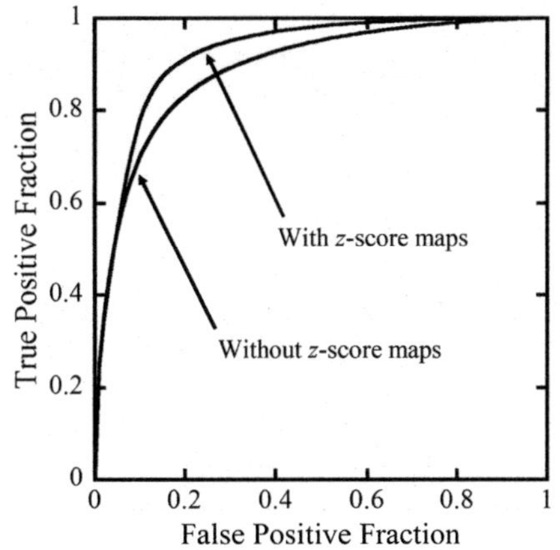

Fig. 15. Average receiver operating characteristic curves for five observers in the detection of focal hypoattenuation without and with the z-score map.

Observer	Without *Z*-Score Maps	With *Z*-Score Maps
A	0.843	0.898
B	0.925	0.955
C	0.925	0.938
D	0.903	0.938
E	0.822	0.894
Mean	0.883	0.924 ($P = 0.01$)

Table 4. AUC values for 5 neuroradiologists in the detection of focal hypoattenuation.

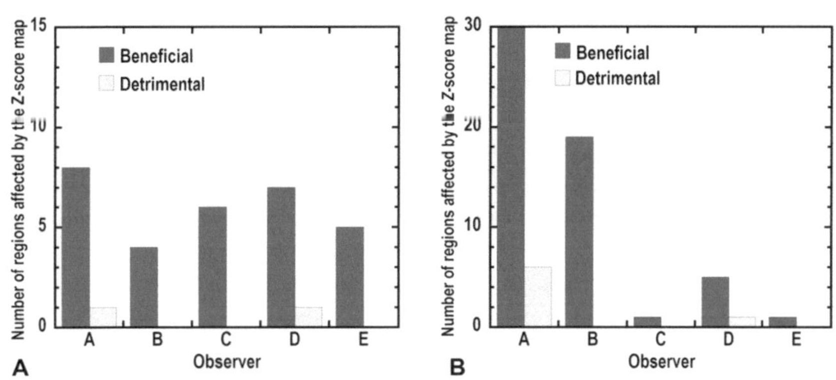

Fig. 16. Number of regions affected by the use of z-score maps in confidence levels with regard to hypoattenuation regions and normal regions. (A) hypoattenuation regions and (B) normal regions. The letters A-E on x-axis represent the five neroradiologists.

The results of the clinically reverse action in confidence levels for the observers are shown in Fig.16. In the hypoattenuation regions, the median number of the regions affected beneficially and that of the regions affected detrimentally were six and zero, respectively, which indicated a significant difference (P=0.04). Similarly, in the normal regions, the median number of the regions affected beneficially and that of the regions affected detrimentally were five and zero, respectively, which indicated a significant difference (P=0.04).

We evaluated the usefulness of the *z*-score mapping method on quantifying the extent of hypoattenuation regions of hyperacute stroke within 3 hours after onset of stroke ictus. The results showed that the neuroradiologists' performance in the quantification of the extent of hypoattenuation regions was improved significantly in patients with the MCA territory infarction by use of the method. So far little work has focused on improving radiologists' performance in the quantification of the extent of hypoattenuation areas by an image-processing approach. Until recently, a noise reduction filter for the increase in visualization of subtle hypoattenuation on nonenhanced CT images has been reported (Takahashi et al. 2007, 2008,; Lee et al. 2007). As a result, the performance of radiologists in the detection of hypoattenuation could be improved. However, not only the detection of hypoattenuation, but the quantification of the extent of hypoattenuation areas is important for the diagnosis and management of acute ischemic stroke. When the ASPECTS method is applied to quantify the extent of hypoattenuation regions, the existence of focal hypoattenuation at each of the 10 ASPECTS-defined locations needs to be accurately identified. Our observer performance test results indicated that the *z*-score map could significantly improve neuroradiologists' confidence levels in identifying the existence of focal hypoattenuation. This result may be an evidence to support the fact that the *z*-score mapping method would enable the neuroradiologists to improve the accuracy for the quantification of the extent of hypoattenuation regions.

The results of the clinically reverse action in confidence levels showed that the number of regions affected beneficially was significantly larger than that affected detrimentally in both the hypoattenuation regions and the normal regions. This result indicated that the use of *z*-score map could be useful in helping interpreters avoid miss interpretation of focal hypoattenuation. Figures 17 and 18 demonstrate two examples of the use of the *z*-score maps. In the case of Fig.17, the use of *z*-score maps prevented three of the five neuroradiologists from missed identification of focal hypoattenuation. Similarly, in the case of Fig.18, four of the five observers avoided the missed identification when using the *z*-score maps. Thus, we believe that the method could help neuroradiologists much in quantifying the extent of hypoattenuation of hyperacute stroke in this study.

There were differencies between our observer test and the clinical environment. First, No patients with old cerebral infarction were included in this study. No matter whether a low-density area of infarcts on unenhanced CT images is fresh or not, the area becomes a high-signal area on *z*-score maps. Therefore, recognizing a recent hypoattenuation area among high-signal areas on *z*-score maps is considerably difficult. However, since high-signal areas on *z*-score maps make interpreters aware that the corresponding areas on the unenhanced CT images might indicate the presence of low density areas, then the interpreter would observe the specific areas on the CT images to justify whether they are acute infarct areas or not. Next, only one patient with leuko-araiosis was included in this study, although many elderly patients with leuko-araiosis are examined by emergency CT scans in a clinical setting. In general, distinguishing a hypoattenuation area of embolic infarction involving cerebral cortex from leuko-araiosis would not be difficult, because low-density areas of leuko-araiosis appear in the cerebral white matter. In this observer test, patients with embolic infarction were treated. Therefore, we believe that leuko-araiosis would not affect the observers' performance in the quantification of the extent of hypoattenuation regions in this study. However, the differentiation between leuko-araiosis and thrombotic infarction might be difficult, because thrombotic infarction often tends to spare the cortices. To further clarify the usefulness of *z*-score mapping, a study including patients with leuko-araiosis and thrombotic infarction will be needed. Practically, imaging studies in acute stroke may be interpreted by non-experts in emergency departments. It has been reported that both the sensitivity for the detection of acute stroke and the inter-rater homogeneity for the identification of lesion extent by non-experts were lower than those by experts in unenhanced CT imaging in the clinical situation (non-experts/experts: sensitivity, 41/61%; κ=0.38/0.51) (Fiebach et al. 2002). We examined the validity of the *z*-score mapping method in the interpretation by neuroradiologits but not by non-experts.

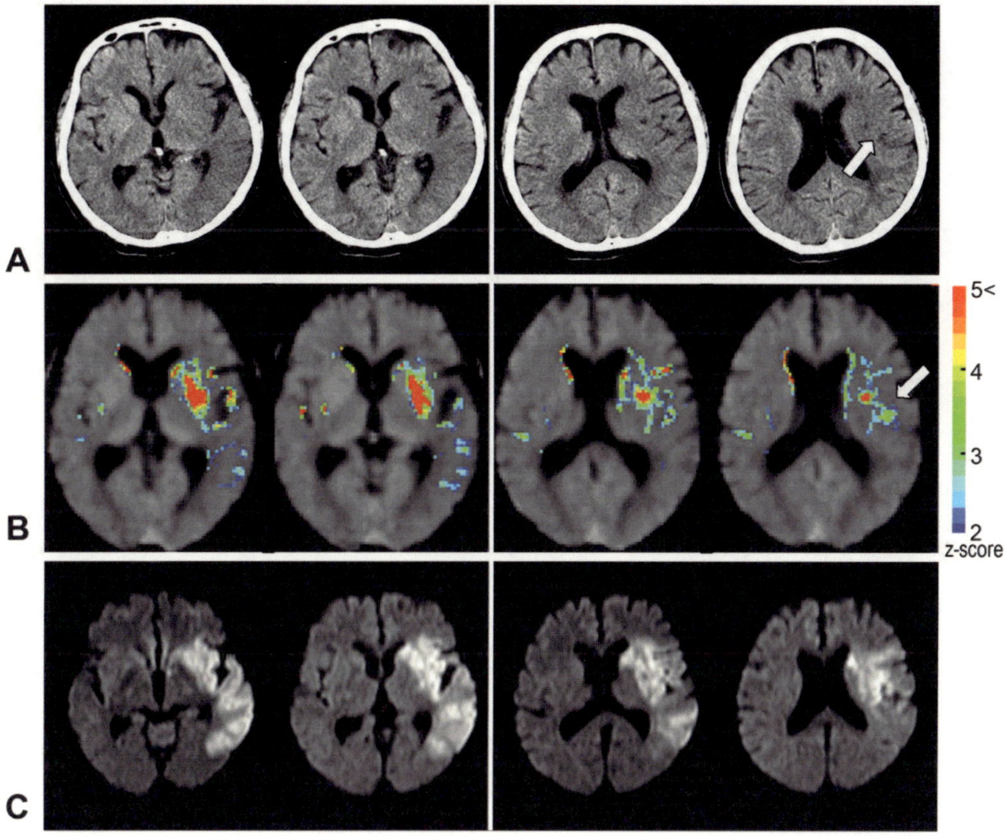

Fig. 17. 62-year-old-man with the right hemiplegia at 3 hours after stroke onset. (A) Unenhanced CT images show that parenchymal hypoattenuation at the left lentiform nucleus, caudate nucleus, temporal lobe, inferior parietal and posterior temporal lobe, and, precentral and superior frontal lobe (an arrow). (B) Z-score maps prevented three observers from missed identification of hypoattenuation at precentral and superior frontal lobe (an arrow); *z*-scores are indicated by a color bar (*right*). (C) Diffusion-weighted MR images taken after the first CT scan reveal hyperintense areas in the left MCA distribution.

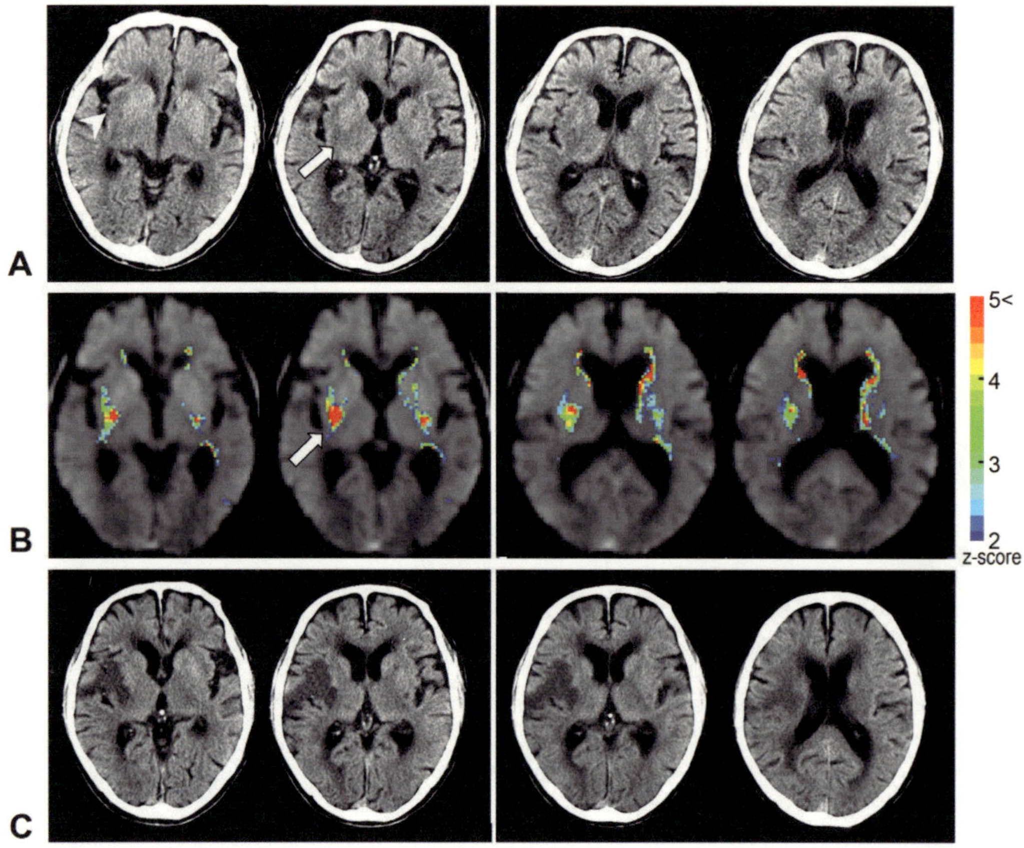

Fig. 18. 92-year-old-man with left hemiplegia at 1.3 hours after stroke onset. (A) Unenhanced CT images show that parenchymal hypoattenuation at the right lentiform nucleus (an arrow) and insula (an arrow head). (B) The *z*-score maps enabled four observers to avoid missing hypoattenuation at the right lentiform nucleus (a white arrow). A high-signal area is also seen within lacunar infarct in the left lentiform nucleus on the *z*-score maps, and moreover, a high-signal area which might be due to inaccurate normalization of enlarged cerebral ventricle appears at the left periventricular region on the *z*-score maps. Z scores are indicated by a color bar (*right*). (C) Follow-up CT images obtained one day after ictus demonstrate hypodense areas in the right MCA distribution.

In consideration that the method could improve the performance of the neuroradiologists who are expert in the diagnosis of acute stroke, we suppose that it might improve even better non-experts' performance in the quantification of the extent of hypoattenuation regions, and might serve as a useful tool for the diagnosis of acute stroke in emergency departments, but this issue remains to be studied further. The execution time required for processing of *z*-score mapping, including normalization, image processing and map display with a personal computer, was approximately six minutes. Data transfer implementations for the processing were performed manually in this study. We are working on constructing a fully automated *z*-score mapping system to further reduce the execution time. Indeed, it might take a longer time for the diagnosis with *z*-score maps in a clinical

situation. However, interpreters review mainly original, unenhanced CT images and refer the z-score maps as a "second opinion". We believed that the use of the z-score mapping method would not significantly increase the reading time.
In conclusion, the z-score mapping method has the potential to assist neuroradiologists to quantify the extent of hypoattenuation regions of hyperacue stroke on unenhanced CT images.

4. Conclusion

Two fundamental schemes to enhance/detect early CT signs were introduced. The enhancement technique was based on adaptive partial medial filter (APMF). The APMF was compared to 14 conventional denoising filters, and the results clearly demonstrated the superiority of the APMF. An observer test was performed to evaluate clinical value of whether the APMF was able to enhance hypoattenuation regions in nonenhanced CT images. As a result, all observers could improve their diagnostic performances, when the APMF image was used. The detection technique of early CT signs was based on z-score mapping method. The z-score mapping was able to distinctly visualize/detect hypoattenuation regions in CT images. Five neuroradiologists observed CT images together with the z-score mapping images to diagnose hyper acute stroke. As a result, the diagnostic accuracy was significantly improved when they referred to the z-score mapping images. In conclusion, the introduced two schemes would aid the clinical diagnosis of hyper acute stroke using nonenhanced CT images. In future works, we will introduce a knowledge based classification technique such as artificial neural network, fuzzy logic, etc., in order to develop intelligent computer-aided diagnosis system for cerebral acute stroke. We hope that the current and future techniques contribute to the improvement of diagnostic accuracy for acute stroke.

5. References

(2002). *The World Health Report 2002*, World Health Organization, pp. (186-191), ISBN 9241562072, Retrieved from < http://www.who.int/whr/2002/en/>

(2004). *Journal of Health and Welfare Statistics*, Health and Welfare Statistics Association, Vol.51, No.12, (October 2004).

Adams, H.; Adams, R.; Brott, T.; Zoppo, G.; Furlan, A.; Goldstein, L.B.; et al. (2003). Guidelines for the early management of patients with ischemic stroke: A scientific statement from the Stroke Council of the American Stroke Association. *Stroke*, Vol.34, pp. (1056-1083)

Adams, H.; Adams, R.; Zoppo, G. & Goldstein L.B. (2005). Guidelines for the early management of patients with ischemic stroke: 2005 guidelines update a scientific statement from the Stroke Council of the American Heart Association/American Stroke Association. *Stroke*, Vol.36, pp. (916-923)

Kummer, R.; Allen, K.L.; Holle, R.; Bozzao, L.; Bastianello, S.; Manelfe, C.; et al. (1997). Acute stroke: usefulness of early CT findings before thrombolytic therapy. *Radiology*, Vol.205, pp. (327-333)

Wardlaw, J.M.; Dorman, P.J.; Lewis, S.C. & Sandercock P.A. (1999). Can stroke physicians and neuroradiologists identify signs of early cerebral infarction on CT ?. *Journal of Neurology, Neurosurgery & Psychiatry*, Vol.67, pp. (651-653)

Barber, P.A.; Demchuk, A.M.; Zhang, J. & Buchan A.M. (2000). Validity and reliability of a quantitative computed tomography score in predicting outcome of hyperacute stroke before thrombolytic therapy. ASPECTS Study Group. Alberta Stroke Programme Early CT Score. *Lancet*, Vol.355, pp. (1670-1674)

Tomura, N.; Uemura, K.; Inugami, A.; Fujita, H.; Higano, S. & Shishido F. (1988). Early CT finding in cerebral infarction: obscuration of the lentiform nucleus. *Radiology*, Vol.168, pp. (463-467)

Truwit, C.L.; Barkovich, A.J.; Gean-Marton, A.; Hibri, N. & Norman D. (1990). Loss of the insular ribbon: another early CT sign of acute middle cerebral artery infarction. *Radiology*, Vol.176, pp. (801-806)

Schriger, D.L.; Kalafut, M.; Starkman, S.; Krueger, M. & Saver J.L. (1998). Cranial computed tomography interpretation in acute stroke: physician accuracy in determining eligibility for thrombolytic therapy. *Journal of American Medical Association*, Vol.279, pp. (1293-1297)

Wardlaw J.M. & Mielke O. (2005). Early signs of brain infarction at CT: observer reliability and outcome after thrombolytic treatment-systematic review. *Radiology*, Vol.235, pp. (444-453)

Kalender W.A. (2000). *Computed Tomography: Fundamentals, System Technology. Image Quality and Applocations*, Wiley-VCH, ISBN 3895780812, Munich, Germany

Kalra, M.K.; Maher, M.M. ; Sahani, D.V. ; Blake, M.A. ; Hahn, P.F. ; Avinash, G.B. ; et al. (2003). Low-dose CT of the abdomen: evaluation of image improvement with use of noise reduction filters-pilot study. *Radiology*, Vol.228, pp. (251-256)

Kachelriess, M.; Watzke, O. & Kalender W.A. (2001). Generalized multi-dimensional adaptive filtering for conventional and spiral single-slice, multi-slice, and cone-beam CT. *Medical Physics*, Vol.28, pp. (475-490)

Lee, Y.; Takahashi, N.; Tsai, D.Y. & Ishii, K. (2007). Adaptive partial median filter for early CT signs of acute cerebral infarction. *International Journal of Computer Assisted Radiology and Surgery*, Vol.2, No.2, pp. (105-115)

Guis, V.H.; Adel, M.; Rasigni, M. & Rasigni G. (2003), Adaptive neighborhood contrast enhancement in mammographic phantom images. *Optical Engineering*, Vol.42, pp. (357-366)

Tsai, D.Y.; Takahashi, N. & Lee Y. (2005). An Adaptive Enhancement Algorithm for CT Brain Images. *Proceedings of the 2005 IEEE Engineering in Medicine and Biology 27th Annual Conference*, paper #124

Lee, Y.; Takahashi, N.; Tsai, D.Y. & Fujita H. (2006). Detectability improvement of early sign of acute stroke on brain CT images using an adaptive partial smoothing filter. *Proceedings of SPIE Medical Imaging*, Vol.6144, pp. (2138-2145)

Takahashi, N.; Lee, Y.; Tsai, D.Y. & Ishi, K. (2007). A novel noise reduction filter for improving visibility of early CT signs of hyperacute stroke: evaluation of the filter's performance - preliminary clinical experience-. *Radiation Medicine*, Vol.25, No.3, pp. (247-254)

Russ, J.C. (1995). *The Image Processing Handbook* (2nd edition), pp. (155-178), CRC Press, ISBN 0849325323, Boca Raton, USA.

Tukey, J.W. (1971). *Exploratory Data Analysis*. Addison Wesley, ISBN 0201076160,

Davis, L.S. & Rosenfeld, A. (1978). Noise cleaning by iterated local averaging. *IEEE Transactions on Systems, Man and Cybernetics*, Vol.SMC-8, pp. (705-710)

Wu, W.Y.; Wang, M.J J. & Liu, C.M. (1992). Performance evaluation of some noise reduction methods. *Comput Vision Graphics and Image Processing*, Vol.54, pp. (134-146).

Ehrich, R.W. (1978). A symmetric hysteresis smoothing algorithm that preserves principal features. *Comput Graphics and Image Processing*, Vol.8, pp. (121-126)

Lev, A.; Zucker, S.W. & Rosenfeld, A. (1977). Iterative enhancement of noisy images. *IEEE Transactions on Systems, Man and Cybernetics*, Vol.SMC-7, pp. (435-442)

Wang, D.C.C.; Vagnucci, A.H., & Li, C.C. (1981). Gradient inverse weighted smoothing scheme and the evaluation of its performance. *Comput Vision Graphics and Image Processing*, Vol.15, pp. (167-181)

Nagao, M. & Matuyama, T. (1978). Edge Preserving smoothing. *Comput Graphics and Image Processing*, Vol.9, pp. (394-407)

Zamperoni, P. (1990). Some Adaptive Rank Order Filters for Image Enhancement. *Pattern Recognition Letters*, Vol.11, pp. (81-86)

Xu, X.; Miller, E.L.; Chen, D. & Sarhadi, M. (2004). Adaptive Two-Pass Rank Order Filter to Remove Impulse Noise in Highly Corrupted Images. *IEEE Transactions on Image Processing*, Vol.13, No.2, pp. (238-247)

Kuan, D.T.; Sawchuk, A.A, Strand, T.C & Chavel, P. (1985). Adaptive Noise Smoothing Filter for Images with Signal-Dependant Noise. *IEEE Transactions on Pattern Analysis and Machine Intelligence*, Vol.7, No.2, pp. (165-177)

Centeno, J.A.A & Haertel, V. (1997). An Adaptive Image Enhancement Algorithm. *Pattern Recognition*, Vol.30, No.7, pp. (1183-1189)

Fischl, B. & Shwartz, E.L. (1999). Adaptive Nonlocal Filtering: A Fast Alternative to Anisotropic Diffusion for Image Filtering. *IEEE Transactions on Pattern Analysis and Machine Intelligence*, Vol.21, No.1, pp. (42-48)

Westin, C.F.; Richolt, J.; Moharir, V. & Kikinis, R. (2000). Affine Adaptive Filtering of CT Data. *Medical Image Analysis*, Vol.4, No.2, pp. (161-177)

Schilham, A.M.R.; Ginneken, B.V. ; Gietema, H. & Prokop, M. (2006). Local Noise Weighted Filtering for Emphysema Scoring of Low-Dose CT Images. *IEEE Transactions on Medical Imaging*, Vol.25, No.4, pp. (451-463)

Gijbels, I.; Lambert, A. & Qiu P. (2006). Edge-Preserving Image Denoising and Estimation of Discontinuous Surfaces. *IEEE Transactions on Pattern Analysis and Machine Intelligence*, Vol.28, No.7, pp. (1075-1087)

Lev, M.H.; Farkas, J.; Gemmete, J.J., Hossain, S.T. ; Hunter, G.J.; Koroshetz, W.J. & Gonzalez, R.G. (1999). Acute stroke: improved nonenhanced CT detection-benefits of soft-copy interpretation by using variable window width and center level settings. *Radiology*, Vol.213, pp. (150-155)

Dolfman, D.D.; Berbaum, K.S. & Metz C.E. (1992). ROC rating analysis: generalization to the population of readers and cases with the jackknife method. *Investigative Radiology*, Vol.27, pp. (723–731)

Kalafut, M.A.; Schriger, D.L.; Saver J.L. & Starkman, S. (2000). Detection of early CT signs of >1/3 middle cerebral artery infarctions: interrater reliability and sensitivity of CT interpretation by physicians involved in acute stroke care. *Stroke*, Vol.31, pp. (1667-1671)

Fiebach, J.B.; Schellinger, P.D.; Jansen, O.; Meyer, M; Wilde, P.; Bender, J.; Schramm, P.; Juttle, E.; Oehler, J.; Hartmann, M.; Hahnel, S.; Knauth, M.; Hacke, W. & Sartor, K. (2002). CT and diffusion-weighted MR imaging in randomized order: diffusion-weighted imaging results in higher accuracy and lower interrater variability in the diagnosis of hyperacute ischemic stroke. *Stroke*, Vol.33, pp. (2144-2155)

Camargo, E.C.S.; Furie, K.L.; Singhal, A.B.; Roccatagliata, L.; Cunnane, M.E.; Halpern, E.F.; Harris, G.J.; Smith, W.S.; Gonzalez, R.G.; Koroshetz, W.J. & Lev, M.H. (2007). Acute brain infarct: detection and delineation with CT angiographic source images versus nonenhanced CT scans. *Radiology*, Vol.244, pp. (541-548)

Takahashi, N.; Tsai, D.Y.; Lee, Y.; Kinoshita, T. & Ishii, K. (2010). Z-score mapping method for extracting hypoattenuation areas of hyperacute stroke in unenhanced CT. *Academic Radiology*, Vol.17, No.1, pp. (84-92)

Takahashi, N.; Tsai, D.Y.; Lee, Y.; Kinoshita, T.; Ishii, K.; Tomaru, H. & Takahashi, S. (2010). Usefulness of z-score mapping for quantification of extent of hypoattenuation regions of hyperacute stroke in unenhanced computed tomography: analysis of radiologist's performance. *Journal of Comupter Assited Tomography*, Vol.34, No.5, pp. (751-756)

Friston, K.J.; Ashburner, J.; Frith, C.D.; Poline, J.B.; Heather, J.D. & Frackowiak, R.S.J. (1995). Spatial registration and normalization of images. *Human Brain Mapping*, Vol.3, No.3, pp. (165-189)

Ashburner, J. & Friston, K.J. (1999). Nonlinear spatial normalization using basis functions. *Human Brain Mapping*, Vol.7, No.4, pp. (254-266)

Uozumi, T.; Nakamura, K.; Watanabe, H.; Nakata, H.; Katsuragawa, S. & Doi, K. (2001). ROC analysis on detection of metastatic pulmonary nodules on digital chest radiographs by use of temporal subtraction. *Academic Radiology*, Vol.8, No.9, pp. (871-878)

Metz, C.E.; Herman, B.A. & Shen, J.H. (1998). Maximum likelihood estimation of receiver operating characteristic (ROC) curves from continuously-distributed data. *Statistics in Medicine*, Vol.17, No.9, pp. (1033-1053)

Takahashi, N.; Lee, Y.; Tsai, D.Y. & Ishii, K. (2008). Improvement of detection of hypoattenuation in sensitive ischemic stroke in unenhanced CT using an adaptive smoothing Filter. *Acta Radiologica*, Vol.49, No.7, pp. (816-826)

2

3D-CT Mammary Lymphography Facilitate the Endoscopic Sentinel Node Biopsy

Koji Yamashita, Shunsuke Haga and Kazuo Shimizu
Nippon Medical School
Japan

1. Introduction

In early breast cancer, the presence of metastasis in axillary lymph nodes is an important factor in prognosis and further treatment. However, axillary lymph node dissection causes many complications such as contracture of the shoulder joint, lymph edema, and paralysis of the upper extremities (Ernst, 2002). Convention holds that there is no need to dissect axillary lymph nodes for node-negative patients. To avoid unnecessary axillary lymph node dissection, sentinel node biopsy (SNB) has been performed (Veronesi, 1997; Schrenk, 2000). Sentinel node (SN) is defined as the first lymph node drained of lymph flow from the tumor (Schwartz, 2002; Kuehn, 2005). SNB can detect such metastases and provide information that may obviate the need for axillary lymph node dissection. The most commonly used methods to identify the SN are dye-staining (Giuliano, 1994; Borgstein, 1997) and radioisotope incorporation (Krag, 1993; Giuliano, 1994). Multidetector-row three-dimensional computed tomography (3D-CT) mammary lymphography (LG) can be used to mark the precise location of the SN on the skin before the operation (Suga, 2003; Tangoku, 2004; Minato, 2004).
The detailed relations between lymph nodes and lymph flow in the breast and the axilla can be clarified using 3D-CT LG (Yamashita, 2008, 2009). We have developed this 3D image processing system to depict more precise anatomical structure of mammary lymphovascular system. It enables us to perform systematic collection of axillary lymph nodes including SNs, and will decrease unnecessary lymph node dissection, even if the SNs have metastasized, and can decrease complications.
Previously, we devised an endoscopic surgical procedure for breast diseases; video-assisted breast surgery (VABS) (Yamashita, 2006). VABS is a less invasive and esthetically a better operation for benign and malignant breast diseases In this study, we assessed the validity of 3D-CT LG in SNB of 186 patients, investigated the extent of metastasis style in 40 patients who were metastasis-positive based on the novel technique, and applied the technique to SNB using the dye-staining method and 3D-CT LG guidance.

2. Patients

Since July 2002, SNB was performed in 186 patients, with SNB using VABS and 3D-CT LG being performed in 146 of these. Patient characteristics are shown in Table 1.

	Mean	Range
Age (y/o)	52.7	26 - 85
Tumor size (cm)	2.2	0.1 - 10
	Number	%
Tis	3	1.6
T1a / T1b / T1c	3 / 20 / 86	1.6 / 10.8 / 46.2
T2 / T3 / T4	53 / 9 / 12	28.5 / 4.8 / 6.5
Lymph node metastasis (N)	40	21.5
Distant metastasis (M)	9	4.8
ER (+/-)	122 / 64	65.6
PgR (+/-)	98 / 88	52.7
HER2 (+/-)[a]	44 / 142	23.7
Total	186	

ER, estrogen receptor; PgR, progesterone receptor; HER, human epidermal growth factor receptor
[a] Modified from reference 14.
[b] HER2: human epidermal growth factor receptor type 2; HER2 + means Herceptest 3+ and 2+; HER2 – means Herceptest 1+ and 0

Table 1. Patient Characteristics [a]

3. 3D-CT lymphography

Interstitial 3D-CT LG was performed using a 16-channel multidetector-row helical 3D-CT scanner (Toshiba Aquilion 16; Toshiba Medical Systems Corporation, Tochigi, Japan). Patients were placed in the supine position with arms positioned in the lateral abduction direction, suitable for the operating position. After local anesthesia by subcutaneous injection of 0.5 ml of 1% lidocaine, 2 ml of iopamidol (Iopamiron 300; Nihon Shering, Osaka, Japan) was injected intracutaneously into the periareolar skin and the skin above the tumor. At 1 and 3 min after injection (sometimes 5 min for observing advancement of lymph flow), a CT image was taken with a 3 mm slice thickness. SNs were identified on transaxial CT images, and their location was marked on the skin surface with an oil-painting pen using a laser pointer of CT on the day before the surgery. 3D-CT images were then reconstructed from transaxial enhanced CT images, which clearly showed the lymph ducts and SNs.

4. SPECT

On the day before surgery, 74 MBq technetium 99m (99mTc) phytate (FUJIFILM RI Pharma Co., LTD., Tokyo, Japan) in sterile saline (total volume 1 mL) was injected intradermally into two different sites of the skin above the tumor and around the periareola. Lymphoscintigraphy and SPECT were performed 2 hours after injection of radio colloid. If one or more focal accumulations of radioactivity (hot spots) were visualized, these were assumed to be SNs. Small amount of RI markers were positioned on the jagular notch of sternum and the xiphoid process to correct the fusion points. We used the image fusion software Syntegra (Philips Medical Systems, Eindhoven, The Netherlands) and Real INTAGE (KGT, Tokyo, Japan) to fuse SPECT data with 3D-CT LG.

5. Surgical methods

VABS has been described in detail previously (Yamashita, 2006). The operative procedures were as follows: skin incision in the axilla and/or periareola, skin flap formation via the tunnel method (Yamagata, 2002), pectoral muscle fascia dissection, vertical section of the mammary gland, SNB by the dye-staining method guided by preoperative 3D-CT LG marking, and axillary lymph node dissection (levels I and II). Radiotherapy and chemotherapy were performed for malignant diseases.

SLNB was performed by the dye-staining method using a part of VABS technique at the beginning of the operation, before gland resection. In the periareolar region and over the tumor, 2 ml of 1% indocyanine green was injected subcutaneously. A 1-cm long skin incision was made along wrinkles in the axilla at the position marked by 3D-CT LG. A Visiport optical trocar (Tyco Healthcare Japan, Tokyo, Japan) was inserted into the incision after 20 min. The endoscopic view was observed through Visiport with a 10 mm diameter, straight-angled rigid endoscope (Olympus Optical, Tokyo, Japan), and the stained lymph nodes were found by following the dye in the lymph ducts. The lymph nodes were sampled and metastasis was determined on fast frozen sections. Axillary lymph node dissection was performed at levels I and II with bipolar scissors through the same incision that was lengthened to 2.5 cm. The inferior pectoral nerve, long thoracic nerve, second and third intercostobrachial nerves, thoracodorsal nerve, artery, and vein were observed and preserved. The lateral pectoral artery was preserved for the lateral tissue flap. After surgery, SNs and axillary lymph nodes were pathologically examined by standard H&E staining.

Informed consent to the procedure was obtained from all the patients before surgery.

6. Lymph flow from tumor to sentinel node (Yamashita, 2008)

The lymph flow of the whole breast has been reported to collect into a subareolar plexus and then drain towards the axilla via lymph collecting ducts, by human cadaver studies (Delamere, 1993; Standring, 2005). It became the theoretical basis for the subareolar injection of dye and/or isotope for lymphatic mapping as part of the SN biopsy for breast cancer (Kimberg, 1999; Kern, 1999). On the other hand, the individual lymphatic flow is not identical in each living patient studies of SN biopsy.

3D-CT LG showed the precise lymphatic flow from the tumor to the SN (Fig. 1). In Figure 1a, the lymphatic flow from the tumor was divided to the periareola and directly to the axilla. The periareolar lymphatic flow was draining from the tumor and circling around the nipple and went to the axilla. This lymph duct to the axilla was separated from the direct duct from the tumor. In Figure 1b, the lymphatic flow was multiple and complicated, but the basic structure was same as that of Fig. 1a.

We classified the relationship between the lymph ducts and drained SNs into four patterns (Yamashita, 2008) (Fig. 2), according to the classification by Suga et al. (Suga, 2005). A single duct to single node pattern was observed in 88 cases (60.2%), multiple ducts to a single node in 29 cases (19.9%), single duct to multiple nodes in two cases (1.4%), and multiple ducts to multiple nodes in 27 cases (18.5%).

The internal mammary SN was also detected in five patients, but the rate was lower than that of the peritumoral injection (Shimazu, 2003). We are trying to improve it by the injection of the contrast medium iopamidole into the retromammary space behind the tumor. The peritumoral injection, which is recommended in radioisotope technique, is not suitable for 3D-CT LG, because the contrast medium is needed to use much volume as 1 ml and it may flow into surrounding mammary duct systems.

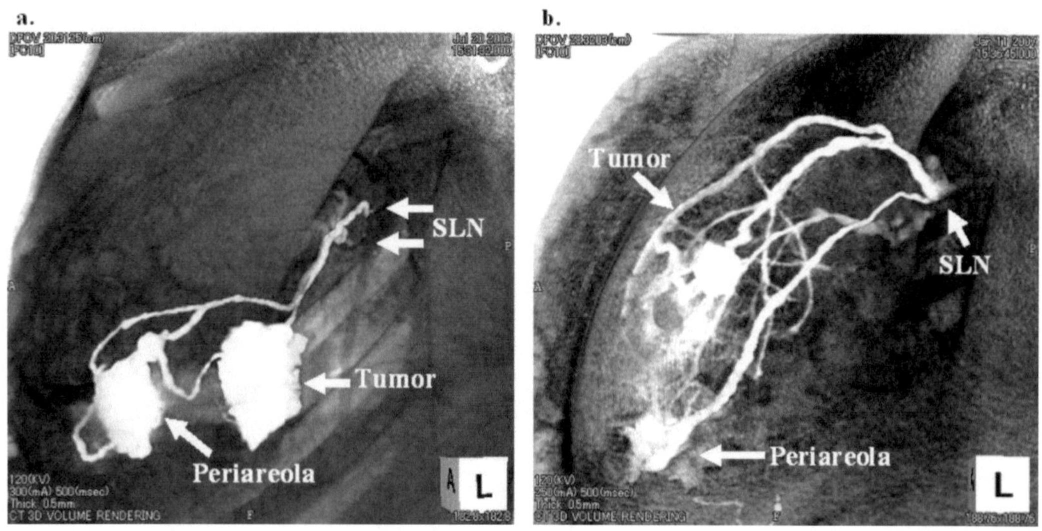

Fig. 1. Visualization of SNs and lymph ducts (LD) using 3D-CT LG *(13)*.
Iopamidol was injected intracutaneously into the periareolar skin and the skin above the tumor. a) Two LDs draining into two SNs. b) Multiple LDs draining into a single SN.

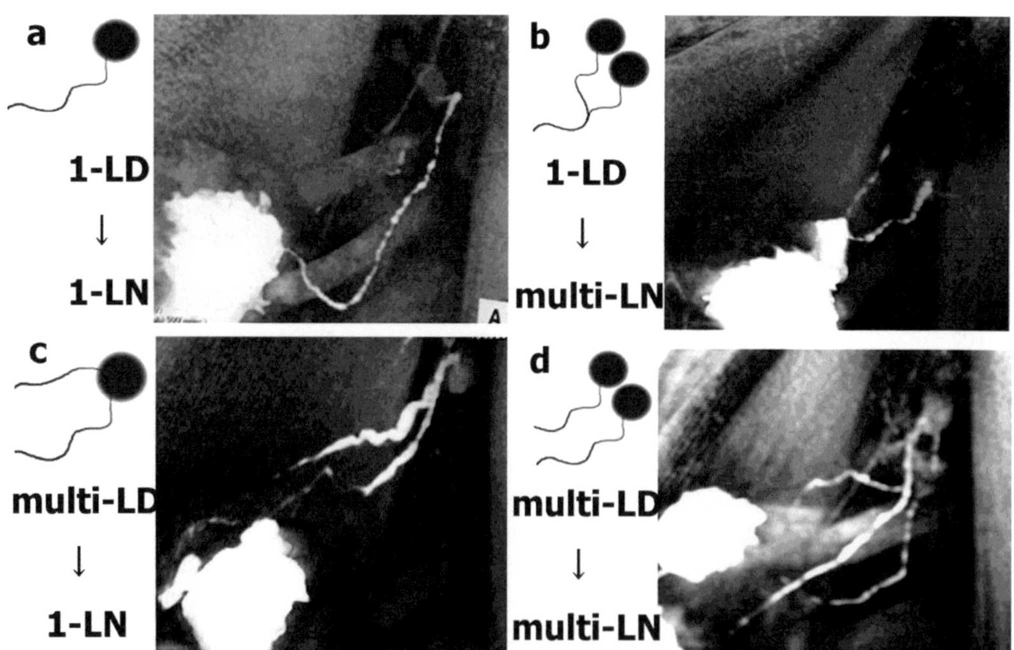

Fig. 2. Four patterns of relationship between the lymph duct and the sentinel lymph node (Yamashita, 2009).
The lymph flow pattern can be classified into these four types.

SN is typically detected using dye-staining or radioisotope incorporation. However, the tract from the tumor to the SN cannot be observed clearly by either methods (Mariani, 2001; Giuliano, 1997). We cannot detect whether dye-stained or hot-spotted nodes are really the first lymph nodes. This may be the basis for false negatives in SN biopsy. Lymphoscintigraphy may only show the main negative lymph node, and cannot clearly visualize the direct connection of SN and their afferent lymph ducts, because of slow lymphatic migration of radiocolloids, and because of the limitation of spatial resolutions and the lack of anatomic landmarks. In contrast, 3D-CT LG can demonstrate the precise route of the lymph duct and the exact location of the SN with the detailed surrounding anatomic structures, and since it does not involve the use of radioisotopes, it can be done at any institution that is equipped with a CT scanner. Therefore, 3D-CT LG is a very useful examination, which is essential for SNB.

Interstitial injection of iopamidol had no adverse effects locally and generally. The pathological metastatic status of SNs and axillary lymph nodes was as follows. No SN was identified in five patients of the 40 SNBs using only the dye-staining method, and the detection rate was 87.5%. However, all SNs were identified in 146 SNBs using the dye-staining method with 3D-CT LG marking. This detection rate was 100%. Backup axillary dissection was performed in each of the 40 SNB patients in the early phase according to both methods of SNB. One false-negative case occurred only in the dye-staining method (12.5%), but no false-negative case was found in 3D-CT LG (0%). The average sampled number of SNs was 1.7 in the cases without 3D-CT LG and 2.3 in the cases with 3D-CT LG.

Four patterns of lymph ducts and SNs have been revealed using 3D-CT LG (Yamashita, 2008). The lymph ducts to the SN are complicated. For example, in this study, we observed that in over 60% of cases, many ducts joined together into a single duct to form a single SN. However, more than two SNs were shown in 19.9% of the cases. These may have been missed without 3D-CT LG guidance. Figure 4a shows a typical example of a multi-node pattern, in which three different lymph nodes were all SN, each from a different lymph duct. The node from the main thick duct was not metastasized; however, the other two from the narrow collateral duct were metastasized. Thus, the sampling of all three nodes is necessary. The dye-staining method and the isotope method of SNB could not reach such the latter collateral nodes. These might become false negative study. Therefore, 3D-CT LG is effective in raising accuracy of SNB.

7. Lymph flow from sentinel node to axillary angle in axilla (Yamashita, 2009)

The procedure of 3D-CT LG takes only about 1 min after injection of iopamidol subcutaneously over the tumor and around the nipple for representing SN precisely. Examination of iopamidol flow 1, 3, and 5 min after injection revealed that the flow extended over the SN into the next nodes, and into the venous angle in half of the patients examined. Therefore, we can easily ascertain the tracts that cancer cells will spread through during metastasis. We defined these tracts as the second and third SNs. As a representative example, Fig. 3 shows a clear view of five bead-like grouped lymph nodes beyond the SN into the center of the body, and lymph duct plexuses between them. They are thought to imply the order of lymphatic route of metastasis. Fig. 4a shows three separated SNs, which were drained from three different lymph ducts diverging from one duct. Two of three separated SNs were positive for metastasis, but the other SNs from the main lymph duct were negative. Fig. 4b shows two chained SNs. The first SN was positive for metastasis, but the second was negative.

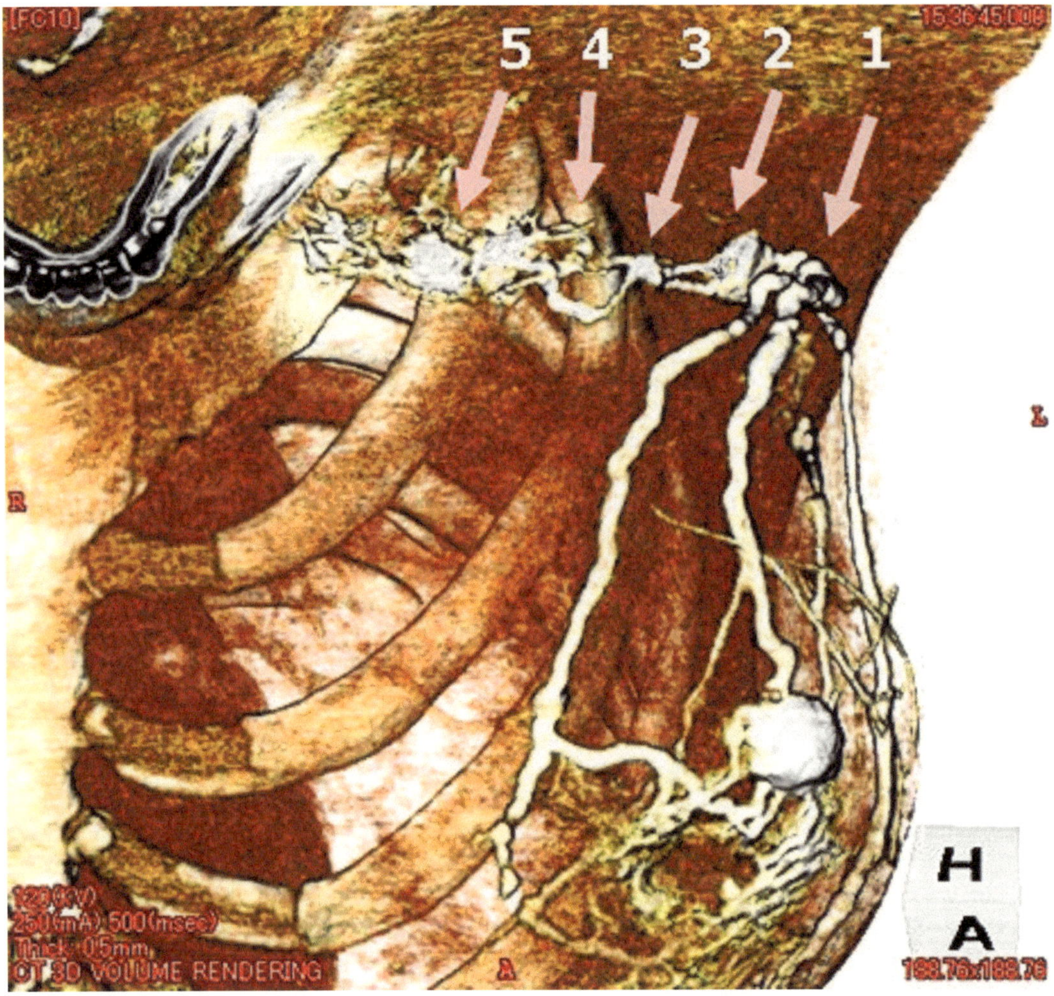

Fig. 3. Chronological examination of 3D-CT LG (Yamashita, 2009).
3D-CT LG was examined 1, 3, and 5 min after iopamidol injection. Iopamidol flowed to extend over the SN into the next nodes. Five bead-like grouped lymph nodes in the axilla can be visualized by partially removing the pectoral muscle in the CT monitor.
These are thought to be the order of lymph metastasis. Arrows point to lymph nodes 1–5 after SN.

Since December 2001, we performed VABS in 230 patients, SN biopsy in 186 patients, and 3D-CT LG in 140 patients. Table 2 shows the pathological status of metastases in SNs and axillary lymph nodes. SN metastasis was positive in 40 patients; of these, 21 patients experienced metastases solely in the SN. Except for SN, only the second axillary lymph node group was metastasized in three patients, the second and the third node groups were metastasized in five patients, and more than three groups were metastasized in eleven patients. It was confirmed that these metastases occurred in order of lymph flow presented by the lymphoid path of these 3D-CT LG (Fig. 3, 4).

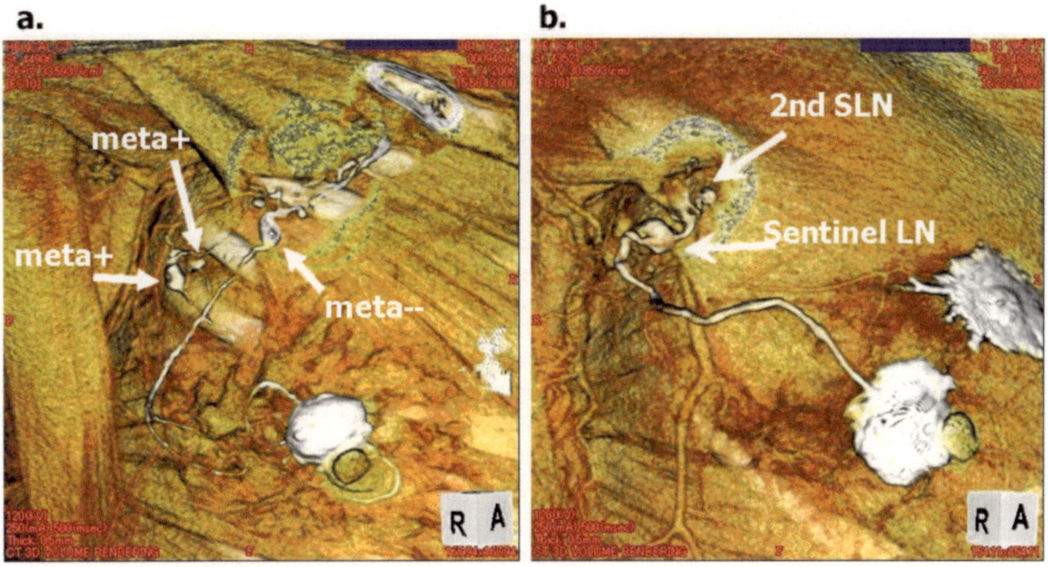

Fig. 4. Detection of SN metastasis (Yamashita, 2009).
a) Three sentinel nodes are recognized by 3D-CT LG. The right node drained from the main lymph duct was not metastasized. On the other hand, the other two nodes drained from the narrow collateral duct were metastasized. Dye and isotope could not reach such the latter collateral nodes. These might become false negative study. Therefore, 3D-CT LG is effective in raising accuracy of SNB.
b) The sentinel node was metastasized, but the second node and the other nodes were all negative.

The second and third lymph nodes groups could be recognized by 3D-CT LG and selectively removed by VABS. Table 2 shows the pathological status of their metastases and the other axillary lymph nodes in 40 SN metastasized patients. If second and third lymph node group biopsy was performed, it was prognostic for other axillary lymph node metastasis. Its accuracy, sensitivity, and false negative rate were 100%, 100%, and 0%, respectively.

Status of 2nd and 3rd Sentinel LN metastasis		Status of Axillary LN metastasis*	
		Negative	Positive
Positive	19	8	11
Negative	21	21	0
Total	40	29	11

Table 2. Metastatic relations of 2nd and 3rd SN to the other axillary nodes [a]
LN: lymph node
* Number of Axillary LN metastasis: Primary, and 2nd, and 3rd Sentinel LN is not included.
2nd and 3rd Sentinel LN biopsy: Accuracy = 100 %, False negative rate = 0 %, Sensitivity = 100 %

Even if the patients presently examined had metastasis of SN, about half of them had no metastasis in axillary lymph nodes (21 among 40 patients, 52.5% in Table 3). In these patients presenting with only SN metastasis, sufficient information can be obtained regarding the lymph node status of cancer staging to plan primary therapy after surgery, avoiding axillary lymph node dissection. Since the absence of other metastases is crucial to this approach, we need to analyze how it would be possible to conclude that SLN metastasis is unique. We suggest that this can be confirmed by collecting lymph nodes systemically based on the 3D-CT LG-acquired map of lymph nodes and ducts beyond SN. Histological examination of fast-frozen sections of the second and third lymph nodes during the operation will provide the information to omit axillary lymph node dissection.

Sentinel LN metastasis		No. of Axillary LN metastasis*			
		2nd	3rd	4th<	Sum
Positive	40	19	16	11	19
Negative	141				
Not detected	5	0	0	0	0
Total	186	19	16	11	19

Table 3. Metastatic status of sentinel and the other axillary nodes
[a] Detection rate 97.3% (without 3D-CT 88% / 40, with 3D-CT 100% /146
Average LN number 2.0, Only SLN metastasis 21 (52.5%)
LN: lymph node, 3D-CT: 3-dimensional computed tomography, LG: lymphography
* Axillary LN metastasis: Sentinel LN is not included*

8. Metastatic evaluation by 3D-CT LG

3D-CT LG may predict whether SN is metastasizing or not. When occupied with cancer cells, 3D-CT LG shows only the trumpet-like inflow portion of the lymph node, but the node is still recognizable. Sometimes, the lymph duct detours around the metastasized lymph node. However, in partial metastasis of the lymph node, 3D-CT LG shows no apparent difference from normal nodes. We have to examine the pattern of the duct route and the enhanced pattern of lymph node more carefully to predict metastasis. Ultrasonography and magnetic resonance imaging show only morphology and blood flow, and cannot reveal metastasis. While positron emission tomography can detect some metastases, those that are small escape detection. Of all these techniques, 3D-CT LG is superior.

9. Endoscopic SNB guided by 3D-CT LG

We have performed endoscopic surgery, named as video-assisted breast surgery (VABS), for all breast surgical procedures through a small wound port in the inconspicuous axillary area or periareola (Yamashita 2006a, 2006b). VABS is also used for SNB. The incisional wound is only 1 cm long and inconspicuous, without any complications. However, precise information is needed about the location of SN, because the method relies on endoscopic

vision. In five cases, we could not find the SLN using just only the dye-staining method. 3D-CT LG guidance helps in finding the SN easily by giving precise information. The structure of the dye-stained lymph ducts and SN were exactly the same on the endoscopic view as with the 3D-CT LG.
The lymph ducts to the SN are complicated. In most cases, many ducts join together into a single duct to a single SN (60.6 %). However, more than two SNs were shown in 19.7%, and these may have been missed without 3D-CT LG guidance, and hence 3D-CT LG is indispensable for SNB.

10. SPECT-CT

SPECT-CT can show the exact location of the hot spots on the axial view of the CT image, as showing in the figure (Fig. 5). They are always coincided with the axillary nodes. However, it cannot show the lymph ducts and the relations between lymph ducts and nodes either. The number of hot spots was usually only one or two. The average number was 1.2, which was less than the number 2.3 of SN found by 3D-CT LG.

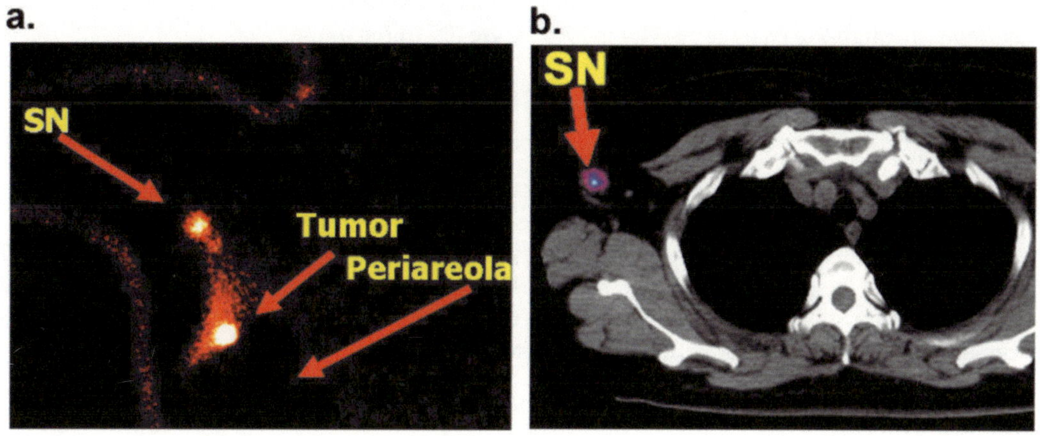

Fig. 5. Lymphoscintigraphy and SPECT-CT
a. Lymphoscintigraphy
The conventional lymphoscintigraphy shows only information about the existence of nodes with an uptake of RI as hot spots
b. Single photon emission computed tomography (SPECT)
SPECT-CT can show the exact location of the hot spots on the axial view of the CT image, as showing in the figure. They are always coincided with the axillary nodes.
SN: sentinel node

We fused the DICOM data of SPECT with 3D-CT LG by using the image fusion software (Fig. 6). The hot spot can be coincided with enhanced SN observed on 3D-CT LG. However, not all of SNs had a hot spot. We call SN with a hot spot as a hot node and SN without a hot spot as a cold node. We can recognize the location of the cold nodes by using the relation to the hot nodes on the map of 3D-CT LG.

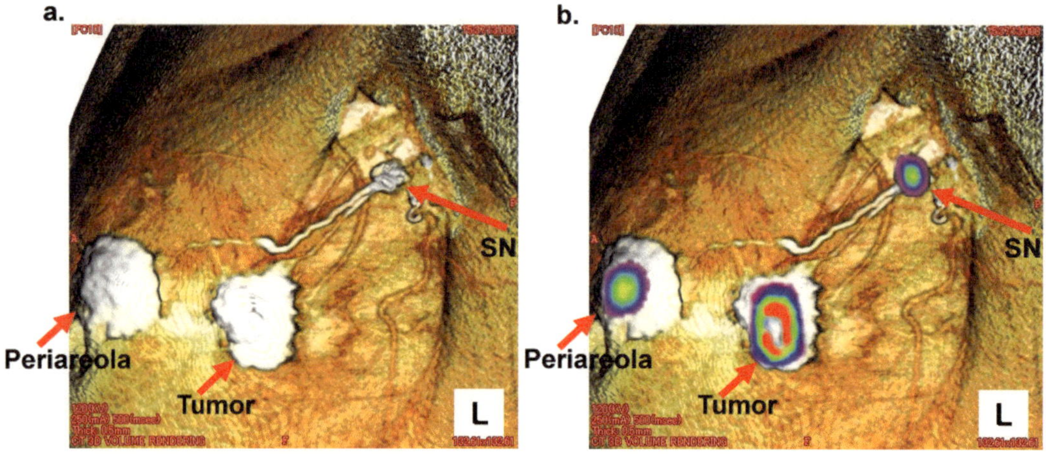

Fig. 6. 3D-CT lymphography and SPECT-fused 3D-CT LG
a. 3D-CT lymphography (LG)
The contrast enhancing materials flow from the injected sites over the tumor and the periareola through the two lymph ducts into single SN in the axilla.
b. SPECT-fused 3D-CT LG
DICOM data of SPECT was projected on 3D-CT LG. The hot spots were coincided with SN detected by 3D-CT LG.

11. Conclusion

By 3D-CT LG, we can recognize the accurate and more precise lymph flow in the breast and the axilla. Even in patients with SN metastasis, if we find no metastatic presence in the second and third SN, the need to dissect more nodes is obviated. In the near future, it will be necessary to omit axillary dissection in such patients.

12. References

Ernst MF, Voogd AC, Balder W. (2002). Early and late morbidity associated with axillary level I-III dissection in breast cancer. *J Surg Oncol*, 79, pp. 151–5.

Veronesi U, Paganelli G, Galimberti V. (1997). Sentinel-node biopsy to avoid axillary dissection in breast cancer with clinically negative lymphnodes. *Lancet*, 349, pp. 1864–7.

Schrenk P, Rieger R, Shamiyeh A. (2000). Morbidity following sentinel lymph node biopsy versus axillary lymph node dissection for patients with breast carcinoma. *Cancer*, 88, pp. 608–14.

Schwartz GF, Giuliano AE, Veronesi U. (2001). Proceedings of the consensus conference on the role of sentinel lymph node biopsy in carcinoma of the breast April 19 to 22, 2001, Philadelphia, Pennsylvania. *Cancer*, 94, pp. 2542–51.

Kuehn T, Bembenek A, Decker T. (2000). A Concept for the Clinical Implementation of Sentinel Lymph Node Biopsy in Patients with Breast Carcinoma with Special Regard to Quality Assurance. *Cancer*, 103, pp. 451–461.

Giuliano AE, Kirgan DM, Guether V. (1994). Lymphatic mapping and sentinel lymphadenectomy for breast cancer. *Ann Surg*, 220, pp. 391–8.

Borgstein PJ, Meijer S, Pijpers R. (1997). Intradermal blue dye to identify sentinel lymph-node in breast cancer. *Lancet*, 384, pp. 149–57.

Krag DN, Weaver DL, Alex JC. (1993). Surgical resection and radiolocalization of the sentinel lymph node in breast cancer using a gamma probe. *Surg Oncol*, Vol.2, No. 6, pp. 335–9.

Giuliano AE, Kirgan DM, Guenther JM. (1994). Lymphatic mapping and sentinel lymphadenectomy for breast cancer. *Ann Surg*, Vol.220, No.3, pp. 391–8.

Suga K, Ogasawara N, Okada M. (2003). Interstitial CT lymphography-guided localization of breast sentinel lymph node: preliminary results. *Surgery*, 133, pp. 170–179.

Tangoku A, Yamamoto S, Suga K. (2004). Sentinel lymph node biopsy using computed tomography-lymphography in patients with breast cancer. *Surgery*, 135, pp. 258–265.

Minato M, Hirose C, Sasa M. (2004). 3-Dimensional computed tomography lymphography-guided identification of sentinel lymph node in breast cancer patients using subcutaneous injection of nonionic contrast medium. A clinical trial. *J Comput Assist Tomogr*, 28, pp. 46–51.

Yamashita K, Shimizu K. (2008). Video-assisted Breast Surgery and Sentinel Lymph Node Biopsy guided by 3D-CT lymphography. *Surg Endosc*, 22, pp. 392-397

Yamashita K, Shimizu K. (2009). Evaluation of sentinel lymph node metastasis alone guided by three-dimensional computed tomographic lymphography in video-assisted breast surgery. *Surg Endosc*, 2008; DOI 10.1007/s00464-008-9809-z. 23, pp. 633–640, 2009

Yamashita K, Shimizu K. (2006). Endoscopic Video-Assisted Breast Surgery: Procedures and Short-Term Results. *J Nippon Med Sch*, 73, pp. 193–202.

Yamagata M, Takasugi T, Takayama T. (2002). Partial mastectomy by the periareolar incision. *Geka Chiryo*, 86, pp. 932–940.

Delamere G, Poirier P, Cuneo B. (1903). The lymphatics. In: Charpy PP eds. A trearise of human anatomy. Westminster: Archibald Constable.

Susan Standring (2005), Editor in Chief, Gray_s Anatomy: The Anatomical Basis of Clinical Practice. 39th Ed. Elsevier Churchill Livingstone.

Kimberg VS, Rubio IT, Henry R, et al. (1999). Subareolar versus peritumoral injection for location of the sentinel node. *Am Surg*, 6, pp. 860–5.

Kern KA. (1999). Sentinel lymph node mapping in breast cancer using subareolar injection of blue dye. *J Am Coll Surg*, 189, pp. 539–45.

Suga K, Yamamoto S, Tangoku A, Oka M. (2005). Breast sentinel lymph node navigation with three-dimensional multidetector-row computed tomographic lymphography. *Invest Radiol*, 40, pp. 336–342.

Shimazu K, Tamaki Y, Taguchi T, et al. (2003). Lymphoscintigraphic visualization of internal mammary nodes with subtumoral injection of radiocolloid in patients with breast cancer. *Ann Surg*, 237, pp. 390–8.

Mariani G, Moresco L, Viale G. (2001). Radioguided sentinel lymph node biopsy in breast cancer surgery. *J Nucl Med*, 42, pp. 1198–1215.

Giuliano AE, Jones RC, Brennan M. (1997). Sentinel lymphadenectomy in breast cancer. *J Clin Oncol*, 15, pp. 2345–2350.

Yamashita K, Shimizu K. (2006). Video-Assisted Breast Surgery: Reconstruction More than 33% Resected Breast. *J Nippon Med Sch*, 73, pp. 320-327.

3

CT Aided Postoperative Breast Conservation Brachytherapy Irradiation

D. O. Odero
Department of Physics and Astronomy, University of Ohio, Athens, Ohio
Radiation Oncology, Raleigh Regional Cancer Center, Beckley, West Virginia
USA

1. Introduction

Breast cancer, with its uncertain causes and confusion over the best treatments, has intrigued the scientific community for years. Numerous resources have been and continue to be devoted to research and technical developments to understand its causes, prevention and treatment. Despite this, breast cancer still remains the most common malignancy and dreaded disease in women in the United States (American Cancer Society [ACS], 2003). Progress has been made, nevertheless, in humanizing the horrors that formerly devastated the body and psyche (Andersen et al., 2008).

Anatomically, breasts are hemispherical in shape and are made up of glandular tissues embedded in connective tissue which lie over the pectoral muscles. Adipose tissues lie between the skin and the glandular tissues, and the size of breasts depend on the adipose tissues. As a woman ages, the adipose tissues of the breasts may become more prominent than the glandular tissues, and the breasts may become softer and begin to be flaccid. Breast cancer is more prevalent in elderly women as they age. The challenges that come with age and the aforementioned breast structure complicates the treatment of breast cancer particularly with radiation.

The most common site of breast cancer is the upper outer quadrant followed by the central area.

Curative treatment of breast cancer include combined modality treatment, which incorporates surgery (radical or conservative) and adjuvant treatments such as chemotherapy, hormonal therapy, external beam irradiation and brachytherapy implantation. The selection of a particular procedure or a combination of procedures depends on established prognostic factors such as stage, grade and extension. In general, surgery is indicative if the tumor is confined to the breast with no extension through the lymphatic system. Brachytherapy implants are used for early stage cancers, either alone or in conjunction with external beam radiation therapy. Patients who require breast conservation using surgical procedures are often potential candidates for brachytherapy as well (Calle et al., 1978; Fisher et al., 1977; Harris et al., 1981; Levene, 1977; Pierquin et al., 1980; Prosnitz et al., 1977); however, patients with extensive tumors are not good candidates for brachytherapy implantation.

Many women with early-stage breast cancer are treated with breast-conserving surgery (lumpectomy) followed by external-beam radiation. The typical radiation course is delivered five days a week for six to seven weeks. A standard "boost" or increased dose to the lumpectomy site usually takes an additional one and one-half to two weeks after the whole breast is treated with a standard radiation regimen. For the external beam radiation treatment to be effective, the geometric location of the affected breast needs to be reproducible (Byhart et al., 1978). Unfortunately, flaccid breasts and the proximity to critical healthy organs such as heart and lungs present a great technical challenge even with superior immobilization tools (Van Arsdale & Greenlaw, 1971). Postoperative intracavitary brachytherapy, delivered twice a day for five days circumvent the technical problems experienced with external beam irradiation. This type of treatment is recommendable for patients with large breast and/or deep-seated tumors although the available data is not yet enough for analysis to conclusively predict the long term outcomes.

Volumetric imaging technology with fast automated visualization and geometric measurement tools has greatly influenced the current practice of breast brachytherapy. Precise details of the tumor or tumor bed help to delineate the area to be treated and to determine the necessary margins around the tumor in breast cancer as well as in other malignancies (Ricke et al., 2004; Manning, 2001).

Details of the clinical aspects of breast cancer and its treatment are beyond the scope of this chapter. This chapter discusses the physical and technologic aspects of the CT aided breast implants using high dose rate (HDR) Iridium-192 afterloading techniques.

2. Breast cancer diagnosis and tumor localization

Mammography remains the major and most reliable imaging method used in breast mass detection. On a mammogram, breast cancer typically appears as an ill-defined, opacified lesion with or without speculated margins (see Figure 1). It can detect small, discrete lesions and chest wall involvement. Unfortunately, mammography presents some challenges such as discomforts when the breast is compressed between positioning paddle and image receptor (see Figure 2), potential image artifacts associated with different breast structures overlying each other rendering the tumor difficult to discern, non-differentiation between tumor and malignancy, and limitation to only two-dimensional (2D) interpretation of images.

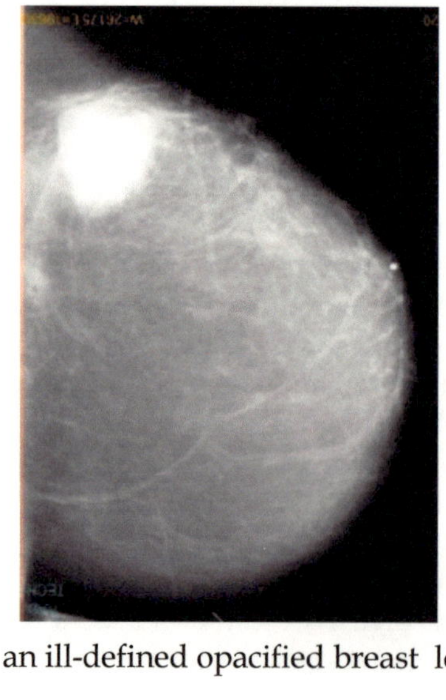

Fig. 1. Mammogram showing an ill-defined opacified breast lesion

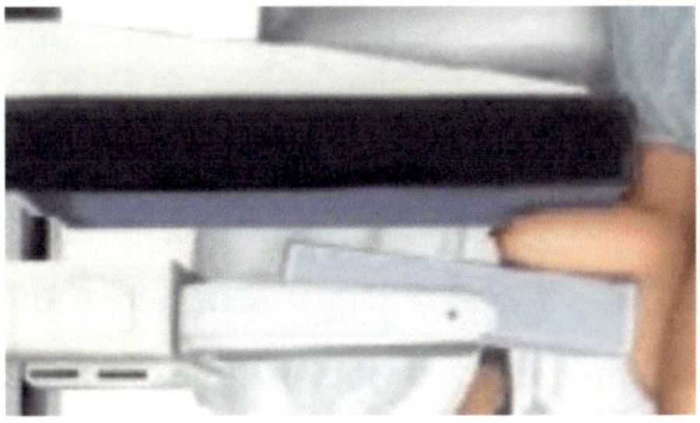

Fig. 2. Mammography - breast compressed on image receptor

CT imaging presents a better three-dimensional (3D) understanding of pathological lesions when they are present, eliminates the compression and can distinguish between the image artifacts and true abnormalities. It is an important tool for the evaluation of local and regional disease in selected patients who have an established diagnosis of breast cancer. However, CT scanners use x-rays at higher energies than do mammograms, reducing the contrast of the images and the ability to distinguish the calcification. For this reason, a CT scanner is less efficient than regular mammography at detecting the tiny clusters of calcium (or microcalcifications) that can sometimes be indicative of breast cancer (Zwicker et al., 1985). CT scanners also have an extra disadvantage of emitting unnecessary radiation exposure to the non-targeted parts of the patient.

A definitive diagnosis of breast cancer can only be made through a microscopic examination of breast tissue obtained from a biopsy. As has been aforementioned, breast cancer is currently the most common malignancy in women; consequently, development of robust screening and detection techniques that can provide earliest diagnosis is necessary since that can lead to cure (Henderson, 1980; Schottenfeld et al., 1976). Such systems should be accurate, cost effective, and non-invasive and should present three-dimensional visualization of the diseased area. A prototype dedicated breast CT has recently been presented (Lindfors et al., 2008).

3. Postoperative breast brachytherapy irradiation

Postoperative irradiation of the breast following a breast-conserving surgical procedure to remove gross tumor is an example of combined surgical and radiation therapy management of local disease. Surgery removes gross tumor while irradiation eradicates subclinical disease in the tumor bed (Calle et al. 1986; Fisher, 1986) to reduce local recurrence (Holland et al., 1985).

The disadvantages of external beam irradiation include the time required for protracted course of treatment, which can last up to seven weeks, as well as radiation exposure to the heart, lung, and normal breast tissue. The development of high activity artificial isotopes (International Atomic Energy Agency [IAEA], 1967; Nath, 1983; Trott 1988), afterloading techniques (Almond, 1983; Delcos, 1980; Delcos, 1992; Glasgow,1995; Henschke et al., 1963; Hillaris, 1975; Pain, 1972; Syed & Feber 1977; Syed et al., 1977), and automated devices with remote control has stimulated renewed interest in brachytherapy.

Brachytherapy can be performed using external surface molds, intracavitary, interstitial, or intraluminal techniques or a combination of these methods. Brachytherapy allows delivery of high dose radiation to the tumor while minimizing radiation exposure to normal tissues by eliminating the unavoidable transit irradiation occurring with external irradiation, and by allowing a highly conformal dose delivery. The radioactive materials used in brachytherapy are of high activity. To allow normal tissue sublethal damage repair, high dose rate brachytherapy is generally fractionated. Before each fraction, images are obtained to determine the geometry of the radioactive sources and their relationship to anatomic targets.

4. Three-dimensional brachytherapy treatment-planning system

Treatment planning is often characterized by the dimensionality of the calculation algorithm. Two-dimensional algorithms have limited anatomy considerations with limited evaluation tools, and in some cases are single point calculations. Three-dimensional algorithms depend upon CT-acquired 3D data sets with comprehensive anatomy, can model 3D dose corrections and use volumetric evaluation tools. 2D calculations represent the dose seen in a single cross sectional slice in an ellipsoid of infinite length and of uniform electron density, while 3D algorithms model the dose obtained in actual patient CT data sets. 3D treatment planning in brachytherapy is therefore the process by which 3D visualization, dose calculation, and plan evaluation tools are used to optimize treatment. Tumor size and shape, as well as outlines of anatomic structures, are adequately established by the use of CT. Tumors of unusual shape or that are located adjacent to radiosensitive tissues benefit from CT based computerized treatment planning.

The development of 3D brachytherapy treatment planning tools has lagged behind that of external beam planning tools. Target definition has traditionally been applicator oriented. Technical developments in brachytherapy treatment planning have been mainly oriented towards conventional x-ray films and very little towards volumetric sectional imaging. The present movement towards 3D image based brachytherapy has been influenced less by the procedure itself and largely by the advancements in the 3D imaging equipment and computer technology that offers the physicians and the planning team the flexibility of understanding the physical aspects of the treatment. McGee and McShan (McGee & McShan, 1988) claimed that the breast brachytherapy based on sectional imaging provides a major contribution to brachytherapy procedure giving examples of potential impacts based on their clinical experience. This experience did not include 3D assessment of anatomy, target, critical organs and 3D image based 3D dose calculations with corresponding display and evaluation capabilities according to ICRU report, 50 (ICRU, 1983). Presently, there has not been similar frame to what ICRU put down in the report 50 (ICRU, 1983) for breast brachytherapy. Calculations based on 2D algorithms ignore the inhomogeneities associated with different composition of human tissue, but with appropriate electron density conversions, CT data can be used to perform bulk dose inhomogeneity corrections in 3D planning (Almond, 1983).

The optimal radioactive source dwell locations and dwell durations can be calculated with the aid of a treatment planning computer based on the prescribed dose. The treatment planning software can optimize these variables once the tumor volume and normal tissues and their dose constraints have been delineated by the radiation oncologist.

3D planning software uses sophisticated Sievert integral algorithms that break a linear radioactive source into tiny components, calculates the dose at every point in the patient from every component, and sums these values to get the final result (Edmundson, 1994).

In keeping with the principles used in 3D external beam radiation planning, breast brachytherapy planning begins by delineating the applicator, air pockets and seroma, and other critical normal organs such as chest wall, heart, lungs, and skin. Planning treatment volume (PTV) in breast brachytherapy using inflatable balloon applicators requires coverage of 1 cm to 2 cm from the applicator which can be constructed using a uniform ring around the applicator.

5. Quality assurance for 3D computer treatment planning system and CT

It is valuable to scan a simple geometric phantom and send this data through the planning process on a weekly or monthly basis. A known phantom geometry should be aligned using lasers, scanned, and the images transferred to the computer planning system. Simple measuring tools in the planning system can serve as a quick check for geometric distortions, image scale, and orientation.

6. CT based accelerated partial breast irradiation

To demonstrate the benefits of the CT image based 3D treatment planning and breast brachytherapy, a MammoSite RTS single channel spherical balloon applicator (Cytyc Corporation, Hologic LP, Marlborough, MA 07152 USA) with Varian Brachyvision 3D treatment planning system together with Varian GammaMed Plus ix (Varian Medical Systems, Inc, Charlottesville, VA 22903) high dose rate (HDR) afterloader is illustrated.

6.1 Intraoperative applicator insertion

MammoSite radiation therapy is a form of accelerated partial breast irradiation (APBI), where an afterloading balloon applicator (Figure 3) is inserted directly onto the lumpectomy cavity (MammoSite, 2010).

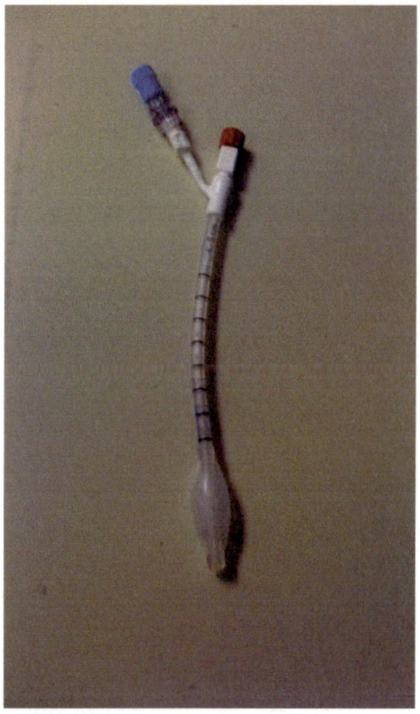

Fig. 3. Deflated MammoSite balloon applicator
Blue -Fluid port for balloon water mixture inflation
Red - Source port for radioation source wire connector

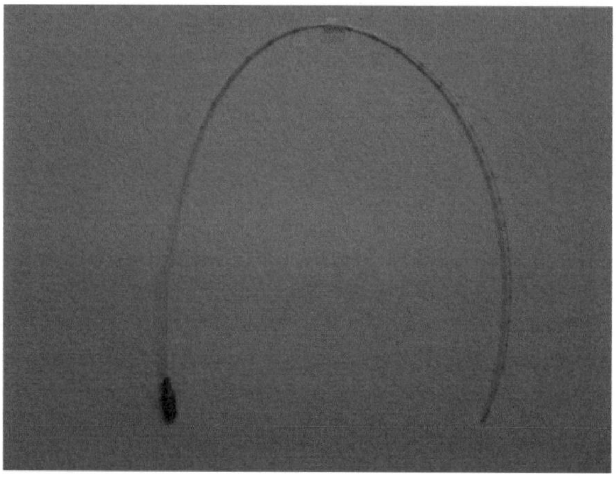

Fig. 4. Dummy source wire with dummy sources

MammoSite RTS is suitable for ductal carcinoma *in situ*, as well as invasive carcinoma (Besaleh et al., 2009). The location of the tumor and post-surgical seroma determine whether a patient is a candidate for this treatment. The balloon must be at least 5 to 7 mm away from the skin, so the technique may not be suitable for small breasted women, or for tumors found near the edge of the skin. The lumpectomy cavity must be spherical, or nearly so, in order for the balloon to conform to the seroma without air pockets. The cavity must also be large enough to allow a balloon volume of at least 30 cc. The balloon is inflated with a dilute mixture of iodinated contrast media to allow CT evaluation of balloon position (Souba et al., 2007).
The MammoSite placement procedure begins by performing the lumpectomy and surgically preparing the cavity for MammoSite balloon applicator. The applicator can then be implanted at the time of the lumpectomy or post lumpectomy.

6.2 Breast brachytherapy treatment planning CT images

Patient data acquisition is an important part of the treatment simulation process, since reliable data is required for computerized treatment planning purposes and allows for a treatment plan to be properly carried out.
The patient should be scanned in supine position with hand over the head unless the chest wall is involved or is less than 7 mm to the balloon surface. Ideally, the treatment CT scanning should be performed 48 hours after the balloon insertion.
Transverse CT scans contain all information required for complex treatment planning in radiation therapy treatment.
Breast CT scan, with radiographic markers (see figure 4 with dummy sources) in place, is required to verify the patient's appropriateness for treatment with brachytherapy and to proceed with 3D planning . A slice width of 3 mm is recommended for adequate resolution of the applicator and surrounding breast tissue on the acquired axial images as well as coronal and sagittal reconstructions. Pilot or scout films relate CT slice position to anterior-posterior and lateral radiographic views of the patient at the time of scanning. They are obtained by keeping the x-ray source at a fixed position and moving the patient (translational motion) through the stationary slit beam. The result is a high definition radiograph which diverges on the transverse axis, but does not diverge on the longitudinal axis (see Figure 5). The patient image data is then transmitted to the treatment planning

computer via either network or portable media using DICOM 2 format or DICOM RT format (ICRU, 1999). It is advisable to archive these images as secondary backup should the treatment planning computer images be corrupted or be unusable. The conformance of the cavity to applicator surface, distance from the balloon applicator surface to skin, and the diameter and symmetry of the applicator then needs to be evaluated either at the CT computer or at the treatment planning computer to determine if the treatment can be delivered. Ideally, this process should be performed while the patient is still on the CT table so that if it is necessary to adjust the balloon volume, this can still be easily done with a follow up CT to confirm the change.

The minimum balloon's surface to chest wall/ ribs distance should also be checked to be not less than 7 mm. If it is less than 7 mm, then the patient should be rescanned and treated in prone position with the aid of customized breast board immobilizer.

Figures 6 through 8 and tables 1 through 5 illustrate these parameters for MammoSite RTS applicator.

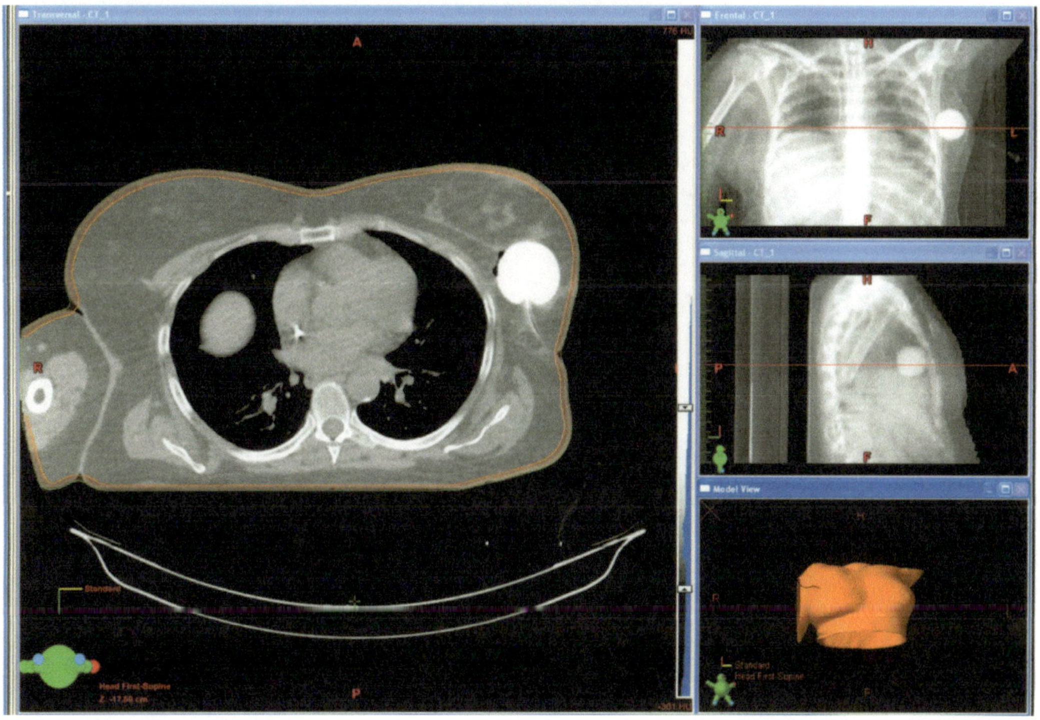

Fig. 5. Breast topogram

Orientation	Measured, x (mm)	x within or greater than (5 mm - 7 mm)? Pass/Fail
Transverse	11.8	Pass
Frontal	9.7	Pass

Table 1. Minimum balloon's surface to skin distance after consideration of all the CT slices. The measurements are a pass if they are within or greater than 5 mm - 7 mm and a Fail otherwise.

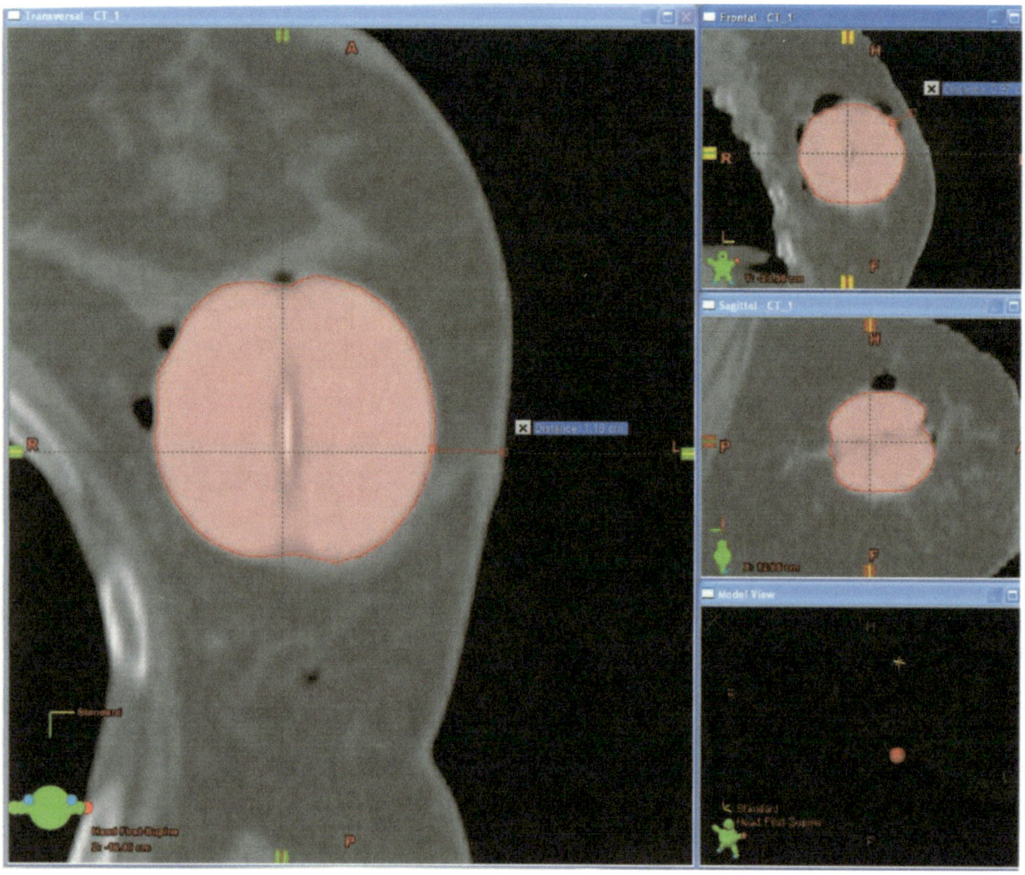

Fig. 6. This figure shows the measured distances from the balloon's surface to the skin in three different orientations. Shown are the CT slices with the shortest distances. Frontal view shows the shortest distance of 9.7 mm which is beyond the acceptable minimum distance of 5 mm.

Orientation	Diameter, d1 cm	Diameter, d2 cm	4.0 ≤ d ≤ 5.0 cm Pass/Fail
Transverse	4.76	4.73	Pass
Frontal	4.18	4.55	Pass

Table 2. Inflated 4.0 - 5.0 cm MammoSite RTS. The transverse diameter, d cm should range between 4 cm to 5 cm to be considered a pass. d1 and d2 represent measurements in different directions

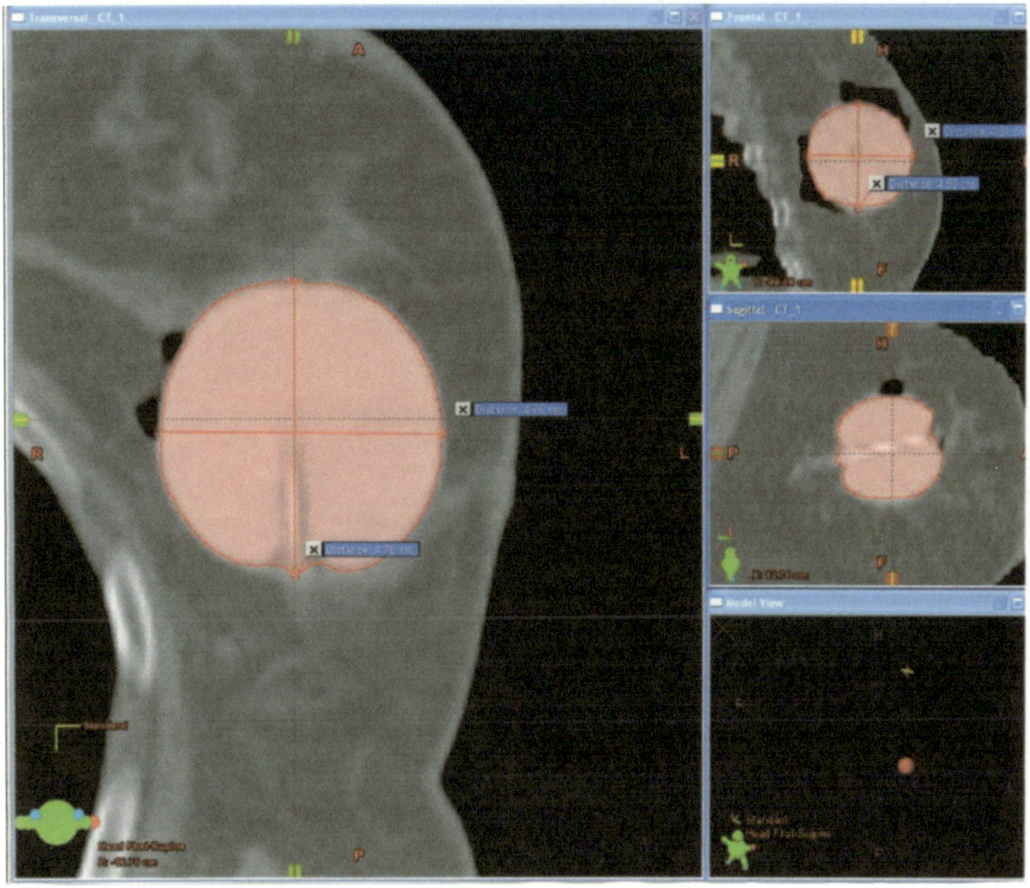

Fig. 7. This figure shows the measured diameters in three different orientations. Shown are the central CT slices with the longest diameters. In this figure, the diameters in all the CT views and directions are between 4.0 cm and 5.0 cm and therefore meets the requirements for the 4 .0 - 5.0 cm diameter fluid inflated balloon.

Orientation	r1 cm	r2 cm	I r1 - r2 I cm	I r1 – r2 I ≤ 0.2 cm Pass/Fail
Transverse	2.23	2.40	0. 17	Pass
Frontal	2.29	2.46	0.17	Pass
Sagittal	2.17	2.09	0 .08	Pass

Table 3. Evaluation of central lumen asymmetry. r1 and r2 represent opposing radii. The magnitude of the difference should not be more than 0.2 cm to be considered a pass.

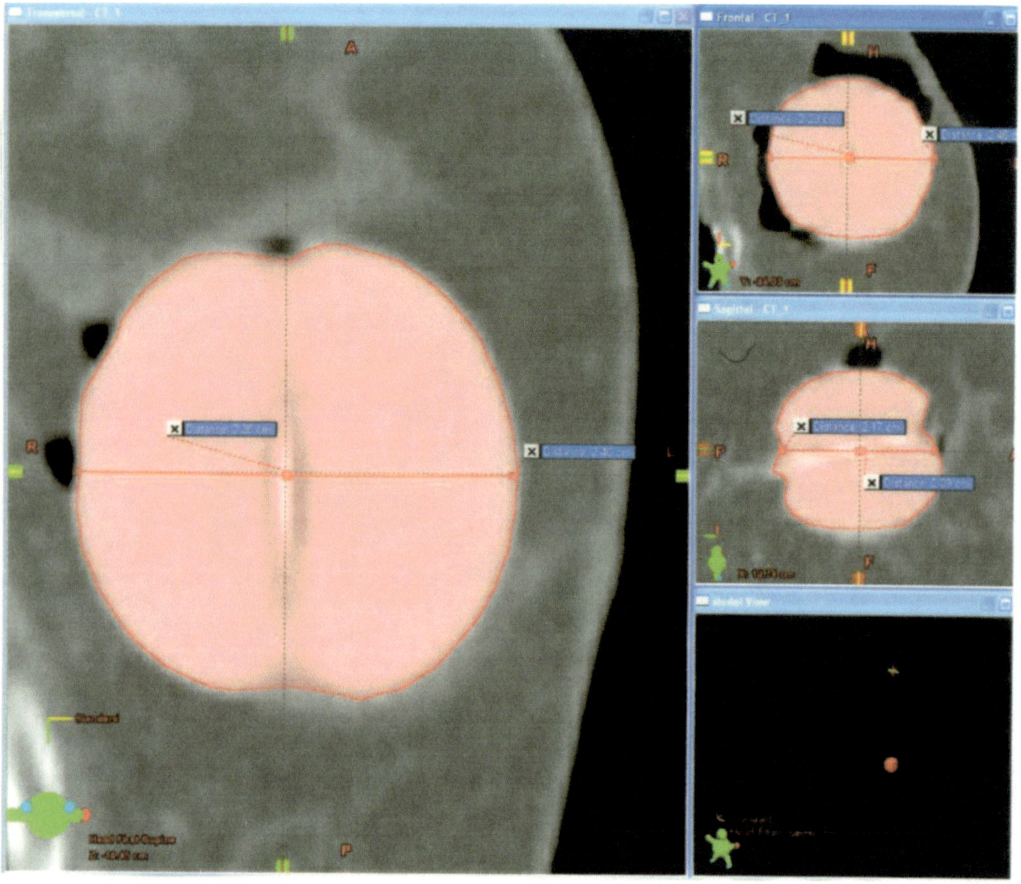

Fig. 8. This illustration is for the CT slices showing delineated balloon in three different views with the largest diameters. The measurements are made for the opposite radii. The maximum differences in the magnitude between the opposing radii in the transverse orientation is 1.7 mm which is less than 2.0 mm as required. The bottom right diagram exhibits a nearly spherical shape 3D model view of the balloon.

Balloon (cm^3)	Air (cm^3)	PTV (cm^3)	Air/PTV (R)	$R \leq 0.1$ Pass/Fail
56.9	6.17	164.47	0.038	Pass

Table 4. Balloon, Air and PTV computed volumes. R should be less or equal to 0.1 to pass.

From table 4, the 3D computed volume is 56.9 cm^3 of a nearly spherical balloon. This gives a spherical radius of 2.386 cm. From table 3, the average measured radius is 2.27 cm. Consequently the measured radius compared to the computed radius differs only by 1.13 mm which is acceptable.

6.3 Radiation dose prescription

MammoSite RTS allows patients to receive their entire treatment in a week, rather than six or seven weeks. Patients have two treatments per day with a minimum 6 hour interfraction interval, over five treatment days (Radiation Therapy Oncology Group [RTOG], 2009). A total dose of 34 Gy is typically prescribed 1 cm from the surface of the balloon. Figure 5 demonstrates a CT scan which is taken each day of treatment in order to obtain the balloon radius, symmetry, and distance from the balloon's surface to the skin's surface.

6.4 3D Computerized treatment planning

The anatomy based 3D treatment planning is performed using the CT images. These images can be fused with images obtained from other modalities such as MRI and PET to clearly define the treatment target. The PTV is obtained by first delineating the balloon using planning system software tools. The balloon surface is then expanded by 1 cm to obtain an expanded volume. Other regions of interest within this expanded volume such as air pockets, ribs, lungs, and muscle are then delineated (see figure 9). Skin is created by extracting the segmentation from the inner wall of the body by 0.5 cm. These regions together with expanded volume lying outside the skin are then removed from the expanded volume to obtain the PTV (see Figure 10).

The air volume within the PTV and PTV volume are then computed. The ratio of the air volume to PTV volume should not be more than 0.1. See table 4 for an example on the patient specific values.

The dummy sources in the CT images are also used to determine the single central dwell position of the radioactive source in the central lumen (see figure 11).

This position should be within 2 mm of the balloon center in order to achieve the precision of dose to the prescription point within 15% (American Association of Physicists in Medicine [AAPM], 1995). Inverse treatment dose computation is then performed on the 3D images where prescription volume is used to optimize the source dwell position and duration. Figure 12 shows the dose-rate distribution and the dose volume histogram (DVH) that is helpful in evaluating the acceptability of the obtained treatment plan. The blue line represents 34 Gy prescription isodose line. The DVH (top right portion of figure 12) indicates that 34 Gy covers 99.6% of the PTV. It can be noticed from the frontal view that part of the skin, which is a normal organ at risk is receiving 39 Gy, more than the prescribed dose because of its proximity to the PTV. The ribs and skin should not receive more than 145% of the prescribed dose. This is an undesirable, but important information that can only be obtained from the CT based 3D treatment plan evaluation.

6.5 Daily quality control and treatment delivery

Once an acceptable computerized treatment plan is obtained, a second independent point dose is calculated to validate the treatment planning computer generated radioactive source dwell durations (American Association of Physicists in Medicine [AAPM], 1995). The treatment parameters such as the treatment machine channel number, radioactive source dwell positions and dwell durations are then exported to the treatment delivery computer and then checked for deliverability before the patient is actually treated. In the example considered above, the measured radius of the balloon is 2.27 cm. The HDR afterloader machine used has a combined MammoSite source train (radioactive source transfer tube) length of 130.0 cm with 0.5 cm reserved for the catheter tip. This is the combined length of the balloon catheter and source guide tube. Therefore the central lumen single dwell position is expected to be located at 127.73 cm. However, for a dwell step size of 0.5 cm, this location would be at 127.5 cm. This value should be compared with the value generated by the afterloader remote control computer before activating the treatment delivery.

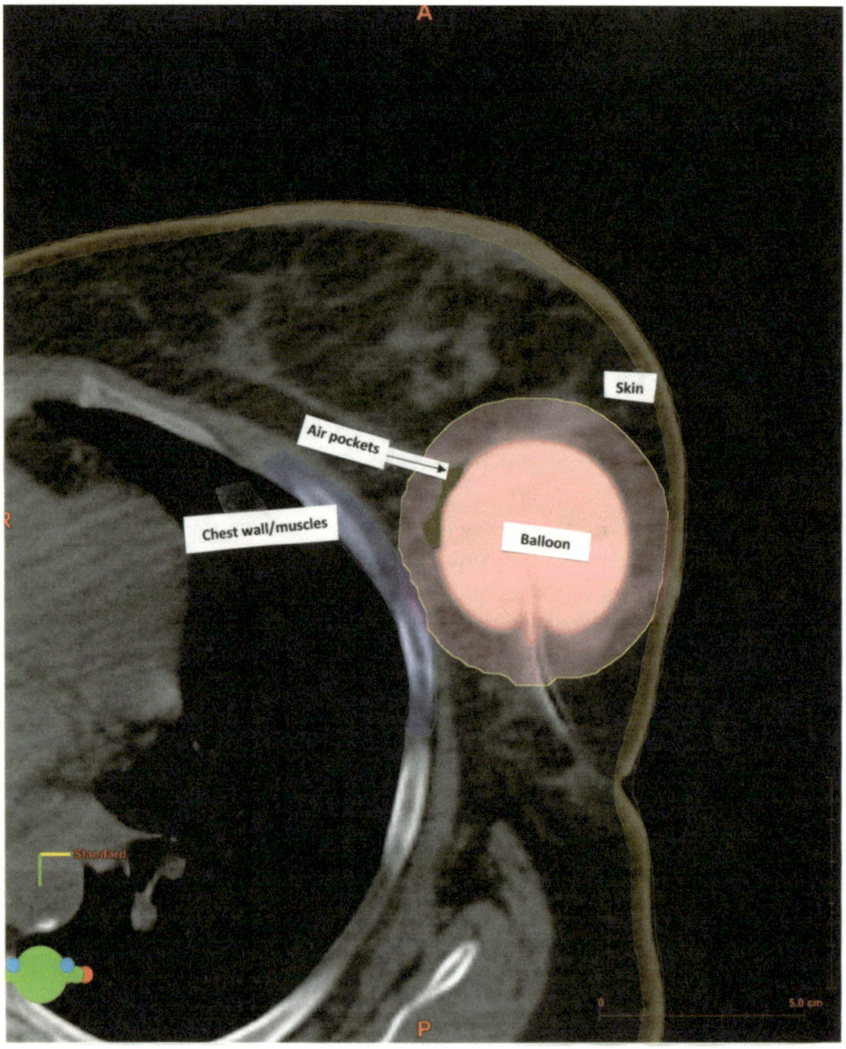

Fig. 9. The figure illustrates the delineated regions of interest. Blue- chest wall, red balloon, green- air gap, orange- skin, purple- expanded balloon.

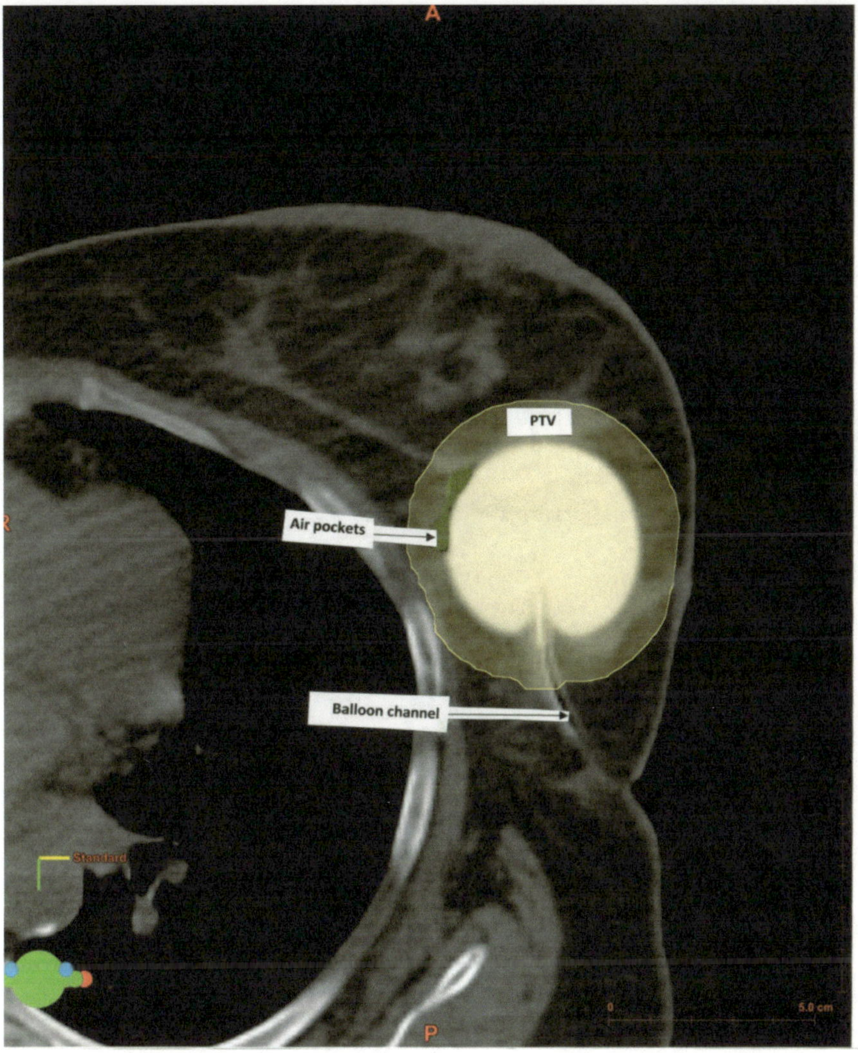

Fig. 10. This figure illustrates PTV with air pockets and a balloon catheter channel. The PTV is formed by removing all the regions of interest within the expanded balloon except the air pockets.

Before the first treatment of each day, CT imaging should be repeated to verify balloon position and its diameter. If balloon diameter changes by 10% (MammoSite, 2010), balloon

integrity must be examined, and a new computerized treatment plan may have to be generated.
The mechanically- controlled motion of the radioactive source from the remote afterloader to the balloon applicator is sensitive to the condition of the transfer tube and applicator. Daily imaging also aids to assure that there are no kinks or obstructions along the transfer tube and applicator situated on the breast to preempt any potential radiation safety issue.
The length and the orientation of the portion of the balloon applicator lying outside the skin surface should be checked to be constant before every treatment. Extra syringe should be available among the emergency kit to be used for draining and deflating the balloon in case of emergency or at the end of the final treatment delivery. The radioactive source transfer tube should not pass through the bed rail and the applicator connectors must be thoroughly cleaned after every usage following the manufacturers guidelines.
Figure 13 shows the treatment delivery system which is remotely controlled by the treatment delivery computer.

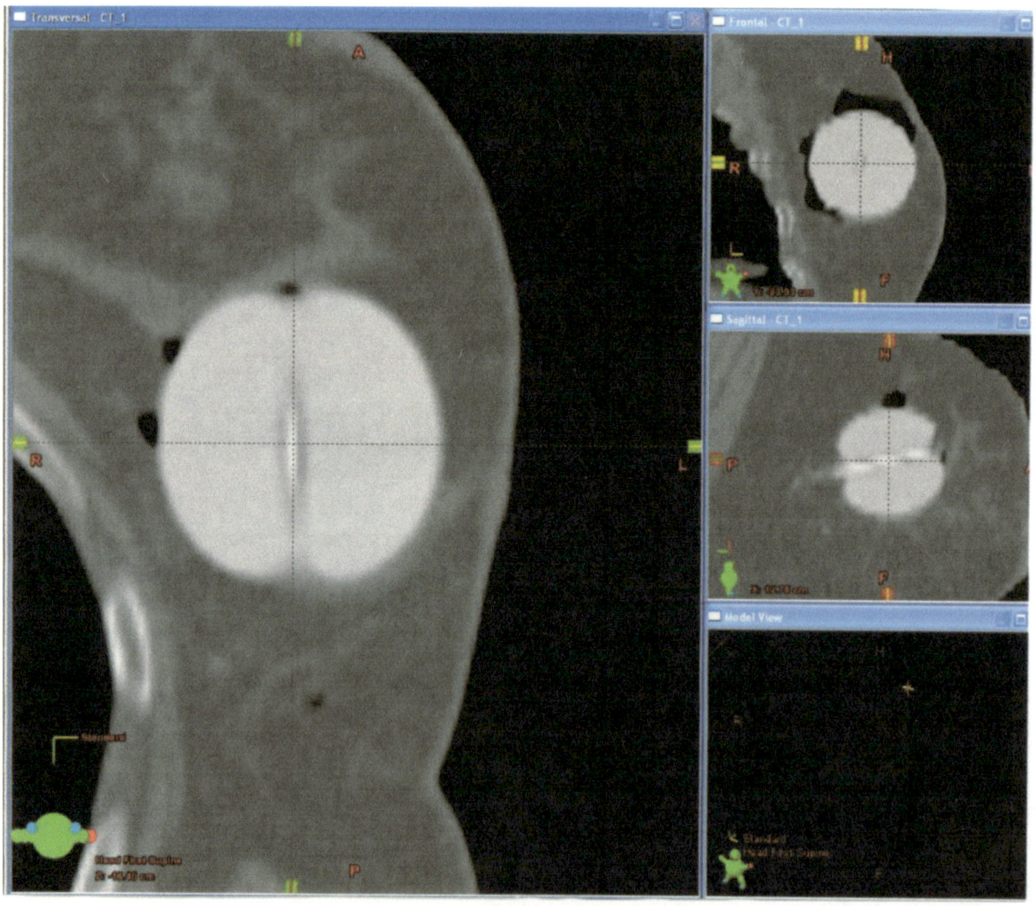

Fig. 11. The central radiographic marker (dummy source) is used to determine the central location of the single dwell source MammoSite RTS.

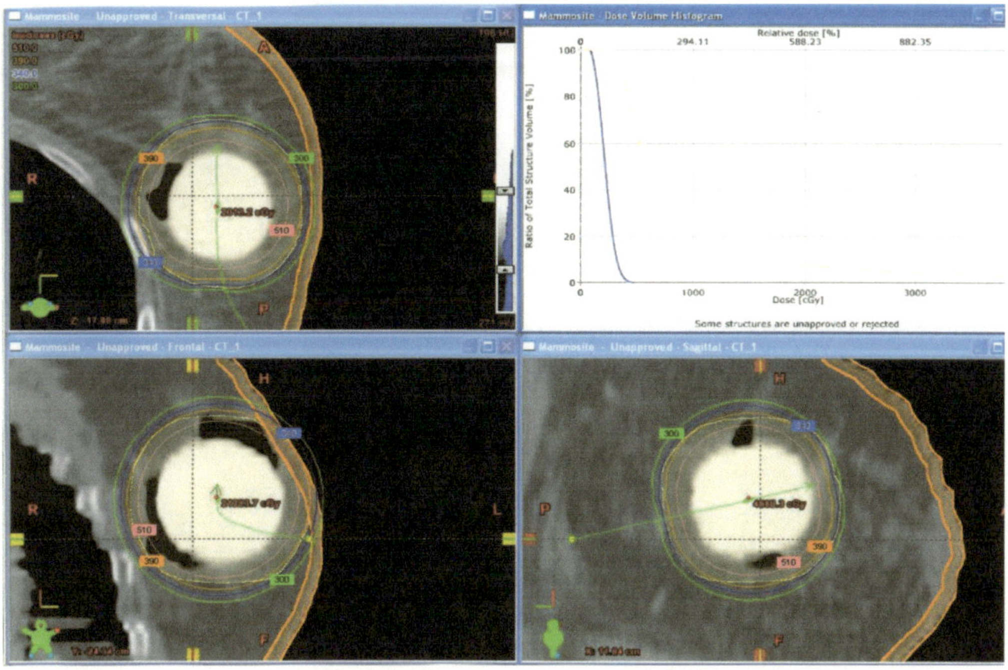

Fig. 12. 3D Treatment plan evaluation. Central bold green is the simulated radioactive source dwell position. Blue line is the 34 Gy prescribed isodose line

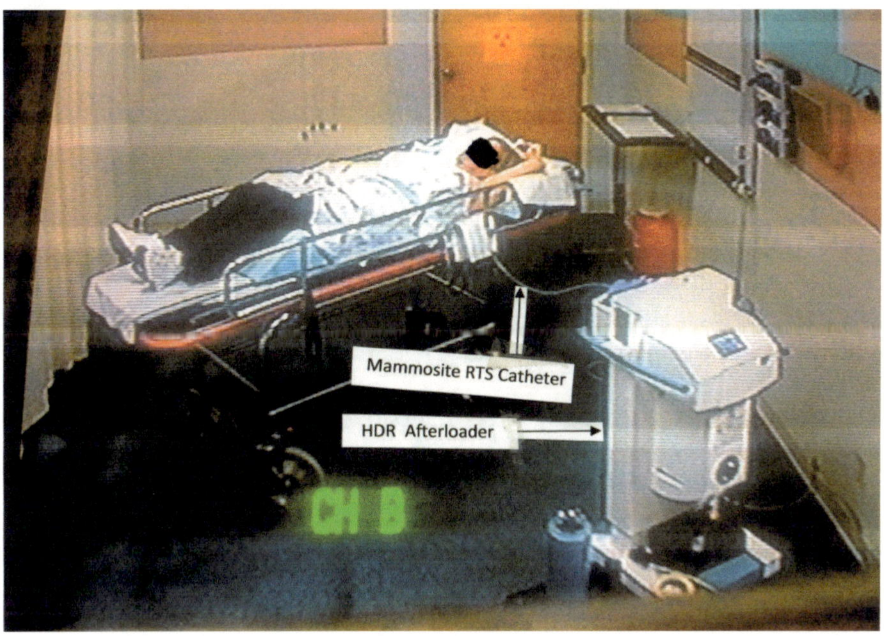

Fig. 13. Patient undergoing left breast Accelerated Partial Breast Irradiation using remotely computer controlled Varian Gammamed plus ix HDR afterloader via MammoSite RTS delivery system.

7. Conclusion

CT aided brachytherapy planning provides advantages over plain radiograph-based brachytherapy planning, as individually customized treatment can be obtained with organs at risk spared from unnecessary radiation exposure. CT based 3D treatment planning software has improved brachytherapy treatment planning because dose in the target and critical organs can be predicted better. CT imaging is also superior when it comes to APBI pre-treatment appropriateness evaluation. However, despite the apparent dosimetric benefits, there is not yet clear clinical data demonstrating an improved therapeutic ratio. Since CT images provide tissue electron density information that can be incorporated into 3D planning systems, the brachytherapy dose calculation algorithms can now be developed further to correct for the tissue heterogeneities to provide more accurate treatments using the electron densities.

8. References

Almond, P. (1983). Remote afterloading, Chapter 8, In: *Advances in Radiotherapy Treatment Planning*, A.E. Wright, and A.L. Boyer (Eds.), pp. 601-619, American Institute of Physics, New York.

America Association of Physicists in Medicine (AAPM), (1995). Dosimetry of brachytherapy sources, AAPM task Group 43 Report, *Med Phys*. Vol.22, pp. 209-239.

American Cancer Society. (2003). Cancer facts and figures-2003, American Cancer Society, Atlanta.

Andersen, B.; Yang, H; Farrar, W.; Golden-Kreutz, D.; Emery, C.; Thornton, L.; Young, D. & Carson, W. (2008). Psychological intervention improves survival for breast cancer patients: A randomized clinical trial, *Cancer*, Published Online: November 17, (DOI: 10.1002/cncr.23969); Print Issue Date: December 15, 2008

Besaleh, S.; Bezak, E. & Bor,g M. (2009). Review of MammoSite brachytherapy: Advantages, disadvantages and clinical outcomes, *Acta Oncol.* Vol.48, No.40, pp. 487-494.

Byhart, R;, et al. (1978). Weekly localization films and detection of field placement errors, *Int J Radiat Oncol Biol Phys Vol*.4, pp. 881-887.

Calle, R.; Pilleron J.; Sclienger P. & Vilcoq J. (1978). Conservative management of operable breast cancer: Ten years' experience at the Foundation Curie, *Cancer,* Vol.42, pp. 2045.

Calle, R.; Vilcoq, J.; Zafrani, B.; Vielh, P. & Fourquest, A. (1978). Local control and survival of breast cancer treated with limited surgery followed by irradiation, *Int J Radiat Biol Phys,* Vol.12, pp. 873-878.

Delcos, L. (1980). Afterloading methods for interstitial .gamma-ray therapy. Chapter 1, In: *Textbook of Radiotherapy*, G.H. Fletcher (Ed.), pp. 84-92, Lea & Febiger, Philadelphia.

Delcos, L. (1992). Afterloading interstitial irradiation techniques, Chapter 11, In: *Levitt and Tapley's Technological Basis of Radiation Therapy, Practical Clinical Applications*, S.L. Levitt, F.M. Khan, F.M., and R.A. Potish (Eds.), pp. 123-154, Lea & Febiger. Philadelphia.

Edmundson, G. (1994). Volume optimization: An American viewpoint, In: *Brachytherapy from irradium to optimization*. R.F. Mould (Ed.), Veenendaal, Nucletron Intl BV.

Fisher, B.; Montague, E.; Redmond, C.; & other NSABP investigators. (1977). Comparison of radical mastectomy with alternative treatments of primary breast cancer; a first report of results from a prospective randomized clinical trial, *Cancer,* Vol.39, pp. 2827.

Fisher, E.; Sass, R.; Fisher, B.; Gregorio, R.; Brown, R. & Wickerham, L. (1986). Pathologic findings from the National Surgical Adjuvant Breast Project (protocol 6) II. Relation of local breast recurrence of multicentricity, *Cancer,* Vol.57, pp. 1717-1724.

Glasgow, G. (1995). Principals of remote afterloading devices. In: *Brachytherapy Physics,* J. Williamson , B. Thomadsen & R. Nath (Eds), Medical Physics Publishing, Madison, Wisconsin.

Harris, J.; Botnick L.; Bloomer W., et al. (1981). Primary radiation therapy for early breast cancer: The experience of the Joint center for radiation Therapy, *Int J Radiat Oncol Biol Phys. Vol.7*, pp. 1549.

Henderson, I. & Canellos, G. (1980). Cancer of breast: the past decade, *N Engl J Med.* Vol.30, pp. 17-30.

Henschkle, U.; Hilaris, B. & Mahan, G. (1963). Afterloading in interstitial and intracavitary radiation therapy, *AJR,* Vol.90, pp. 386.

Hillaris, B. (Ed.). (1975). Afterloading, 20 Years of Experience 1955-1975, *Proceedings of the II International Symposium on Radiation Therapy,* American Institute of Physics, Memorial Sloan-Kettering Cancer Center, New York.

Holland, R.; Veling, S.; Mravunac, M. & Hendricks, J. (1985). Histologic multifocality of Tis T1-2 breast carcinomas, *Cancer,* Vol.56, pp. 979.

Internationl Atomic Energy Agency (IAEA). (1967). Physical Aspects of Radioisotope Brachytherapy, technical Report Series No. 75, International Atomic Energy Agency, Vienna.

ICRU Report No. 50. (1983). Prescribing recording, and reporting photon beam therapy, T. Landberg et al (Eds), International Commission on Radiation Units and Measurements, Bethseda.

ICRU Report No. 62. (1999). Prescribing recording, and reporting photon beam therapy, (supplement to ICRU report 50), T. Landberg (Eds), International Commission on Radiation Units and Measurements, Bethseda.

Levene, M. (1977). Interstitial therapy of breast cancer, *Int J Radiat Oncol Biol Phys. Vol.2*, pp. 1157.

Lindfors K.; Boone J.; Nelson T.; Yang K.; Kwan A. & Miller D. (2008). Dedicated Breast CT, Initial Clinical experience, *Radiology,*Vol.3, pp. 725-733.

MammoSite RTS (2010). Private communication.

Manning, M.; Zwicker, R.; Arthur, D., et al. (2001). Biologic treatment planning for high-dose-rate brachytherapy, *Int J Radiat Oncol Biol Phys.* Vol.49, pp. 839-884.

McGee, J. & McShan, D. (1988). Computerized Tomography for Ir 192 Iridium breast implants, In: *Fortschritte in der interstitiellen und intrakavitaren Strahlentherapie,* Karcher & Hammer (Eds), pp. 105-109, W. Zuckschwerdt Verlag, Munchen, Bern, Wien.

Nath, R. (1993). New directions in radionuclide sources for brachytherapy, *Semin. Radiat. Oncol.*, Vol.3, pp. 279-289.

Paine, C. (1972). Modem afterloading methods for interstitial radiotherapy, *Clin. Radiol.*, Vol.23, pp. 263-272.

Pierquin, B.; Owen, R.; Maylin, C., et al. (1980). Radical radiation therapy of breast cancer. *Int J Radiat Oncol Biol Phys. Vol.*6. No.17.

Prosnitz, L.; Goldenburg, I.; Packard, R., et al. (1977). Radiation therapy as initial treatment for early stage cancer of the breast without mastectomy, *Cancer* Vol.39, pp. 917.

Radiation Therapy Oncology Group (RTOG), NSABP B-39/RTOG 0413: A Randomized Phase III Study of Conventional Whole Breast Irradiation (WBI) versus Partial Breast Irradiation (PBI) for Women with Stage 0, I, or II Breast Cancer. Nov. 2, 2009, Available from: 208.251.169.72/members/protocols/0413/0413.pdf

Ricke, J.; Wust, P.; Stohlmann, A.; et al. (2004). CT-guided interstitial brachytherapy of liver malignancies alone or in combination with thermal ablation: phase I/II results of a novel technique, *Int J Radiat Oncol Biol Phys.* Vol.58, pp. 1496-1505.

Schottenfeld, D. et al. (1976). Ten-years results of treatment of primary operable breast carcinoma, *Cancer*, Vol.38. pp. 1005.

Souba, W.; Frank, M.; Jurkovich, G.; et al. (2007). ACs Surgery: principles and practice. New York: WebMD.

Syed, A . & Feber, B. (1977). Technique of afterloading interstitial implant, *Radiol. Clin.*, Vol.46, pp. 458-475.

Syed, A; Nisar, S. & Feber, B. (1977). Techniques of afterloading interstitial implants. in Renaissance of Interstitial Brachytherapy, *Proceedings of the 12th Annual San Francisco Cancer Symposium, California*, pp. 119-135, Frontiers of Radiation Therapy Oncology, Vol.12, J.M. Vaeth,. (Ed.), S. Karger, Basel, 1978.

Trott, N. (Ed). (1988). Radionuclides in Brachytherapy, Radium and After, *Br. J. Radiol.*, Suppl. 21, British Institute of Radiology, London.

Van Arsdale, E. & Greenlaw R. (1971). Formalized immobilization and localization in radiation therapy, *Radiology* Vol. 99, pp. 697-698.

Zwicker, R.; Schmidt-Ullrich, R. & Schiller, B. (1985). Planning of Ir-192 seed implants for boost irradiation of the breast, *Int J Radiat Oncol Biol Phy. Vol.* 11, pp. 2163.

4

Application of CT Scanning in the Studies of Minimal Invasive Thoracoscopic Surgery of Adolescent Idiopathic Scoliosis

Yong Qiu
Spine Surgery, The Affiliated Drum Tower Hospital of Nanjing University Medical School
China

1. Introduction

Adolescent idiopathic scoliosis (AIS) is a structural, lateral, rotated curvature of the spine that arises in otherwise healthy children at or around puberty, for which no cause has be established. (Lowe TG, *et al.* 2000, Weinstein SL, *et al.* 2008, Wang WJ, *et al.* 2011) The diagnosis is one of clinical and radiographic exclusion, and is made only when other causes of scoliosis, such as vertebral malformation, neuromuscular disorder, syndromic disorders, connective tissue disorders and genetic syndromes, have been ruled out. Spinal deformity is usually noted by a school screening examination, a pediatrician, or a family member observant to the changes seen in the trunk including: unlevel shoulders, waistline asymmetry, and thoracic or lumbar prominences. The diagnosis is confirmed on long-cassettal coronal and lateral radiograph of the spine, with a Cobb measurement greater than or equal to 10°. In addition, the radiographs should exclude congenital anomalies of the spine and atypical curve patterns, such as left thoracic curves that may be associated with syringomyelia. With this definition, epidemiological studies estimate the prevalence of 1-3% in the at-risk population (children aged 10-16 years). In these patients, the most common type of AIS is main right thoracic curve (RT).
The size of the curve tends to increase over the entire lifetime, but the fastest progression happened during pubertal growth. Female showed a significant higher tendency of progression than male AIS patients, with the ratio of 9:1 or 10:1 with curves greater than 40°, at which a surgical intervention would be recommended with the aim of arresting progression, achieving maximum permanent correction of the deformity in three dimensions, improving appearance by balancing the trunk, and keeping short-term and long-term complications to a minimum. Both posterior and anterior instrumentation methods have been used successfully in surgical treatment of AIS. The AIS patients with a primary thoracic curve have the highest prevalence of progression. When the curve pattern is such that only thoracic instrumentation is required, the choice between anterior and posterior surgical approach exists. Segmental posterior spinal instrumentation and fusion has been accepted as the gold standard method in treating RT-AIS, for the consistent correction rate in short and long term, and low incidence of complication. (Weinstein SL, *et al.* 2008) In contrast, anterior scoliosis surgery was introduced with the ability to create thoracic kyphosis and better correct vertebral rotation and torsion, and with the fusion of

fewer motion segments when compared to posterior approach. The procedure, however, traditionally has required a thoracotomy, which has approach-related morbidity, such as significantly reduced pulmonary function with slow recovery after operation, large skin scar with massive wound injury which results in the postoperative pain.

Two decades ago, a video-assisted thoracoscopic surgery (VATS) was developed for intervention of spinal deformation, firstly for anterior release of severe and rigid RT-AIS, and then successfully used for instrumentation and correction of well-chosen patients with RT-AIS. This approach obviates many of the disadvantages of the traditional open anterior thoracic approach. The morbidity associated with a thoracotomy is limited because of the requirement of minimal skin and chest wall dissection by this method, hence the approach showed less detrimental to pulmonary function and more favorable in terms of postoperative pain and appearance.

The fundamental aims of AIS instrumentation and fusion are safe and efficient curve correction and solid fusion to maintain the long term correction. In anterior spinal instrumentation, ideal discectomy with auto bone graft is important for bony fusion. In addition, bi-cortical vertebral screw projecting one or two threads outside the vertebra was recommended to reinforce pull out strength (Lowe T, *et al.* 2002, Huang TJ, *et al.* 2003). However, it was in concern that during the procedure of discectomy, instrumentations may penetrate into spinal canal and lead to spinal cord injury. In addition, the bi-cortical inserted screws could result in vascular injury or neurological complications. Furthermore, comparing with the control subjects, the thoracic aorta in patients with RT-AIS was found to shift more posteriorly and closely to the vertebra because of the vertebral rotation and morphological anomaly at the vertical plane.(Sevastik B, *et al.* 1996, Sucato DJ and Duchene C 2003a, Maruyama T, *et al.* 2004) When correcting RT-AIS with VATS, it's challenge for surgeons to work with this minimal invasive approach by long-arm instruments based on two-dimensional vision on fluoroscopy, instead of managing under direct view through free hand. (Sucato DJ, *et al.* 2004, Grewal H, *et al.* 2005, Lonner BS, *et al.* 2005, Newton PO, *et al.* 2005a) For these reasons, the placement of the screws in these patients thoracoscopically was subject to the complication of aorta injury and the penetration of the spinal canal.(Dunn HK 1986, Ohnishi T, *et al.* 2001, Parent S, *et al.* 2002, Bullmann V, *et al.* 2005, Kuklo TR, *et al.* 2005, Huitema GC, *et al.* 2006) Hence a well knowledge on the anatomic relationship between the para spinal tissues and the thoracic vertebral bodies, and the dynamic changes of the relationship during operation is critical for accurate screw insertion and the other procedures so that a satisfied instrumentation and fusion could be achieved in patients with RT-AIS.

With these objectives, a series computed tomography (CT) based studies were carried out in our centre. Firstly, with the concern of aortic and neurological complications caused by screw insertion, morphometric comparison of the spatial relationship between thoracic aorta and thoracic vertebrae in patients with RT-AIS and that in control subjects were carried out to find the safe entry point, trajectory, and length of screw for Chinese AIS as well as provide the anatomic reference data for correct screw placement under thoracoscopy. Secondly, during curve correction, thoracic pleura would be dissected for discectomy and anterior release of thoracic spine, and sometimes thoracic aorta would be released as well. Some surgeons close the pleura to minimize the drainage, while others would not with the aim to save operation time. Whether the anatomic relationship between thoracic aorta and vertebrae would be changed during surgical procedures is also critical for screw insertion. Hence the dynamic changes of this relationship during operation were investigated. With the knowledge, VAST and VAST associated mini-open thoracotomy approaches were used in correcting RT-AIS, then the accuracy of instrumentation was investigated on CT scan images.

2. Methods and results

2.1 Anatomical relationship between the aorta and thoracic vertebral bodies in RT-AIS

2.1.1 Methods

2.1.1.1 Subjects

Thirty cases of RT-AIS including 8 males and 22 females, with an average age of 15.7 years (range 13–20 years) were recruited. Posteroanterior and lateral radiographs and pan spinal cord MRI were performed to ensure that the scoliosis was idiopathic. Patients with proven or suspected congenital, muscular or neurological scoliosis were excluded.
Sixty-four patients without any spinal deformity who had axial thoracic CT because of non-vertebral pathology were chosen as the control group. Patients with any congenital malformation or other diseases which may affect the normal anatomy of thoracic vertebrae and aorta were excluded. There were 28 males and 36 females with an average age of 13.3 years (range 15–20 years) in the control group. The patients in both groups were from mainland China.

2.1.1.2 CT scans and analysis

Spiral scans were obtained on a 16-multidetector-spiral CT (MDCT) scanner (LightSpeed, GE Healthcare) with the following parameters: 320 mAs, 120 kvP, 10 mm slice thickness. Images showing bilateral rib heads and costevertebral joints were selected for measurement. The transverse CT images from T4 to T12 in both groups were measured with conimeter, vernier caliper and compasses with respect to the following parameters (figure 1): (1) the angle for safety screw placement (β): angle formed by the line that passed the anterior edge of the bilateral rib heads(Line RR) and the line from the anterior edge of the right rib head to the posterior wall of the aorta, (2) the angle of the aorta relative to the vertebral body (α): angle composed by Line RR and another line from the anterior midpoint of the spinal canal to the center of the aorta, (3) the vertical distance from the line RR to the anterior wall of the spinal canal (*RV*), (4) the distance from the anterior edge of the left rib head to the posterior wall of the aorta (*a*), (5) the vertebral body transverse diameter (c), (6)vertebral rotation (γ) i.e. RAsag angle. (Krismer M, *et al.* 1992)

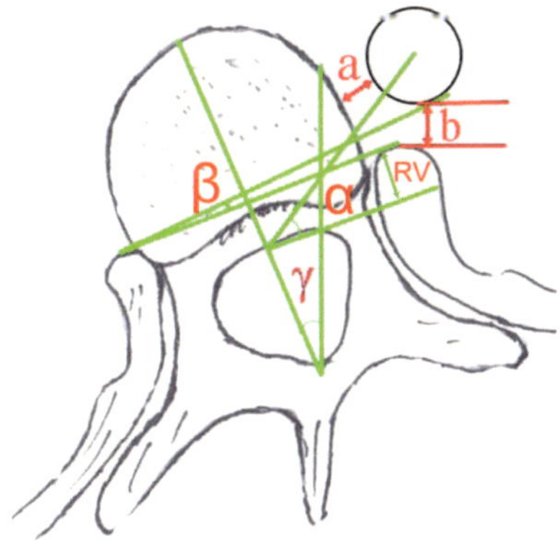

Fig. 1. Illustration of parameters measured on the CT images.

2.1.1.3 Statistical analysis

Statistical analysis was performed with the use of SPSS software (version 11.5, America). Mean values ± standard deviations were calculated for all variables at each level. Comparisons were made between the two groups with the use of the student t test. Significance was defined as a $p< 0.05$.

2.1.2 Results

No significant differences were found between the two groups with respect to age or gender distribution. In the scoliosis group, Cobb angles ranged from 40° to 70° with an average of 54°. No anomaly of thoracic vertebrae and aorta were found except scoliosis, and the most common apical vertebra was eighth thoracic vertebra. A total of 403 vertebrae in the control group and 266 vertebrae in the scoliosis group were measured. The measurement results in the control group and the scoliosis group were summarized in Table 1. The β angle, α angle and a value had a tendency to decrease and then increased from T4 to T12, and values were generally lower in the scoliosis group than that in the control group. The β angle from T7 to T10, α angle from T5 to T10 and a values at T9, T10 were significantly lower in the scoliosis group. The RV value decreased steadily from the cephalic to the caudal aspect of the spine in both groups and became negative at T11 and T12 in the scoliosis group, while the values were significantly lower in the scoliosis group from T4 to T11. The c value of both groups increased gradually from T4 to T12, however, no significant difference was found at any segment level other than T7. The γ angle in the scoliosis group also had a tendency to increase and then decrease from T4 to T12, while the value was larger at the periapical levels. At the periapical levels, there were significant negative corrections between the vertebral rotation and the α angle($R = -0.765$, $p< 0.05$).

Level	n	β(°)	α(°)	RV (mm)	a (mm)	c (mm)
T4	44	27.5±8.9	60.8±8.2	6.4±2.6	17.8±5.8	26.2±2.4
T5	44	13.4±9.3	47.0±9.5	5.9±2.4	8.1±5.5	27.1±2.0
T6	45	9.2±7.9	43.0±9.3	5.1±1.9	5.5±4.9	28.0±2.1
T7	44	11.5±8.7	45.2±10.6	4.7±2.2	7.3±5.2	29.2±2.3
T8	46	18.4±9.2	50.3±10.2	3.6±2.4	11.5±5.7	30.1±2.4
T9	48	21.8±9.7	54.8±12.6	3.4±2.3	14.0±6.3	31.5±2.7
T10	49	26.9±8.6	59.2±15.8	3.3±2.4	18.0±6.0	33.1±2.9
T11	42	31.7±7.3	67.0±9.4	2.3±2.1	21.6±6.3	35.2±2.1
T12	39	35.9±6.1	70.8±7.6	0.2±2.5	26.4±5.2	37.9±2.2

Table 1. Quantitative measurements of relationship between aorta and vertebrae in control

2.2 Dynamic changes of the relationship between thoracic aorta and vertebrae in RT-AIS underwent thoracic associated mini-open thoracotomy Instrumentation with pleura closure

2.2.1 Methods

2.2.1.1 Surgical technique

Fourteen patients treated with mini-incision thoracoscopic anterior fusion with CDH-TSRH instrument (Medtronic Sofamor Danek, Memphis, TN) were recruited. The operation was done under general anaesthesia with routine endotracheal intubation. The patient was

Level	n	β(°)	α(°)	RV (mm)	a (mm)	c (mm)	γ(°)
T4	30	29.1±13.0	61.1±19.1	3.7±2.0*	17.3±7.6	26.2±2.2	-13.0±6.0
T5	30	10.1±11.3	38.5±17.7*	2.4±2.2*	6.8±6.8	27.6±2.8	-10.3±7.9
T6	30	5.8±9.7	32.6±14.7*	1.8±1.9*	4.0±6.2	28.9±3.8	–3.3±8.9
T7	30	5.2±7.8*	26.9±12.2*	1.4±1.7*	4.8±5.9	30.4±4.2*	7.1±7.3
T8	30	10.5±8.9*	31.5±13.5*	1.2±1.4*	8.5±8.1	30.9±3.2	13.4±5.3
T9	30	12.7±9.1*	37.6±12.3*	0.6±2.4*	8.4±5.5*	32.1±3.6	13.4±6.8
T10	30	17.8±11.5*	43.6±15.2*	0.5±3.0*	13.0±7.5*	33.1±3.1	11.6±9.0
T11	29	26.6±11.5	68.5±55.2	-1.4±1.9*	20.5±7.7	34.8±3.7	4.2±11.6
T12	27	35.4±12.1	69.0±18.7	-1.6±3.3	26.7±7.9	37.1±4.0	-2.8±15.3

*: the difference was significant when comparing with the control group ($p<0.01$).

Table 2. Quantitative measurements of relationship between aorta and vertebrae in RT-AIS

placed in lateral decubitus position with the convexity up. The superior and the inferior vertebrae in the fusion segments as well as their skin projections were determined with the help of a C arm X-Ray. A 10 cm incision was done parallel to the sixth or seventh rib ending 2–4 cm anterior to the anterior axillary line and 2–3 cm posterior to the posterior axillary line. The thoracotomy was made by removing 10–12 cm of rib.

Elevate the parietal pleura along the thoracic spine with Adsons and open it with Metzenbaum scissors. Extend the opening of the parietal pleura in a cephalad and caudad direction till upper and lower instrumented level. Bluntly dissect the cut edges of the parietal pleura off the spine with a sponge. Elevate it on the discs and lift it off the vessels on the vertebral body. Dissection started over the discs was less likely to cause bleeding. Segmental vessels were clamped and ligated. After division of the segmental vessels, bluntly expose the out surface of the spine. Periosteal elevator was used to expose the entire disc and vertebral column. On the convex side of the curve, the parietal pleura were elevated from vertebral body laterally till right rib head. On the concave side of the curve, the swabs were inserted under the parietal pleura to bluntly push the aorta away from vertebrae and the parietal pleura were peel off the vertebral bodies to the opposite side.

Disectomy at periapical vertebral were done through the incision. Then CDH vertebral screws (6.5 mm in diameter and 3.0–3.5 mm in length) were inserted into the four apical vertebrae, with the similar techniques as conventional anterior open surgery. Two portals with 2.0 cm diameter were made on the middle axillary line at the interval of two intercostals spaces above and below the incision, respectively. These two portals were used as working portals for thoracoscopic procedures. Under direct and thoracoscopic observation, two more intervertebral discs above and below the apical area was removed. Through the portals, CDH or TSRH screws (6.5 mm in diameter and 2.5–3.0 mm in length) were placed into the target vertebrae. At the cephalad thoracic spine (T4–T6), the ventral excursion angle was 15°, the entry-point of the screw should be close to the rib head. For apical vertebrae (T7–T9), the ventral excursion angle should be 10°. At the caudal thoracic spine (T10–T12), the ventral excursion angle was 15°, the entry-point should shift 5 mm ventrally. Morserized autogenous ribs grafts were packed into intervertebral discs for fusion and followed by the placement of the previously bent rod into the CDH or TSRH screws. Without derotation manoeuvre, only compression was applied on adjacent screws from the apex to the upper and lower end vertebrae. The correction of the deformity was

checked under C arm X-ray and finished by wrench out self-breaking nuts. The parietal pleura covering the vertebrae were thoroughly sutured, haemostasis was confirmed and a chest tube was placed through the inferior portal.
All patients were operated on by the same team of surgeons (Y.Q and B.W). Somatosensory evoked potential (SEP) was used for intra-operative neurological monitoring. The pre- and post-operative thoracic coronal curves, kyphosis between T5 and T12 and apical vertebral translation (AVT) were measured on standard standing posterior-anterior and lateral X-ray using the Cobb method.

2.2.1.2 CT scan and analysis

All recruited subjects underwent spiral CT of the spine before and one week after operation. Axial images from T5 to T12 were obtained with the subjects in supine position. The CT examinations were performed by a spiral CT scanner (LightSpeed GE Healthcare) with the following parameters: 320mAs, 120kvP, and 5mm thicknesses, with 5mm gap between slices. Pre- and post-operative CT images with most similar morphology of vertebrae and bilateral rib heads were selected for analysis. A number of parameters were measured using PacsClient software (PACS) on workstation, which included (1) Angle α, the angle subtended by the line joining left and right rib heads and the line from anterior midpoint of vertebral canal to midpoint of the aorta showing the relative position of aorta to the vertebrae, (2) Vertebral rotation angle γ, similar to the Rasag angle,(Krismer M, *et al.* 1992) (3) Distance a, defined as the distance from posterior wall of the aorta to anterior edge of the left rib head, and (4) Distance b defined as the distance from aorta to the closest point of the cortex of the vertebral body (figure 1). The screw position was analyzed on CT images based on the following criteria. The vertebral screw had a bi-cortical penetration which did not encroach on the spinal canal and had at least 1mm distance from aorta. This was defined as satisfactory screw position.(Sucato DJ, *et al.* 2004, Bullmann V, *et al.* 2005, Kuklo TR, *et al.* 2005) All the measurements were taken by an independent observer.

2.2.1.3 Statistical analysis

The data was statistically evaluated using SPSS software for Windows (10.0, Chicago). Related two sample test (Wilcoxon signed ranks test) was used to determine the difference between vertebral levels pre- and post-operation and also differences between the two groups. The Pearson correlation analysis was used to evaluate the relationship between the aorta shifting and curve correction. Significance was defined as a $p<0.05$.

2.2.2 Results

The average age was 14.3±1.7 (12~18) years. The Cobb angle, the curve pattern, thoracic kyphosis and flexibility of main thoracic curve were listed in Table 3. All patients were treated with selective spinal instrumentation (Lenke LG, *et al.* 2001) with an average fusion level of 8.2±0.4 (8~9). The average immediate postoperative MT curve magnitude was 9.6°, showing an average curve correction rate of 78.6%. The thoracic kyphosis was restored. Significant improvement of the apical vertebral translation was achieved (Table 3). No intro-operative SEP monitoring abnormality was found and no neurologic deficits were occurred after operation. All patients were followed up for a minimum of one year. No obvious complications were found during the operation and follow up.

		Pre-OP	Post-OP
N (F)		14 (13)	
Riser sign		3.4 (2~4)	
Main thoracic curve			
Cobb angle (°)		44.9±5.8 (40~55)	9.6±3.6 (4~15)
Flexibility (%)		59.6±13.2 (40.5-69.4)	78.6±7.2 (69~90)
Kyphosis Cobb angle (T5-T12) (°)		12.6±9.5(-4~22)	19.3±11.3 (2~40)*
Apical vertebral translation (mm)		3.50±1.14 (0.70~5.10)	0.53±0.55 (0~1.68)**
Lenke classification		-	N
	1A	3	5
	1B	1	2
	1C	1	2

Significant difference was found when compared with pre-operation: *: $p<0.05$; **: $p<0.01$
Significantly higher curve correction rate was achieved in group A: ††: $p<0.01$

Table 3. The pre-operative and post-operative information of patients

2.2.2.1 The changes in the relative anatomical position of the thoracic aorta with the vertebral body postoperatively

In total, 111 thoracic vertebrae were instrumented and measured. The results were summarized in Table 4. By curve correction, the angle α increased at T6-T12 with maximum found at T8 and T9 measuring 11.7°. The increments were 44.8%. The distance between the left rib head and the thoracic aorta also increased from T6 to T10 with the most significant increase at T9 (31.3%, $p<0.05$). These increments showed that the aorta had shifted anteriorly relative to the vertebrae after curve correction (figure 2). Significant derotation was also found in the periapical vertebrae. Further analysis revealed that the increase of angle α and distance were significantly correlated with the decrease of angle γ ($p<0.01$). The most significant aortic shifting was found at the periapical vertebral levels. The increase of angle α and distance were negatively correlated with the decrease of AVT ($p<0.05$). The distance b decreased post-operatively with the maximum decrease at T9 (27.0%, $p<0.05$), which meant aorta moved closely to the vertebral body following curve correction. The decrease also correlated significantly with the increase of thoracic kyphosis ($p<0.05$).

	α(°)		γ(°)		a(mm)		b(mm)	
	Preop	Postop	Preop	Postop	Preop	Postop	Preop	Postop
T5	40.8±22.3	38.9±11.5	1.1±14.0	-1.6±4.1	7.6±8.4	7. 4±5.1	3.1±1.5	2.9±2.3
T6	31.0±25.7	34.4±14.0	4.2±10.0	1.1±4.3	5.1±8.2	6.6±6.4	3.5±2.8	2.7±1.0
T7	28.4±21.8	32.5±14.7	8.1±10.5	4.5±5.4	5.4±8.2	6.0±6.3	3.6±2.7	2.8±1.5
T8	26.1±22.5	37.8±14.9**	12.2±7.8	4.7±5.2**	6.4±8.1	9.2±7.4	3.8±3.1	3.3±1.1
T9	32.7±23.4	42.3±16.0*	12.1±9.7	6.0±5.9**	9.6±8.1	12.6±6.6*	3.7±2.4	2.7±1.7*
T10	44.4±22.4	48.5±13.9	10.9±13.5	7.0±7.1	14.7±8.1	15.7±7.6	3.2±1.3	2.9±1.5
T11	53.8±24.9	56.5±13.8	8.3±18.3	4.0±8.9	19.5±7.4	18.5±9.1	2.5±1.4	2.0±1.1
T12	65.8±23.2	67.8±15.2	4.2±20.3	1.4±9.7	26.6±7.0	25.2±8.3	2.0±1.4	1.3±1.2

Significant difference was found compared with the pre-operation: *$p<0.05$, ** $p<0.01$
Related two sample test: Wilcoxon Signed Ranks Test

Table 4. The average measurements of CT scans

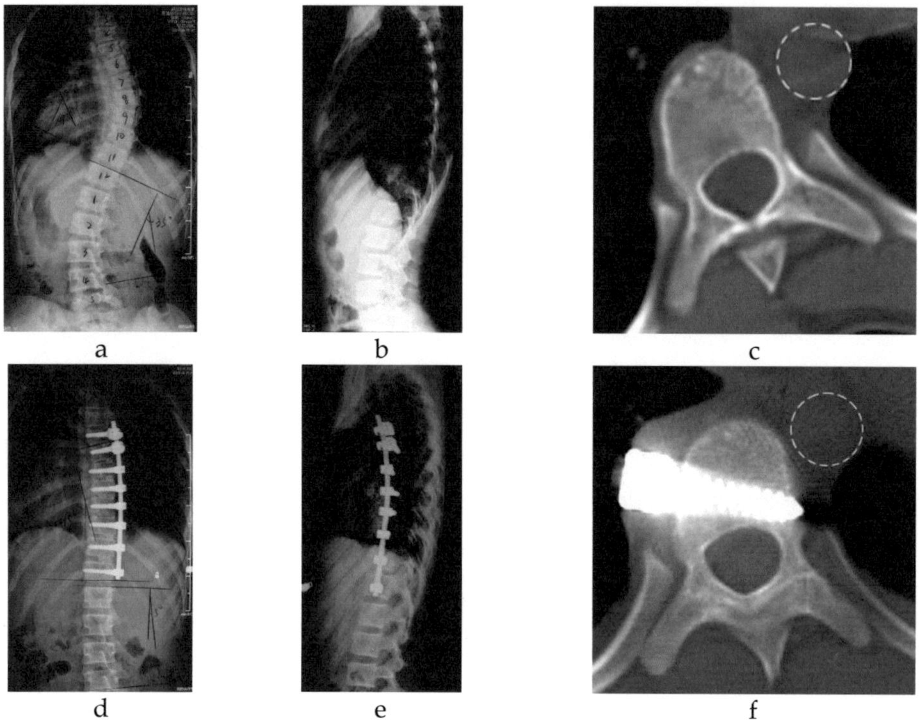

Fig. 2. A 12-year-old girl with AIS Lenke Type 1BN was operated by mini-incision thoracotomic anterior approach. a & d: Pre and Post-operative anteroposterior X-ray; b & e: Pre and Post-operative lateral X-ray ; c & f: CT images of T8, the aorta shift antero-medially after curve correction compared with the preoperative CT images

2.3 Migration of thoracic aorta after the anterior correction of RT-AIS without parietal pleura closure

2.3.1 Methods

2.3.1.1 Subjects

Thirty one patients with the diagnosis of RT-AIS who underwent anterior instrumentation in our institute were recruited. Of which fifteen cases (10 females and 5 males) met the following criteria were recruited into this prospective study. The inclusion criteria were: (1) the Cobb angle less than 60°, (2) apex between T8~T9, (3) the thoracic kyphosis less than 40°, (4) pre-operative and one week post-operative spiral CT scanning available for the same patient. The exclusion criteria were: (1) CT scanning did not clearly show the aorta and bilateral pedicles in interest levels, (2) previous spinal surgery, (3) previous intra-thoracic surgery, (4) pleural adhesions found during surgery, (5) thoracolumbar junctional kyphosis. The average age was 15.9±3.6 years (range, 12~20 years). The average Cobb angle was 45.8°±6.3° (range, 40°~60°) and thoracic kyphosis from T5 to T12 was 13.7°±12.4° (range -2°~25°) . The apex vertebra ranged from T8 to T9 and the AVT was 3.62±1.84 cm (0.81 cm ~5.22 cm). The curve type was classified as Lenke type 1A in eight cases, type 1B in three cases and type 1C in four cases21 (Table 5). The pre- and post-operative thoracic coronal curves, kyphosis between T5 and T12 and AVT were measured on standard standing whole spine X-ray films. The study was approved by a university based Institutional Research Ethics Committee.

		Pre-OP	Post-OP
N (F)		15 (10)	
Riser sign		(3.8)2~5	
Main thoracic curve			
Cobb angle (°)		45.8±6.3 (40~60)	10.9±5.7 (6–18)
Flexibility (%)		64.5±10.4(45.0-70.3)	75.0±8.4 (70~85)
Kyphosis Cobb angle (T5-T12) (°)		13.7±12.4 (-2-25)	22.4±10.8 (10~40)
Apical vertebral translation (mm)		3.62±1.84 (0.81-5.22)	0.78±0.65 (0~1.75)
Lenke classification		-	N
	1A	4	4
	1B	2	1
	1C		4

Table 5. The pre- and post- operative general information of patients

2.3.1.2 Surgical techniques

The anterior mini-open instrumentation was performed by the same team of surgeons (Y.Q and B.W) at a single institution. The surgical procedures were same as the one described previously. The only difference was that the dissected parietal pleura was not sutured and kept free from any tension on it after correction.

2.3.1.3 CT scans and analysis

Same as the methods described in previous part, CT scans were carried pre-operation and oen week post-operation. Then the relative position of the aorta to the vertebral body was evaluated on CT images as in the previous study.

2.3.1.4 Statistical analysis

All data were expressed as mean ± standard deviation (SD). SPSS/PC 13.0 (SPSS Inc., Chicago, USA) was used on all statistical computation. Comparisons between the pre- and post-operative parameters were analyzed by related two sample test (Wilcoxon signed ranks test). The Pearson correlation analysis was used to evaluate the relationship between the aorta shifting and curve correction. A value of $p<0.05$ was considered statistically significant.

2.3.2 Results

2.3.2.1 Clinical and radiographic data

The thoracic curve was instrumented from upper to lower end vertebrae which were T5~T12 in 11 cases, T5~T11 in 2 cases and T6~T12 in 2 cases. The post-op Cobb angle of the thoracic curve on average was 10.9°±5.7° (range, 6°–18°) with 75% curve correction. AVT was corrected to 0.78 cm±0.65 cm (range, 0 cm - 1.75 cm). Normal kyphosis was restored in all patients (Table 5). The total thoracic drainage ranged from 260ml to 600ml (average 450ml). The chest tube was removed once the drainage was less than 50 ml per 24 hr and the mean duration of chest tube stay was 3.1 days (ranged 2 to 4 days). There was no intra-operative fracture of vertebrae body and aortic injury. No complication of pneumonia, effusive pleuritis, pulmonary atelectasis, pneumothorax or respiratory tract obstruction was observed. All patients were followed up for a minimum of one year (ranged 12~38 months). There was no neurological or vascular complication, nor instrumentation failure.

2.3.2.2 CT-based analysis

In CT measurement, the average preoperative angle α decreased from 39.8° at T5 to 28.9° at T8, then gradually increased to 68.3° at T12. After surgery, the angle α became smaller at all levels with an average value of 34.7°, 18.8° and 63.2° at T5, T8 and T12, respectively. The distance a decreased from 7.0 mm at T5 to 8.1 mm at T8 then increased to 28.1 mm at T12 before surgery. After operation, the distance a was smaller at all levels with an average of 5.8 mm, 3.7 mm and 24.3 mm at T5, T8 and T12, respectively. The pre-operative distance b increased from 3.2 mm at T5 to 4.3 mm at T7 then decreased to 1.9 mm at T12. The distance b increased in all levels after surgery with an average of 3.9 mm at T5, 8.0 mm at T8 and 2.3 mm at T12, respectively. All the post-operative parameters were significantly different from the pre-operative ones (p<0.05) except in T5, T11 and T12 (Table 6). The post-operative decrease of angle α and the distance a indicated that the aorta migrates posteriorly after surgery, while the increase of distance b indicated the lateral migration of the aorta relative to the vertebrae (figure 3).

level	Angle *a*(°)		Distance *a* (mm)		Distance *b* (mm)	
	Pre-op	Post-op	Pre-op	Post-op	Pre-op	Post-op
T5	39.8±9.8	34.7±13.0	7.0±6.1	5.8±4.4	3.2±0.9	3.9±3.3
T6	36.0±13.0	28.0±9.6	6.3±4.9	3.5±3.1*	3.5±2.9	5.7±3.9*
T7	35.5±15.0	23.2±10.2*	5.6±4.8	2.3±2.2*	4.3±2.8	7.9±2.7*
T8	28.9±12.7	18.8±10.3*	8.1±5.5	3.7±3.1*	4.1±3.3	8.0±2.0*
T9	35.3±13.2	26.2±10.4*	12.6±6.3	5.0±3.2*	2.2±1.8	6.9±2.4*
T10	53.1±10.4	38.5±11.2*	16.8±5.7	10.5±4.1*	1.7±1.2	4.1±1.5*
T11	58.1±18.3	53.6±13.7	20.9±5.4	18.1±5.6	2.0±1.5	2.3±1.1
T12	68.3±17.5	63.2±14.6	28.1±7.9	24.3±6.9	1.9±1.6	2.3±0.7

Significant difference was found compared with the pre-operation: *p<0.05. Related two sample test: Wilcoxon Signed Ranks Test.

Table 6. Average Measurement results of CT scans in patients (Average ± SD, n=15)

Further analysis revealed that the most significant aortic shifting was found at the periapical vertebral levels with the maximum decrease of angle α at T8 (34.9%) and increase of distance b at T9 (213.6%). The changes of angle α, the distance a and distance b didn't correlate with coronal curve correction, the decrease of AVT and the increase of thoracic kyphosis.

2.4 Accuracy of thoracic vertebral screw in rt-ais inserted through thoracoscopic and mini-open thoracotomy approaches

2.4.1 Methods

2.4.1.1 Subjects

Patients with right thoracic AIS treated with thoracoscopic or mini-open anterior instrumentation from June 2002 to December 2005 in one center were reviewed retrospectively. Those with post-operative CT scanning on instrumented vertebrae were

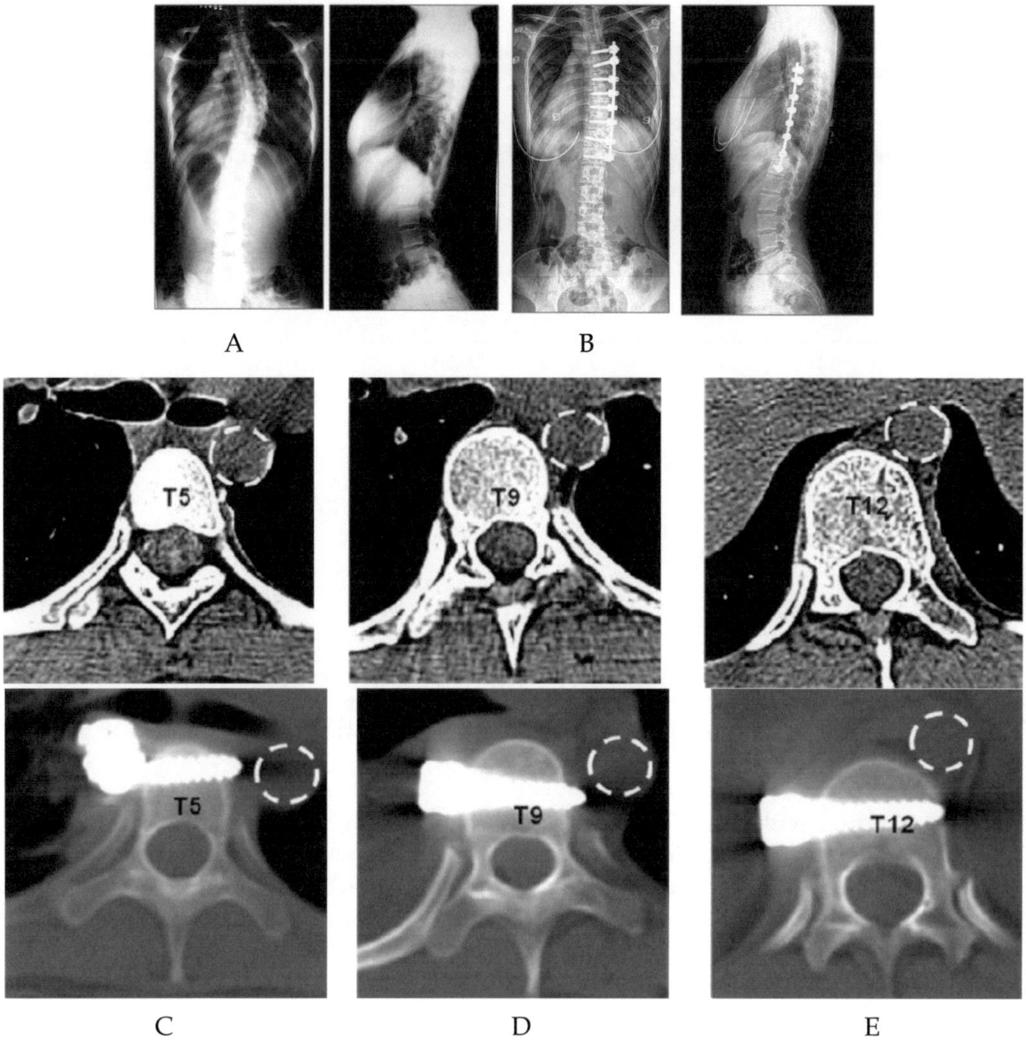

Fig. 3. A 17-year-old girl with IS Lenke Type 1A- was operated by mini-open thoracotomic anterior approach. A: Pre-op anteroposterior and lateral X-ray, Cobb angle 40°; B: Post-operative anteroposterior and lateral X-ray show the Cobb angle corrected to 10°; pre and post-op CT images of T5 (C), T9 (D), T12 (E), the aorta shift posterolaterally after curve correction.

recruited into the study. To lessen the learning curve effect of thoracoscopic technique on screw positioning,(Lonner BS, *et al.* 2005, Newton PO, *et al.* 2005a) the first 20 patients were excluded from the study. To allow better comparison, the first 27 patients treated with mini-open thoracotomy within the same period were also excluded. In this series, a total of ten girls treated with thoracoscopic instrumentation and twenty-one patients (19 female and 2 male) with instrumentation through mini-open thoracotomy were recruited as Group A and Group B respectively. The general clinical information of these patients was listed in Table 7. The curve types were classified according to the Lenke classification.(Lenke LG, *et al.* 2001)

In Group A, two patients were classified as 1A-, three as 1B-, the remaining five were classified as 1AN, 1BN, 1B+, 1CN, 2AN, respectively. In Group B, there were five patients with Lenke type 1A-, six as 1AN, three as 1B-, three as 1BN, two as 1C- and two as 1CN. Eight patients in Group A were treated with *Eclipse* instrumentation (Medtronic Sofamor Danek, US) and the latter two with *Frontier* instrumentation (Johnson & Johnson, US). All patients in Group B were corrected with CDH-TSRH instrumentation (Medtronic Sofamor Danek, US). The instrumentation and fusion techniques were described in previous studies.

	Thoracoscopy (Group A, n=10)	Mini-open thoracotomy (Group B, n=21)
Age (yr)	14.4 (11.5-16.3)	14.4 (11.8-17.2)
Riser grade	2.5 (0-4)	3.5 (2-5)
Pre-operation		
Thoracic curve (°)	52.9 (45-70)	45.4 (40-55)
Flexibility (%)	50.8 (37-73)	57.2 (28.9-87.5)
lumbar curve (°)	30.1 (15-37)	26.5 (16-41)
Post-operation		
Fusion level	7.3 (6-8)	8.1 (8-9)
Thoracic curve (°)	14.3 (5-24)	10.0 (4.3-15.0)
Correction rate (%)	73.6 (66.0-100)	77.9 (66.7-89.2)

Table 7. The pre- and post-operative general clinical information of patients in both groups

2.4.1.2 Surgical techniques

In patients treated with mini-open thoracotomy approach, the sixth or seventh rib was removed through a 10-12cm incision parallel to the rib with its center in the median axillary line. Screws for the four vertebrae at the apical region could be inserted through the incision similar to the conventional anterior thoracotomy approach. The vertebral levels were confirmed by lateral fluoroscopy. For girls with AIS, 30mm-length screws were used for T7, T8 and T9 and 35mm-length screws for T10 vertebrae. The screws were inserted into the vertebral bodies 5mm anterior to the right rib head with a 10° ventral excursion. Two portals with 2.0cm diameter were made on the median axillary line with an interval of two ribs above and below the incision respectively. Screws with 25mm length were selected for proximal vertebrae (often T5, T6). The screws were inserted through the upper portal with the help of thoracoscopic equipments under direct visualization through the thoracotomic incision. The entry points were close to the right rib heads while the ventral excursion angle is no more than 5°. Screws for distal vertebrae (often T11, T12) were inserted with similar technique. 35mm-length screws were used for these lower vertebrae. The entry-point should move 10mm anteriorly away from the rib head with the ventral excursion angle around 15-20°.(Qiu Y, *et al.* 2007) In boys with AIS, the screw length was determined according to preoperative CT scans. The bio-cortical purchase of screw was confirmed by palpating the contralateral tips. Further more, the proper screw placement was confirmed by anteroposterior and lateral fluoroscopy.

In patients treated with thoracoscopic approach, surgery was performed under single-lung ventilation. As proposed by Newton *et al.*(Newton PO, *et al.* 2000) and Mehlman *et al.*,(Mehlman CT, *et al.* 1997) the first portal (2cm in diameter) was established in the anterior axillary line at the sixth or seventh intercostal space. After confirming deflation of the lung, three additional portals were placed gradually in the median axillary line under thoracoscopic visualization. The first screw was inserted into the apical vertebra using thoracoscopic instruments under fluoroscopic image guidance with guide wire. The position was confirmed with anteroposterior and lateral fluoroscopic images. The other screws were inserted with similar procedures through the four portals and the entry points and trend of screws were same as Group B. Anteroposterior fluoroscopic image was taken on every screw to confirm proper screw placement.

2.4.1.3 CT scan and analysis

Axial spiral images of the instrumented vertebrae were obtained by a 16-multidetector-spiral CT scanner (LightSpeed, GE Healthcare) two weeks after operation with the following specifications: 320mAs, 120kvP, 5mm thickness, with 5mm gap between slices. CT images were then reconstructed at 1.25mm intervals. The images showing bilateral rib heads and screw were selected for analysis with Dicm Pacs Client on workstation. Several parameters were measured as described by other studies:(Sucato DJ, *et al.* 2004, Bullmann V, *et al.* 2005, Vaccaro AR, *et al.* 2005) (1) Distance a: the distance from the anterior edge of the right rib head to the central line of screw, (2) Distance b: the minimum distance of the screw to the anterior cortex of the spinal canal, (3) Distance c: the minimum distance of the screw to the aorta, (4) Length d: the length of screw tips to the contralateral vertebral cortex, (5) Distance e: distance from the aorta to the closest point of vertebral body cortex, (6) Angle α: the angle subtended by the line joining the left and right rib heads and the line parallel to the axis of screw (figure 1). According to previous studies,(Sucato DJ, *et al.* 2004, Bullmann V, *et al.* 2005, Kuklo TR, *et al.* 2005) the closest distance from the screw tip to aorta was measured and the screws were categorized into three different grades (DAC grades, figure 4): D, the screw was distant from the aorta (>1mm); A, the screw was adjacent to the aorta (≤1mm); C, the screw was found to be against the aorta and creating contour deformity. The bicortical purchase of screws was also evaluated. Finally, the screw distant from the aorta and the spinal canal with bicortical purchase was defined to be in a good position and the rate of good position was analyzed.

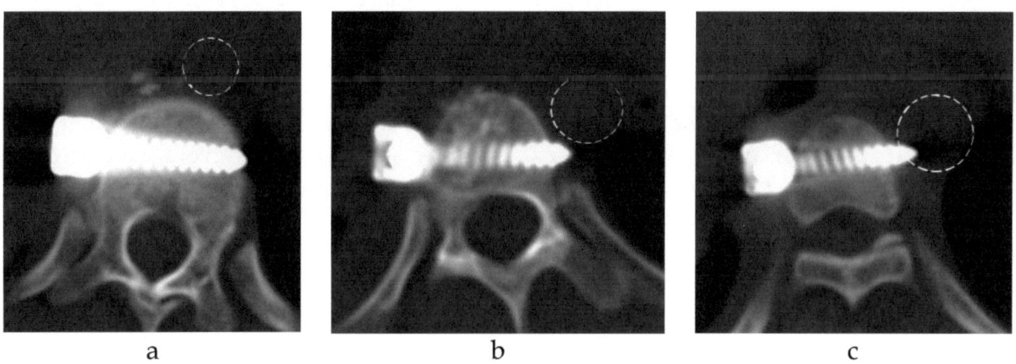

Fig. 4. Relationships between screw tip and aorta. a: the distance between screw tip and the aorta is more than 1mm; b: the screw tip is adjacent to the aorta with the distance no more than 1mm; c: the screw tip shows contour deformity to the aorta.

2.4.1.3 Statistical analysis

The data was analyzed by SPSS software for Windows (10.0, Chicago, IL). Parameters measured at all thoracic instrumented vertebrae in two groups were compared by independent samples t test. The Chi-square test was carried out regarding the DAC grades, bicortical purchase and the good position rate from the thoracic corresponding vertebrae of the two groups. When the cell was less than 5 in number, Fisher exact test was used. Correlation analysis was used to test the relationship between screw insertion accuracy and the Cobb angle of main thoracic curve. The difference was statistically significant when $p<0.05$.

2.4.2 Results

2.4.2.1 Clinical and radiographic data

In Group A, six patients were instrumented from T5 to T12; the other four patients were instrumented from T5 to T10, T6 to T11, T6 to T12 and T7 to T12, respectively. In Group B, instrumented levels were from T5 to T12 in twelve patients, from T5 to L1 in three patients and from T6 to L1 in six patients. The mean operative time averaged 330±65min for Group A and 240±57min for Group B. The difference was statically significant using Student's t test. The saved operative time in Group B was mainly attributing to the faster screw insertion. The main thoracic curve correction rates were 73.6% in Group A and 77.9% in Group B (Table 7). No neurovascular complications were found during the operation and at the last follow-up. Rod breakage was found in one case at two years after operation with Eclipse instrumentation; a 26% loss of curve correction was noted. However, no symptoms were found in this patient. Neither screw loosening nor rod migration was noted. No reversion procedure was needed. There was no implant-related complication in other patients immediately after operation or during follow-up,.

2.4.2.2 CT analysis

Seventy-three thoracic vertebral screws were inserted in Group A while 162 in Group B. The distance a, b, c, d, e and angle α showed no significant difference between the two groups at corresponding vertebral levels. However, length d in Group A was smaller than Group B with significant difference at T7 and T8 ($p<0.05$) (Table 8).
Regarding the location of screws in relation to the aorta, 89.0% of screws in Group A and 80.2% in Group B were at grade D. In Group B, the length d in grade D screws was much less than that in grade A&C screws ($p<0.05$). Significant negative correlation was found between the main thoracic Cobb angle and the percentage of Grade D screws (t=-0.794, $p<0.01$). The bicortical purchase rate was 89.0% and 87.0% in Group A and B respectively. The good position rate was 74.0% and 66.7% in Group A and B respectively. Two screws in Group B penetrated into the spinal canal, the distance c was -0.51mm and -2.06mm respectively. When comparing the DAC grade, bicortical purchase rate and good position rate, no significant difference was found in screws for all corresponding thoracic vertebrae between the two groups (Table 9).

3. Discussion

3.1 Anatomical relationship between the aorta and thoracic vertebral bodies in RT-AIS

At present, the correction of scoliosis under thoracoscopy has been performed on some thoracic AIS patients, especially those with the Cobb angle less than 70° or relatively flexible

	Group	n	a(mm)	b(mm)	c(mm)	d(mm)	e(mm)	α(°)
T5	A	7	8.9±2.0	7.7±3.4	-11.3±3.7	1.9±2.1	5.8±1.9	1.3±5.3
	B	15	5.9±3.4	5.2±3.3	-6.3±8.2	1.8±2.9	3.0±3.4	6.2±7.5
T6	A	9	9.5±2.8	7.8±3.6	-9.0±6.3	2.0±1.8	5.5±1.7	-2.6±9.3
	B	21	6.9±2.8*	4.3±2.2*	-3.8±7.2	1.0±1.4	3.0±1.1*	-1.6±9.5
T7	A	10	11.4±2.4	7.2±3.6	-6.9±8.7	2.1±2.0	4.2±1.8	-4.4±6.5
	B	21	11.4±3.2	5.9±2.9	-2.7±7.1	4.3±2.3*	3.0±1.3	-8.7±6.9
T8	A	10	11.3±3.3	5.5±4.3	-2.6±8.8	1.4±2.0	4.2±1.5	-5.9±11.3
	B	21	12.2±2.7	5.9±2.5	1.2±7.0	3.7±2.8*	2.9±1.3*	-11.6±7.2
T9	A	10	10.9±2.9	5.3±4.4	0.4±8.0	1.2±1.6	3.1±1.2	-4.4±6.6
	B	21	12.6±2.6	6.0±2.7	3.7±7.6	2.8±3.1	2.4±1.1	-8.9±6.2
T10	A	10	10.0±3.1	6.5±2.9	2.7±6.8	1.2±1.4	2.7±1.1	-1.0±6.2
	B	21	12.4±2.4*	5.9±2.7	6.4±5.3	1.7±1.7	2.4±1.0	-7.8±6.6*
T11	A	9	11.2±3.5	7.6±3.6	4.8±6.8	2.2±1.5	2.3±1.1	3.4±4.2
	B	21	13.7±2.2*	6.7±2.6	7.8±4.5	2.1±2.5	1.8±1.2	-5.2±6.7*
T12	A	8	11.4±3.6	9.6±3.0	6.4±5.3	1.8±1.7	2.9±1.0	10.1±7.5
	B	21	14.4±3.4	8.1±2.6	7.4±4.2	3.4±2.8	1.8±1.3*	1.4±7.6*

Data in each group is normally distributed. The difference was significant when compared with corresponding results in Group A (*p<0.05, **<0.01).

Table 8. Results of the parameters measured with CT images between patients operated by thoracoscopic and mini-open thoracotomy approaches.

		DAC grade				Bicortical purchase		Good position rate (%)	
Group	Area	D	A	C	%	n	%	n	%
A	Proximal (T5-T7)	22	2	1	84.6	22	84.6	17	65.4
	Periapical (T8-T9)	18	2	0	90	18	90	15	75
	Distal (T10-T12)	25	2	0	92.6	25	92.6	22	81.5
	Total	65	7	1	89	65	89	54	74
B	Proximal (T5-T7)	40	11	6	70.2	50	87.7	32	56.1
	Periapical (T8-T9)	30	2	10	71.4	36	85.7	25	59.5
	Distal (T10-T12)	60	2	1	95.2	55	87.3	51	81
	Total	130	15	17	80.2	141	87	108	66.7

There was no difference at corresponding area with respect to the DAC grade, bicortical purchase and good position rate.

Table 9. Analysis of accuracy of Screw insertion in patients operated by thoracoscopic and mini-open thoracotomy approaches

curve.(Picetti GD, 3rd, *et al.* 2002) The thoracoscopic technique features minimal injury, fewer complications, faster recovery, reduced pain, fewer respiratory compromises and cosmetically a less prominent surgical scar when compared with the traditional anterior thoracotomic approach.(Picetti G, 3rd, *et al.* 1998, Arlet V 2000, Newton PO, *et al.* 2000, Niemeyer T, *et al.* 2000, Husted DS, *et al.* 2003, Newton PO, *et al.* 2005b) With the increasing popularity of this technique, there has also been an increasing concern over the proximity of the descending aorta to the tips of screws and the possibility of vessel wall erosion over time.(Baker JK, *et al.* 1993, Maruyama T, *et al.* 2004, Sucato DJ, *et al.* 2004, Huitema GC, *et al.* 2006, Zhang H and Sucato DJ 2006) Due to the rotation and distortion of vertebra, the deflected aorta and the deformed morphology of the spinal canal in patients with scoliosis,(Sevastik B, *et al.* 1996, Sucato DJ, *et al.* 2003a, Maruyama T, *et al.* 2004) the insertion of vertebral screws during scoliosis correction may place the patient at risk for aorta injury and violation of the spinal canal. Although no thoracic aorta complication caused by the placement of vertebral screw through thoracoscopic technique in AIS patients has been reported, some aortic complications such as screw penetration,(Matsuzaki H, *et al.* 1993) aortic laceration,(Woolsey RM 1986) false aneurysm of the thoracic aorta(Ahat E, *et al.* 1996, Choi JB, *et al.* 2001) have been found in anterior spinal instrumentation for other diseases.

Proper placement of the screws during anterior corrective surgery of scoliosis showed great importance and challenge to spine surgeons. Picetti *et al.* (Picetti GD, 3rd, *et al.* 2002) suggested usage of capitulum costae and vertebra segment vessel as the position landmark of screw placement. Ebara *et al.* (Ebara S, *et al.* 2000) recommended a new thoracoscopic instrument to measure the transverse diameter of vertebra after removing the intervertebral discs. Despite these studies, there was little information documenting the relationship of the aorta to the thoracic scoliotic spine and little anatomic data based on the pathological morphology of scoliosis. Through analyzing the CT images of the apical vertebra T8 or T9, Sevastik *et al.*(Sevastik B, *et al.* 1996) found that the mean lateral translation distance from the aorta to the mid axis of the vertebral body in the scoliosis group increased, while the vertical distance from the aorta to the mid axis of the vertebral body reduced compared with the adult control group. Liljenqvist *et al.* (Liljenqvist UR, *et al.* 2002) got the same result by measuring the distance from the aorta to the vertebra, without comparing with the normal spine. By analyzing the magnetic resonance images from the fourth thoracic vertebra to the third lumbar vertebra, Sucato *et al.* (Sucato DJ, *et al.* 2003a) found that the aorta was located more laterally and posteriorly relative to the vertebral body in patients with right thoracic idiopathic scoliosis compared with that in patients without scoliosis.

In the present study, the vertebrae from T4 to T12 in patients with scoliosis and age-matched controls were analyzed. A total of 401 vertebrae in the control group and 266 vertebrae in the scoliosis group were measured in the present study, and the parameters of β angle, b value and RV value were taken to ensure the safety of the placement of the screws. The β angle and a value could reflect the safe margin of screw insertion, and the RV value could predict the possibility of spinal cord injury during placement of the screw, then the α angle along with γ angle would show the extent of aortic displacement. The c value provided a reference index in screw length selection.

The displacement of the aorta in patients with scoliosis was expressed as the aorta-vertebral angle or α angle in the present study. Both Sucato *et al.* (Sucato DJ, *et al.* 2003a) and Sevastik *et al.* (Sevastik B, *et al.* 1996) found that the aorta was positioned more posteriorly in patients with AIS than in patients with a normal spine. The present study showed that α angle was smaller in the scoliosis group than that in the age matched control group at every vertebra, and the differences were significant from T5 to T10 ($p<$ 0.01) particularly close to the apex of the curve (T7 to T9), with an angle of 45.2° and 26.9°, respectively, at the seventh thoracic vertebrae in control and scoliosis group; 50.3° and

31.5°, respectively, at the eighth thoracic vertebraae; and 54.8° and 37.6°, respectively, at the ninth thoracic vertebrae. As the rotational deformity increased in the scoliosis group, the α angle relative to the vertebral body decreased, and this negative correlation was significant in the periapical levels. The vertebral rotation was significant in the apex and the γ angle was 13.4°, which was similar with the report of Sucato *et al.* (Sucato DJ, *et al.* 2003a) But at proximal and distal thoracic levels, the vertebrae rotated to the convex side and γ angle turned out to be negative.

The safe margin for screw insertion was affected by the displacement of the aorta. The aorta arch was located more anterior to the vertebra at T4 level (β angle was 29.1°, b was 17.3 mm), which indicated that the screw placement in T4 was safe and unlikely to injure the aorta unless the insertion angle exceeded 29°. From T5 to T12, compared with that in the control group, β angle and a values in scoliosis group were relatively lower, the difference in β angle at T7–T10 levels and a value at T9, T10 levels are significant (Figure 2). It showed that the aorta was positioned more posteriorly to vertebrae and a safe margin for screw insertion decreased especially at the apex of the curve (T7–T10), where the vertebra rotation angel (c) was increased. Sucato *et al.* (Sucato DJ, *et al.* 2004) analyzed the accuracy of the vertebral screw placed following thoracoscopic anterior instrumentation. Fifteen (14.2%) of 106 screw tips were adjacent to the aorta, and there were 13 (12.3%) screws that were thought to create a contour deformity of the aorta. During Maruyama's(Maruyama T, *et al.* 2004) study, the aorta was found to be located posteriorly between T6 and T9 in patients with AIS, at these levels the aorta was found to be crossed by a line that passed the anterior edge of the bilateral rib heads in 33 of 40 vertebrae, so giving up the bicortical screw position at these levels were suggested. In the present study, the a value was minimum (4–8 mm) and from T5 to T9 in the scoliosis group the aorta was very close to the lateral wall of the vertebra. According to β angle, the safe ventral excursion angle couldn't exceed 5° at T6 and T7, 10° at T5 and T8 and 12° at T9, respectively. To get the bicortical fixation without violating the aorta, the screw could run nearly parallel to the posterior wall of the vertebral body directed to the rib head of the opposite side. In addition, the safe ventral excursion angle couldn't exceed 17° at T10 and 20° at T4, T11 and T12 while bicortical fixation was also recommended.

In the study of Sucato *et al.*,(Sucato DJ, *et al.* 2004) four screws at proximal and distal thoracic levels (T5, T6, and two at T12) were found to be violating the posterior cortex of the vertebral body. Zhang and Sucato (Zhang H, *et al.* 2006) have studied the position of the rib head with respect to the spinal canal and vertebral body in both normal patients and those with right thoracic AIS using MRI. They have found that the percent of the vertebra obscured by the rib head significantly decreased from T4 to T12 in both groups and no significant difference was found at the same thoracic levels between the two groups. They concluded that when placing anterior thoracic screws at the caudal thoracic spine (T10–T12), staying anterior to the rib head was important to avoid penetration into the spinal canal. In the present study, the vertical distance from Line RR to the anterior wall of the spinal canal (a) decreased steadily from T4 to T12 in both groups, while it turned out to be negative from T10 to T12 with the minimum negative value, -6 mm in the scoliosis group. The RV value was significantly lower in the scoliosis group at all segment levels but T12, which was opposite to Zhang *et al.* (Zhang H, *et al.* 2006) In the scoliosis group, the RV value was 0.5 ± 3.0 mm at the tenth thoracic vertebrae, -1.4 ± 1.9 mm at the 11th thoracic vertebrae and -1.6 ± 3.3 mm at the 12th thoracic vertebrae. Because the RV value (the vertical distance from the line RR to the anterior wall of the spinal canal) decreased steadily from the cephalic to the caudal levels of the spine in both groups and

became negative at T11 and T12 in the scoliosis group, the risk of screw violating into spinal canal would increase when the screw entry-point was still close to the rib head. Considering the screw was usually 6.5 or 5.5 mm in diameter, we recommend 3–5 mm ventral shift to the rib head at T10–T12 and be parallel to the rib head at T4–T9.
The screw length, which could be estimated by measuring the transverse diameter of vertebra on the CT scanning, was generally longer than that of the reported results.(Liljenqvist UR, *et al.* 2002) The c value at the fourth to the 12th thoracic reported the vertebral deformation of scoliosis, but in the present study the transverse diameter of the vertebral body showed no significant difference at any of the segment levels except for T7 between the two groups. It posed problems with present instrumentation systems that the incremental changes in screw length was 5 mm. Large increments would increase the risk of vascular injuries to the thoracic vertebrae. According to the present results, we suggested that the optimal screw length be 25 mm from T4 to T6 and 30 mm from T7 to T9, 35 mm from T10 toT12.

3.2 Dynamic changes of the relationship between thoracic aorta and vertebrae

3.2.1 Pleura closure

The anatomic relationship between thoracic aorta and vertebrae studied on the preoperative CT scans was static. During operation, the surgical procedures would release the paraspinal tissues which may result in a dynamic change of the relationship and affect the safety of screw insertion. Two studies on aorta shifting following curve correction of thoracic AIS have been reported. By studying the pre- and post-operative CT images, Kuklo *et al.* (Kuklo TR, *et al.* 2005) found the descending aorta moved antero-medially with curve correction. However, because the main emphasis in this study was given to the accuracy of screw placement, the position of the aorta relative to vertebral body was only recorded using a semi-quantitative clock method, and no further analyses were done on the shifting of thoracic aorta postoperatively. Recently, in a prospective study taken by Bullmann *et al.*.,(Bullmann V, *et al.* 2006) the position of aorta in 25 consecutive patients with right thoracic AIS treated with anterior spinal fusion were studied. Base on the preoperative MRI and postoperative axial CT scans, the author concluded that the aorta had migrated from postero-lateral to a more antero-medial position after curve correction. This migration is maximal at the apex vertebra. The patients were scanned in supine position during MRI which differs from the lateral position in CT scanning thus making it difficult to calculate the real changes in aortic position postoperatively.
In the present prospective study, the changes of angle α, distance a and b in anterior instrumentation supported the fact that the aorta shifted antero-medially following curve correction. Same as Bullman, most significant shifting were found in periapical vertebrae. In group B, however, no shifting of aorta was found though the curve was equally well corrected as group A. To minimize the variation between pre- and post-operative images, same scanning technique and patients' position were used. Never the less, the metallic artifacts in some post-operative images would make the margin vertebrae and aorta hard to distinguish. In that case the margin of vertebrae and aorta would be determined by exploring on serial CT images. Another weak point in this study is all the images were parallel to transverse plane. The tilt of vertebrae might be changed by curve correction so it's ideal do measurement on the pre- and post-operative images made exactly through the same plane of each vertebrae. However, it's unavailable for the CT machine used. The images with similar morphology of vertebrae and aorta were selected for measurement to minimize the variation.

Several procedures in anterior spinal instrumentation might be responsible for the antero-medial aorta shifting. Opening and dissecting of the parietal pleura followed by cutting of the right segmental vessels along the periapical vertebrae could mobilize the aorta. Then following disectomy, the partially spontaneous vertebral derotation could contribute in part to the anterior shifting of aorta with increased angle α and distance a. By curve correction after instrumentation, much more aorta shifting would be gain. Moreover, the giving up pleura closure following with curve correction were also thought to help in allowing the aorta to transpose anteriorly by Crawford. (Crawford AH 2004) As the pleura were sutured in all patients in the present study, we would test the hypothesis in further study. In group B, no shifting of aorta was found, which can probably be explained by the absence of soft tissue release and vertebral derotation, and thoracic kyphosis. One of the concerns on the ligation and dissection of the segmental vessels and aorta shifting is the risk of spinal cord ischemia. (Orchowski J, *et al.* 2005) However, these have not been thought as the potential risk factor of neurological deficits of surgical correction for scoliosis in several previous studies. (MacEwen GD, *et al.* 1975, Orchowski J, *et al.* 2005, Coe JD, *et al.* 2006, Qiu Y, *et al.* 2008b) Our previous study (Wu L, *et al.* 2006) has showed that the occlusion of the segmental vessels could cause a temporary change of SEP monitoring but will return to its normal baseline within 17minutes and no neurologic complication was found in all patients. In the present study no abnormality was found by intro-operation SEP monitoring and no neurologic deficit was occurred in all patients after operation.
Since part of vertebral derotation was achieved before screw placement, the maximum ventral excursion angle for screw insertion could be increased slightly. After curve correction, with more anterior shifting of aorta the risk of aorta locating in the axis of screw would be diminished. However, as the distance between aorta and vertebral body was decreased, the bi-cortical inserted screws have higher risk of aorta encroaching if it's located on the screw axis. A feasible way to improve the critical situation is to use screws with shorter increment. Results from previous and present studies have shown that the risk of aorta encroaching by vertebral screws were relatively higher in patients instrumented by screws with 5mm increment(Sucato DJ, *et al.* 2003a, Kuklo TR, *et al.* 2005) when compared with those treated by screws with 2.5mm increment. (Bullmann V, *et al.* 2005) One of the reasons is the increment of vertebral width in thoracic vertebrae was 1.2mm per level.(Sucato DJ, *et al.* 2003a) Moreover, screws with blunt tips would also help to diminish the risk of aorta penetrating.

3.2.2 Pleura in non-closure

It was speculated that leaving the parietal pleura in no closure would allow more freedom for the aorta transposition which would reduce the risk of aortic injuries from screw tips impingement. (Crawford AH 2004) This hypothesis was supported partially by the results of the present study, for it was shown that the aorta located more laterally from the vertebral body after operation. By quantitative analysis of the pre- and post-operative CT scans of the thoracic spine these patients without closure of the pleura, it was found that angle α and the distance between the aorta and rib head decreased while the distance between aorta and vertebrae increased in post-operative CT images, indicating the aorta migrated postero-laterally during and after operation. The increased distance between the aorta and vertebral body lead to an increased safe margin for the bi-cortical penetrated screw tips which would lessen the risk of the late complication of aorta impingement. The posterior migration of the aorta observed in the current study would lead to a smaller safe space of screw tip accommodation between aorta and rib heads (especially in T7 and T8 with angle α less than 25°). The risk of the aorta touching the trajectory of the vertebral screw increased with the decrease of angle α. However, the potential risk maybe diminished by the lateral migration of aorta with the distance b increased to 5.7mm, 7.9mm and 8.0mm in T6, T7 and T8 respectively. Migration of the thoracic aorta in patients with main right thoracic IS treated with posterior spinal instrumentation or anterior spinal instrumentation with pleura closure has been reported previously. (Bullmann V, *et al.* 2006, Wang W, *et al.* 2008) In patients treated with posterior spinal instrumentation only, no change was found on the relative position of the aorta to the vertebrae. However, these studies showed that patients who were treated with anterior curve correction with pleural closure the thoracic aorta migrated antero-medially,(Bullmann V, *et al.* 2006, Wang W, *et al.* 2008) which was attributed to releasing the aorta through pleural dissection and derotation of the curve. By comparing with the study from Wang *et al.*,(Wang W, *et al.* 2008) the clinical data and surgical outcomes were quite similar in terms of pre-op coronal and sagittal Cobb angle, curve flexibility, curve correction rate, pre-op and post-op AVT translation (Table 8 and 9). In the present study, by leaving the parietal pleura in non-closure, the post-operative CT imaging showed that the aorta was in a more postero-lateral position than its pre-operative location. Considering other factors which may be related to the aorta transposition are similar between Wang's and the current study, the contradiction on the direction of aortic migration strongly indicated the effect of pleural closure in affecting the post-operative position of the thoracic aorta. Two factors may contribute to the postero-lateral migration of the aorta in this study. Firstly, the wide range of dissection and stripping of the pleura. The parietal pleura was longitudinally incised from T5 to T12, and was peeled away from the vertebral body. On the convex side, the parietal pleura were elevated from the vertebrae and retracted to the right rib head. On the concave side, the parietal pleura were peeled off from the vertebral body to the contralateral side and swabs were inserted under the parietal pleura to bluntly push away the aorta from the vertebrae. Secondly, the segmental vessels were ligated and cut during surgery which may release the tension on the parietal pleural from restoring to its original position. More importantly, the divided vessels would be pushed laterally apart with their associated parietal pleura to visualize the vertebral body, which may additionally cause the aorta to migrate to a more postero-lateral position. In addition, it has been reported that the aorta would migrate to a more postero-lateral location when the patient is in a supine position and more antero-medial in a prone position.(Sucato DJ and Elerson E 2003b) In the present study, both pre- and post-operative CT scans of all subjects were carried out in a supine position.

One of the concerns of leaving the pleura in a non-closured state is the thoracic drainage.(Newton PO, *et al.* 2000, Sucato DJ, *et al.* 2003a) Increased thoracic drainage was also found in the present study. In previous study, the chest tube drainage in scoliotic patients after anterior instrumentation were 210±90 ml (with parietal pleural closure) and 500±160 ml (without parietal pleural closure), respectively. (Qiu Y, *et al.* 2008a) In the present study, the average thoracic drainage observed in the current study was 450 ml and the duration for chest tube drainage was averaged 3.1 days. But besides the relative increased volume and duration of chest tube drainage, no other related complication occurred in this series. So it is worthwhile to leave the parietal pleural unclosed after anterior corrective surgery in particular patients with relative smaller safe margin for vertebra screw insertion.

The problem of the metallic artifacts can't be denied in current study which would make the margin of vertebrae and aorta hard to distinguish in some post-operative images. In that case the borderline of vertebrae and aorta would be determined by exploring on upper and lower serial CT images.

In order to prevent the potential vascular injury without loss the accuracy of screw insertion, sacrificing bi-cortical penetration or optimal alignment of screws(Maruyama T, *et al.* 2004) and not closing the parietal pleura(Crawford AH 2004) were recommended options. In the case of the aorta being closely adhered to the vertebral body (distance b less than 2 mm) or the aorta closer to the pathway of vertebral screws (angle α less than 45°) on pre-operative CT scanning, the result of the present study suggested to keep the pleura open so as to increase the safe distance between the aorta and vertebrae, which will lessen the risk of screw tip impingement on the aorta. In patients whose aorta are away from the trajectory of vertebral screws (angle α larger than 45°), the pleural closure should be attempted. For patients receiving anterior release surgery, a postero-lateral positioned aorta with the parietal pleura open could decrease the risk of pedicle screw impingement on the aorta during pedicle screw insertion on the concave side of the thoracic curve.

3.3 Accuracy of vertebral screw

In anterior spinal instrumentation through thoracoscopic approach, one of the main concerns is the potential risk of damage to the spinal cord and aorta caused by the vertebral screws. The rotation of vertebrae makes the determination of the direction of screws difficult. In addition, the thoracic aorta was found to displace more laterally and posteriorly in relation to the vertebral body in patients with main thoracic AIS.(Sevastik B, *et al.* 1996, Sucato DJ, *et al.* 2003a, Maruyama T, *et al.* 2004, Qiu Y, *et al.* 2007) Thoracoscopic instrumentation is also technically demanding and requiring a longer duration of surgery with a sharp learning curve.(Grewal H, *et al.* 2005, Lonner BS, *et al.* 2005, Newton PO, *et al.* 2005a) Majority of the reports have found that the curve correction by thoracoscopic anterior instrumentation was as effective as the conventional thoracotomy approach.(Mehlman CT, *et al.* 1997, Picetti G, 3rd, *et al.* 1998, Faro FD, *et al.* 2005, Grewal H, *et al.* 2005) However, whether the vertebral screws inserted through thoracoscopic approach carries the same accuracy rate as the thoracotomy approach has not been properly studied. In the present study, the CT images of vertebral screws inserted through thoracoscopic and mini-open thoracotomy approach were compared. The relative position between the screw and the spinal canal, between the screw and the aorta and the bicortical purchase were quantitatively analyzed and compared.

Migration of vertebral screws into spinal canal has been reported.(Sucato DJ, *et al.* 2004, Huitema GC, *et al.* 2006, Qiu Y, *et al.* 2007) In a consecutive series of 17 patients with thoracolumbar idiopathic scoliosis treated with anterior spinal instrumentation, three vertebral screws were found penetrating into the spinal canal in two patients with three and 15 month postoperative leg pain respectively.(Huitema GC, *et al.* 2006) In patients with right thoracic AIS, the distance from the line joining the left and right rib heads to the anterior wall of the spinal canal was significantly lower from T4 to T11 compared with normal subjects.(Qiu Y, *et al.* 2007) Furthermore, in order to escape from the posteriorly located aorta, the ventral excursion of a screw might be limited or even become negative (dorsally excursion). In the study by Sucato *et al.*,(Sucato DJ, *et al.* 2004) the screw-to-spinal-canal distance averaged at 5.3mm from the coronal axis. Four of 106 screws were found to encroach into the canal by <2mm. In the present study, the minimum distance of the screw to the anterior cortex of the spine canal were 7.05mm and 6.02mm in average in Group A and B respectively, showing adequate safe zone between the screw and the spinal canal in both groups. No significant difference was found between the two groups. In Group B, the spinal canal cortex was found to be penetrated by two screws. One screw at T5 encroached

into the canal by 0.51mm, while the other one at T7 by 2.06mm. There was no neurologic complication observed in these two cases. This might be due to the minor encroachment of screws. It has been suggested that encroachment of less than 4mm into the canal by pedicle screws is probably safe.(Gertzbein SD and Robbins SE 1990, Sucato DJ, *et al.* 2004)
To achieve maximum pullout strength, the bicortical screw fixation with anterior spinal instrumentation was found mandatory in several biomechanical studies.(Lowe T, *et al.* 2002, Huang TJ, *et al.* 2003) In the present study, 89.0% and 87.0% of screws inserted through the thoracoscopic and mini-open thoracotomy approach showed bicortical purchase. The results were comparable with those of Bullmann *et al.*(Bullmann V, *et al.* 2005) in anterior dual rod instrumentation in which 88% of screws were found to have a bicortical purchase. The high rate of bicortical screw fixation might be partly attributed to the good preoperative anatomical assessment of the vertebral diameter.(Qiu Y, *et al.* 2007) In addition, the palpating of the tip of screw from the contralateral side of the vertebra enhanced the accuracy of placement in Group B, while the fluoroscopic guidance during screw insertion raised the rate in Group A. The bicortical screws, however, might result in critical proximity of the screw to the thoracic aorta. The life-threatening aortic complications caused by the penetrating of thoracic vertebral screw into the aorta can be found in the literature. Matsuzaki *et al.*(Matsuzaki H, *et al.* 1993) reported direct aortic screw penetration after anterior spinal fusion from T5 to T10 for thoracic myelopathy. Ohnishi *et al.*(Ohnishi T, *et al.* 2001) reported a case of delayed aortic rupture from pulsation of the aorta adjacent to the plate after anterior instrumentation and fusion from T10 to T12 for a T11 burst fracture via a left thoraco-abdominal approach. In thoracic AIS, Sucato *et al.*(Sucato DJ, *et al.* 2004) found that in 106 vertebral screws inserted thoracoscopically, 15 (14.2%) screws were adjacent to the aorta while 13 (12.3%) were thought to create a contour deformity. According to Kuklo's(Sucato DJ, *et al.* 2004) study the risk was significantly higher (x2=4.897, P=0.027) when compared with the screws inserted through a thoracotomy approach. However, the differences in the experience and technique of different surgeons do not allow any reliable conclusion that the screws inserted by thoracoscopy has runs a higher risk of aortic impingement. The screws were all inserted by the same team of surgeons in the present study, which greatly diminished the variation of surgical techniques. The rate of screw causing contour deformity of the aorta was similar between the two groups. This demonstrated that thoracoscopic approach did not increase the risk of aorta impingement when compared with conventional mini-open thoracotomy approach. It has been a main concern that screws causing contour deformity of aorta could have high risk of aortic complication. From the literature, the actual outcomes has not been well documented. In the studies of Kuklo *et al.*(Kuklo TR, *et al.* 2005) and Sucato *et al.*,(Sucato DJ, *et al.* 2004) no aortic complication caused by these screws was found and the patients remain asymptomatic . In the present study the screws with grade C were followed up regularly and all patients remained asymptomatic. Similar to previous two studies,(Sucato DJ, *et al.* 2004, Kuklo TR, *et al.* 2005) aortography would be recommended for all suspected patients to confirm whether the screws have encroached into the aorta or leading to disruption of the aortic wall which may require removal or shortening. In future operation, measurement of the vertebral diameter on preoperative CT or magnetic resonance images could further help accurate screw length determination.
The impingement of the aorta by screw might be partially attributed to the large increments of screws. Previous studies have shown that the vertebral body width increased gradually from T4 to T12 with an average increment of 1.1mm or 1.2mm.(Sucato DJ, *et al.* 2003a, Bullmann V, *et al.* 2005) However, the screws used at our institution and by Sucato *et*

al.(Sucato DJ, *et al.* 2004) and Kuklo *et al.*(Kuklo TR, *et al.* 2005) have an increment interval of 5mm. The excessive contralateral penetration by screws would increase the risk of aorta impingement. This assumption was also supported by the study of Bullmann et el.(Bullmann V, *et al.* 2005) 226 screws with 2.5mm increment were inserted in standard anterior open dual-rod instrumentation in thoracic AIS while all of them were at least 1mm away from the aorta. In agreement with Sucato *et al.*,(Sucato DJ, *et al.* 2004) we also suggested that screws with smaller increment intervals should be used to get good bicortical screw purchase but at the same time without excessive contralateral penetration. Another reason for screw proximity to the aorta is the migration of the aorta with curve correction. The studies by Kuklo *et al.*(Kuklo TR, *et al.* 2005) and Bullmann *et al.*(Bullmann V, *et al.* 2006) have demonstrated that the posterolateral location of the aorta in thoracic AIS will shift anteromedially with anterior spinal instrumentation. The distance between the vertebrae and the aorta decreased significantly from 5.5mm to 3.7mm at the apical and periapical vertebrae. The curve severity was also found to attribute to the risk of aorta impingement by vertebral screws in the present study. The significant negative correlation between the Cobb angle of thoracic curve and the percentage of Grade D screws indicated that with the increasing of thoracic curve, the vertebral screws have a higher risk of being adjacent to or contouring a deformity of the aorta. This could be explained by the more severe vertebral tilt and rotation in larger curve and much more migration of the aorta after curve correction.
According to previous studies, (Sucato DJ, *et al.* 2004, Bullmann V, *et al.* 2005, Kuklo TR, *et al.* 2005) the screws which were bicortically purchased but away from the aorta and the spinal canal were defined to be in a good position. In the present study, the rate of good position increased from proximal area to distal in both groups, which was thought to be attributed to the increment of vertebral morphology.(Kuklo TR, *et al.* 2005) When compared between the groups, the rate in Group A was higher than that in Group B. This was the same in all corresponding thoracic vertebrae, although the difference was not statistically significant. According to our experience, the higher rate of good position of screw insertion in Group A may be attributed to more frequent and careful fluoroscopic verification during surgery.

4. Conclusion

The advent of CT has revolutionized diagnostic radiology in the past decades. Through the series CT scanning-based studies on the patients with RT-AIS, a systematical understanding on the anatomic relationship between vertebral bodies and paraspinal tissues was achieved.
According to our findings, to place the thoracoscopic vertebral screw safely, at the cephalad thoracic spine (T4–T6), the maximum ventral excursion angle should decrease gradually from 20° to 5°, the entry-point of the screw should be close to the rib head and the optimal screw length was 25 mm. At apical area (T7–T9), the maximum ventral excursion angle should increase gradually from 5° to 12°, and the optimal screw length was 30 mm. At the caudal thoracic spine (T10–T12), the maximum ventral excursion angle increased, the entry-point should shift 3~5 mm ventrally and the optimal screw length was 35 mm.
In addition, dynamic changes of the anatomic relationship between thoracic aorta and vertebrae were identified in RT-AIS during anterior spinal instrumentation and fusion. When the pleura were sutured, significant antero-medial shifting of the thoracic aorta could be achieved. More space would be freed for screw excursion, but the aorta is closer to vertebral body with less safe area for contralateral screw penetration. In contrast, if the pleura were not sutured, the aorta would shift to a more postero-lateral position. In this case, the safe distance between the aorta and vertebrae increased, which will lessen the risk of screw tip impingement on the aorta.

With the knowledge, vertebral screws inserted through thoracoscopical approach could have comparable accuracy with mini-open thoracotomy approach in terms of relative position between the screws and the spinal canal, between the screws and the aorta, the bicortical screw purchase rate and rate of good position. Furthermore, the accuracy could be enhanced by using screws with smaller increments, being aware of the migration of the aorta with anterior spinal instrumentation and keeping the curve severity under consideration.

In addition, the variation of the vertebral rotation and morphology in different patients should also be taken into consideration. A preoperative measurement of CT scanning may be helpful in determining the precise screw selection. However, it should be kept in mind that the radiation exposure during CT scans might do harm to patients especially to children i.e. the radiation-induced carcinogenesis.(Brenner DJ and Hall EJ 2007) Hence the magnetic resonance imaging may serve as an optional media instead of the CT scans in future.

5. References

[1] Ahat E, Tuzun H, Bozkurt AK, et al. False aneurysm of the descending aorta due to penetrating injury. *Injury* 1996;27:225-6.

[2] Arlet V. Anterior thoracoscopic spine release in deformity surgery: a meta-analysis and review. *Eur Spine J* 2000;9 Suppl 1:S17-23.

[3] Baker JK, Reardon PR, Reardon MJ, et al. Vascular injury in anterior lumbar surgery. *Spine (Phila Pa 1976)* 1993;18:2227-30.

[4] Brenner DJ and Hall EJ. Computed tomography--an increasing source of radiation exposure. *N Engl J Med* 2007;357:2277-84.

[5] Bullmann V, Fallenberg EM, Meier N, et al. The position of the aorta relative to the spine before and after anterior instrumentation in right thoracic scoliosis. *Spine (Phila Pa 1976)* 2006;31:1706-13.

[6] Bullmann V, Fallenberg EM, Meier N, et al. Anterior dual rod instrumentation in idiopathic thoracic scoliosis: a computed tomography analysis of screw placement relative to the aorta and the spinal canal. *Spine (Phila Pa 1976)* 2005;30:2078-83.

[7] Choi JB, Han JO and Jeong JW. False aneurysm of the thoracic aorta associated with an aorto-chest wall fistula after spinal instrumentation. *J Trauma* 2001;50:140-3.

[8] Coe JD, Arlet V, Donaldson W, et al. Complications in spinal fusion for adolescent idiopathic scoliosis in the new millennium. A report of the Scoliosis Research Society Morbidity and Mortality Committee. *Spine (Phila Pa 1976)* 2006;31:345-9.

[9] Crawford AH. Position of the aorta relative to the spine in idiopathic scoliosis. *J Bone Joint Surg Am* 2004;86-A:429; author reply -30.

[10] Dunn HK. Anterior spine stabilization and decompression for thoracolumbar injuries. *Orthop Clin North Am* 1986;17:113-9.

[11] Ebara S, Kamimura M, Itoh H, et al. A new system for the anterior restoration and fixation of thoracic spinal deformities using an endoscopic approach. *Spine (Phila Pa 1976)* 2000;25:876-83.

[12] Faro FD, Farnsworth CL, Shapiro GS, et al. Thoracic vertebral screw impingement on the aorta in an in vivo bovine model. *Spine (Phila Pa 1976)* 2005;30:2406-13.

[13] Gertzbein SD and Robbins SE. Accuracy of pedicular screw placement in vivo. *Spine (Phila Pa 1976)* 1990;15:11-4.

[14] Grewal H, Betz RR, D'Andrea LP, et al. A prospective comparison of thoracoscopic vs open anterior instrumentation and spinal fusion for idiopathic thoracic scoliosis in children. *J Pediatr Surg* 2005;40:153-6; discussion 6-7.

[15] Huang TJ, Hsu RW, Tai CL, et al. A biomechanical analysis of triangulation of anterior vertebral double-screw fixation. *Clin Biomech (Bristol, Avon)* 2003;18:S40-5.
[16] Huitema GC, van Rhijn LW and van Ooij A. Screw position after double-rod anterior spinal fusion in idiopathic scoliosis: an evaluation using computerized tomography. *Spine (Phila Pa 1976)* 2006;31:1734-9.
[17] Husted DS, Yue JJ, Fairchild TA, et al. An extrapedicular approach to the placement of screws in the thoracic spine: An anatomic and radiographic assessment. *Spine (Phila Pa 1976)* 2003;28:2324-30.
[18] Krismer M, Bauer R and Sterzinger W. Scoliosis correction by Cotrel-Dubousset instrumentation. The effect of derotation and three dimensional correction. *Spine (Phila Pa 1976)* 1992;17:S263-9.
[19] Kuklo TR, Lehman RA, Jr. and Lenke LG. Structures at risk following anterior instrumented spinal fusion for thoracic adolescent idiopathic scoliosis. *J Spinal Disord Tech* 2005;18 Suppl:S58-64.
[20] Lenke LG, Betz RR, Harms J, et al. Adolescent idiopathic scoliosis: a new classification to determine extent of spinal arthrodesis. *J Bone Joint Surg Am* 2001;83-A:1169-81.
[21] Liljenqvist UR, Allkemper T, Hackenberg L, et al. Analysis of vertebral morphology in idiopathic scoliosis with use of magnetic resonance imaging and multiplanar reconstruction. *J Bone Joint Surg Am* 2002;84-A:359-68.
[22] Lonner BS, Scharf C, Antonacci D, et al. The learning curve associated with thoracoscopic spinal instrumentation. *Spine (Phila Pa 1976)* 2005;30:2835-40.
[23] Lowe T, O'Brien M, Smith D, et al. Central and juxta-endplate vertebral body screw placement: a biomechanical analysis in a human cadaveric model. *Spine (Phila Pa 1976)* 2002;27:369-73.
[24] Lowe TG, Edgar M, Margulies JY, et al. Etiology of idiopathic scoliosis: current trends in research. *J Bone Joint Surg Am* 2000;82-A:1157-68.
[25] MacEwen GD, Bunnell WP and Sriram K. Acute neurological complications in the treatment of scoliosis. A report of the Scoliosis Research Society. *J Bone Joint Surg Am* 1975;57:404-8.
[26] Maruyama T, Takeshita K, Nakamura K, et al. Spatial relations between the vertebral body and the thoracic aorta in adolescent idiopathic scoliosis. *Spine (Phila Pa 1976)* 2004;29:2067-9.
[27] Matsuzaki H, Tokuhashi Y, Wakabayashi K, et al. Penetration of a screw into the thoracic aorta in anterior spinal instrumentation. A case report. *Spine (Phila Pa 1976)* 1993;18:2327-31.
[28] Mehlman CT, Crawford AH and Wolf RK. Video-assisted thoracoscopic surgery (VATS). Endoscopic thoracoplasty technique. *Spine (Phila Pa 1976)* 1997;22:2178-82.
[29] Newton PO, Parent S, Marks M, et al. Prospective evaluation of 50 consecutive scoliosis patients surgically treated with thoracoscopic anterior instrumentation. *Spine (Phila Pa 1976)* 2005a;30:S100-9.
[30] Newton PO, Shea KG and Granlund KF. Defining the pediatric spinal thoracoscopy learning curve: sixty-five consecutive cases. *Spine (Phila Pa 1976)* 2000;25:1028-35.
[31] Newton PO, White KK, Faro F, et al. The success of thoracoscopic anterior fusion in a consecutive series of 112 pediatric spinal deformity cases. *Spine (Phila Pa 1976)* 2005b;30:392-8.
[32] Niemeyer T, Freeman BJ, Grevitt MP, et al. Anterior thoracoscopic surgery followed by posterior instrumentation and fusion in spinal deformity. *Eur Spine J* 2000;9:499-504.

[33] Ohnishi T, Neo M, Matsushita M, et al. Delayed aortic rupture caused by an implanted anterior spinal device. Case report. *J Neurosurg* 2001;95:253-6.
[34] Orchowski J, Bridwell KH and Lenke LG. Neurological deficit from a purely vascular etiology after unilateral vessel ligation during anterior thoracolumbar fusion of the spine. *Spine (Phila Pa 1976)* 2005;30:406-10.
[35] Parent S, Labelle H, Skalli W, et al. Morphometric analysis of anatomic scoliotic specimens. *Spine (Phila Pa 1976)* 2002;27:2305-11.
[36] Picetti G, 3rd, Blackman RG, O'Neal K, et al. Anterior endoscopic correction and fusion of scoliosis. *Orthopedics* 1998;21:1285-7.
[37] Picetti GD, 3rd, Pang D and Bueff HU. Thoracoscopic techniques for the treatment of scoliosis: early results in procedure development. *Neurosurgery* 2002;51:978-84; discussion 84.
[38] Qiu Y, He YX, Wang B, et al. The anatomical relationship between the aorta and the thoracic vertebral bodies and its importance in the placement of the screw in thoracoscopic correction of scoliosis. *Eur Spine J* 2007;16:1367-72.
[39] Qiu Y, Wang B and Zhu F. Comparison of the curative effects of video assisted thoracoscopic anterior correction and small incision, thoracotomic anterior correction for idiopathic thoracic scoliosis. *Chin Med J (Engl)* 2008a;121:1369-73.
[40] Qiu Y, Wang S, Wang B, et al. Incidence and risk factors of neurological deficits of surgical correction for scoliosis: analysis of 1373 cases at one Chinese institution. *Spine (Phila Pa 1976)* 2008b;33:519-26.
[41] Sevastik B, Xiong B, Hedlund R, et al. The position of the aorta in relation to the vertebra in patients with idiopathic thoracic scoliosis. *Surg Radiol Anat* 1996;18:51-6.
[42] Sucato DJ and Duchene C. The position of the aorta relative to the spine: a comparison of patients with and without idiopathic scoliosis. *J Bone Joint Surg Am* 2003a;85-A:1461-9.
[43] Sucato DJ and Elerson E. A comparison between the prone and lateral position for performing a thoracoscopic anterior release and fusion for pediatric spinal deformity. *Spine (Phila Pa 1976)* 2003b;28:2176-80.
[44] Sucato DJ, Kassab F and Dempsey M. Analysis of screw placement relative to the aorta and spinal canal following anterior instrumentation for thoracic idiopathic scoliosis. *Spine (Phila Pa 1976)* 2004;29:554-9; discussion 9.
[45] Vaccaro AR, Yuan PS, Smith HE, et al. An evaluation of image-guided technologies in the placement of anterior thoracic vertebral body screws in spinal trauma: a cadaver study. *J Spinal Cord Med* 2005;28:308-13.
[46] Wang W, Zhu Z, Zhu F, et al. The changes of relative position of the thoracic aorta after anterior or posterior instrumentation of type I Lenke curve in adolescent idiopathic thoracic scoliosis. *Eur Spine J* 2008;17:1019-26.
[47] Wang WJ, Yeung HY, Chu WC, et al. Top theories for the etiopathogenesis of adolescent idiopathic scoliosis. *J Pediatr Orthop* 2011;31:S14-27.
[48] Weinstein SL, Dolan LA, Cheng JC, et al. Adolescent idiopathic scoliosis. *Lancet* 2008;371:1527-37.
[49] Woolsey RM. Aortic laceration after anterior spinal fusion. *Surg Neurol* 1986;25:267-8.
[50] Wu L, Qiu Y, Ling W, et al. Change pattern of somatosensory-evoked potentials after occlusion of segmental vessels: possible indicator for spinal cord ischemia. *Eur Spine J* 2006;15:335-40.
[51] Zhang H and Sucato DJ. Regional differences in anatomical landmarks for placing anterior instrumentation of the thoracic spine in both normal patients and patients with adolescent idiopathic scoliosis. *Spine (Phila Pa 1976)* 2006;31:183-9.

5

Endoscopic Vidian Neurectomy: The Anatomy Consideration and Preoperative Images Analysis

Wan-Fu Su, Shao-Cheng Liu and Hsing-Won Wang
Graduate Institute of Clinical Medicine and Department of Otolaryngology, Taipei Medical University - Shuang Ho Hospital, Taipei, Taiwan Republic of China

1. Introduction

Although surgery is not a primary treatment for manaing rhinitis, it can have some adjuvant benefit in patients with significant nasal congestion or poor pharmacologic response. It is usually performed by surgical approaches to the inferior turbinate, and the more aggressive procedures such as the vidian neurectomy have not been widely applied. Traditional approaches to the vidian canal necessitate larger incisions, including transseptal, transpalatal and transantral methods. These approaches are often not reliable and at the risk of injury to the abutting neurovascular structures. Pioneers in endoscopic surgery are exploring alternatives to these traditional techniques in an attempt to minimize morbidity and the lack of irrelevant incisions. The main difficulties encountered during endoscopic approach are anatomic variations such as canal wall dehiscence, intra-sphenoid septa, pneumatization degree of pterygoid process and the relationship between vidian canal and middle turbinate. Those variations will have effect in determining the surgical success rate and the related complications. Therefore, a powerful tool, in the purpose of identifying the canal location and its surrounding anatomy, is very important to guide the surgeon in preoperative assessment and intraoperative approach. Computed tomography (CT) scanning is superior for the evaluation of the bony confines of the sinonasal tract and skull base. The most minimal recesses of the sinonasal region are easily assessed and it is possible to evaluate the position and configuration of the vidian canal. That valuable information provided by imaging studies enhances the surgical feasibility and offers an alternative for treating the rhinitis. This chapter describes the use of CT images in this capacity. Growing surgical experience and evolving technology will help to advance the feasibility of endoscopic vidian neurectomy and elucidate their indications by using preoperative images.

2. General principles

The term rhinitis refers to an inflammatory disease of the nasal mucosa. This inflammation can be acute or chronic and leads to a cluster of symptoms that may include sneezing, nasal itching, rhinorrhea, impairment in smell, and nasal congestion. A number of discrete mechanisms are involved in the pathogenesis of chronic rhinitis, including both allergic and nonallergic. A recent consensus document has classified rhinitis into one of four categories: (a) structural, (b) infectious, (c) allergic, and (d) other.(Bernstein 2010) These categories can be difficult to apply and overlap between two or more of these classes is quite common, leading to a classification of rhinitis as being "mixed" in a significant proportion of patients complaining of symptoms of nasal inflammation. Furthermore, the lack of clear diagnostic criteria and the absence of reliable diagnostic tests often add to the confusion in reaching a precise diagnosis of the type of rhinitis and its most favorable treatment. (Scadding et al. 2008)

Allergic rhinitis (AR) is an immunologic nasal response, primarily mediated by immunoglobulin E (IgE). It has traditionally been divided into two categories based on the seasonality of the symptoms: seasonal allergic rhinitis, which is defined as AR symptoms triggered by seasonal increases in relevant antigens, such as pollens and outdoor molds, and perennial allergic rhinitis, defined as AR symptoms occurring throughout most of the year, and related to perennial antigens such as animal dander, dust mites, cockroach, and indoor molds.(Broide 2010) In contrast to AR, nonallergic rhinitis (NAR) is a disease that cannot be explained by any uniform pathophysiologic mechanism. It is rather considered a diagnosis of exclusion among patients with allergic symptoms yet negative to allergy testing. The condition exists in a variety of forms that are a function of differing physiologic processes and are considered a syndrome that is broadly referred to as NAR. These various influences include infection, hormonal fluctuations, pharmacological agents, and autonomic dysfunction.(Salib et al. 2008)

Vasomotor rhinitis (VMR) is the most common form of chronic NAR with the clinical presentations including nasal obstruction, postnasal drip, itching, clear rhinorrhea, epiphora, crocodile tears and Sluder syndrome. It has been thought to result from an imbalance in the autonomic input to the nasal mucosa with increased parasympathetic stimulation without adequate sympathetic balance.(van Rijswijk et al. 2005) The vidian nerve, with its autonomic fibers formed by the union of the greater and deep petrosal nerve, is responsible for VMR. This nerve exits the lateral part of the anterior end of the carotid canal, passes along the upper part of the anterolateral edge of the foramen lacerum, courses through the vidian canal, and ends in the pterygopalatine ganglion in the posterior part of the pterygopalatine fossa.(Osawa et al. 2009) Clinically it serves as an important landmark in endoscopic and microsurgical approaches to the cranial base, especially for the lacerum and petrosal segment of the internal carotid artery. Damage to the vidian nerve does not prevent normal mucosal reaction to colds; however, it may reduce lacrimation as measured by Schirmer's test.(Jang et al. 2011) Its surgical role in treating chronic rhinitis is yet to be established since different healing results were reported in the past.

The successful treatment of both AR and NAR is based on the patient's understanding of the nature of the disease, its triggers, and the strategy for its management. Because rhinitis is a chronic condition that requires treatment over time, the complete participation of the patient in treatment is necessary. Education is essential as a component of the overall treatment strategy. The treatment involves mainly stimulant avoidance and pharmacological approaches such as mast cell stabilizers, anti-histamines, decongestants, immunotherapy or corticosteroids. Surgery is not a primary treatment in treating chronic rhinitis. In patients with significant nasal congestion, surgical approaches to the inferior turbinate can have some adjuvant benefit because of the nasal resistance reduction.(Mora et al. 2009) As for other nasal presentations, the vidian neurectomy is an option because it can inhibit the excessive efferent stimulation of the parasympathetic system and interrupt cholinergic innervation to the nasal mucosa. An increased feasibility with the advance in instruments and image analysis is obtained and we believe this surgery plays a role in treating patients with chronic rhinitis who shows poor response to an at least 3-month medical treatment.

3. History of vidian neurectomy

Golding-Wood first described vidian neurectomy (VN) in the early 1960s.(Golding-Wood, 1961) Various approaches were developed thereafter, including transseptal, transpalatal and transantral methods.(Chandra 1969; Gregson 1969; Minnis and Morrison 1971; Nomura et al. 1971) The multitude of proposed surgical approaches to the vidian nerve connotes that none is totally satisfactory, mainly because of difficulties in nerve identifications, highly demanding surgical technique and risk of complication. The vidian nerve is seated deep at the base of the skull, an area which is anatomically difficult to reach and is surrounded by numerous important structures. Therefore, this technique had been largely abandoned for about 20 years after Golding-Wood.

The transnasal approach had been advocated with the help of an operating microscope and diathermy coagulation since the 1980s.(Krajina 1989) It once had been viewed as an ideal technique which was fast, less invasive and associated with a lower complication rate. Most of these approaches obtained their outcome by cauterization of the vidian nerve. It raised a concern of inaccurate or inadequate nerve function block. In the 1990s, the endoscope was introduced and facilitated the same procedures in the pterygopalatine fossa (PPF).(el Shazly 1991; Kamel and Zaher 1991) The use of endoscope led to a precise identification of the vidian nerve and enabled a nerve resection instead of a nerve cauterization. Kamel and Shazly etc were pioneers in this entity with the region targeted confined in the PPF. They approached the anterior opening of vidian canal subperiosteally by carefully pushing the mucoperiosteum and contents of PPF slightly laterally. In their attempts, the brisk bleeding from injury of sphenopalatine artery (SPA) was the major surgical difficulty. Besides, the difficulty to remove sphenoid process of palatine bone between sphenopalatine foramen and anterior wall of sphenoid sinus and its resultant bone oozing usually frustrate frustrated surgeons and reduced their willingness to attempt this process. Shazly etc admitted that two main difficulties were encountered: bleeding and working in a relatively narrow operative field.

Robinson and Wormald were the first ones who took advantage of sphenoid sinus as guidance.(Robinson and Wormald 2006) He claimed that enlargement of the sphenopalatine foramen posteriorly up to the anterior face of the sphenoid to the level of the floor of the sphenoid sinus using a bone punch facilitated the identification of vidian nerve in the PPF. To eliminate the intimidation of vascular risk, the SPA should be cauterized first. Transection of the vidian nerve was performed before its entrance into the PPF. In those above retrograde fashion (from sphenopalatine foramen to anterior opening of vidian canal), the surgical difficulties include failure to find the sphenopalatine artery at the expected site since the relationship between the sphenopalatine foramen and ethmoid crest is so variable. Middle turbinate with large posterior end and unintentional penetration of the posterior ethmoid sinuses also rendered this technique unfit for a precise nerve transection. With better understanding of vidian canal anatomy in the sphenoid sinus and encountering the difficulties in duplicating the retrograde approach, antegrade approach, (from intraspehonid vidian canal to PPF), has been introduced recently in Taiwan.(Liu 2010)

There are two common antegrade nerve resection fashions, which were developed by Su and Wang in 2006. The vidian canal courses in the floor of the sphenoid sinus and may protrude into the sphenoid sinus, especially into the anterior part of a well-pneumatized sinus. If the prominence over the vidian canal in the floor of sphenoid sinus can be unroofed directly in the sinus cavity without resection of the sphenoid body or pterygoid process, this procedure is named type I transsphenoid approach. If the prominence over the vidian canal is absent or it is situated laterally and hampered by the pterygoid process, the vidian nerve management can be achieved via an additional removal of partial sphenoid wall and pterygoid process, and type II transsphenoid approach will be named. The type I maneuver has its advantages, such as less intraoperation bleeding, less risk of important vascular injury, shorter operating time and a minimized wound. But most patients are not good candidates for it, since this approach often failed due to the intrasphenoid septum, the embedded canal and an extreme lateralized position. Therefore, type II approaches are more widely used and usually serves as a rescue after a failure of attempted type I surgery. By using antegrade fashions, the precise intraoperative vidian nerve recognition is no longer a difficulty. However, not all patients with identified nerve can be definitely transacted and still a portion of those required using cauterization as a remedy. Again, the anatomy variances are crucial in determining the appropriate surgical approaches. The preoperative CT images are therefore vital tools for this purpose.

4. Endoscopic vidian neurectomy

4.1 Indications

VN of whatever form is not the first-line management of chronic rhinitis. The vast of majority of both rhinitis can be managed by conservative treatment.(Brozek et al. 2010) Therefore, no absolute indications exist for surgical intervention in chronic rhinitis. However, the surgery should be considered if the symptoms interfere with daytime function, adversely impact sleep or cause a decline in global or specific quality of life despite treatment with corticosteroids and anti-allergy medications. VN (destruction of the vidian nerve) is originally designed to treat patients suffering from VMR. It also has been advocated for the management of AR and nasal polyposis.(Nomura 1974) Recent clinical results show ideal postoperative symptom improvement in patients with allergic and non-allergic rhinitis both. This may be explained by the fact that the pathophysiology of the rhinitis is commonly overlapping between two or more of these classes. Once one of those is intervened, such as the vasomotor component, the threshold for a stimulant to cause symptoms might be elevated and lead to reduced symptoms. A unilateral nerve resection shows adequate symptom relief and this might also be the result of the elevated threshold. The reflex arc is broken by cutting the parasympathetic fibers on one side and the reduction of half the afferent supply leading to a bilateral effect. Some studies shows that the denervation will lead to a significant reduction of stromal edema and eosinophilic cellular infiltration, a reduction in mast cell levels and histamine concentrations and a reduction of the contents of the acini of mucosal glands.(Konno 2010) Because of this, there are also some authors advocating the use of VN for managing nasal polyposis. However, additional research is warranted in the possible role of VN for nasal polyposis and chronic rhinosinusitis.

A variety of headache and autonomic disturbances attributes to impulses transmitted by the vidian nerve have been relieved by its interruption. For example, cluster headache can be treated with lesions in the pterygopalatine ganglion.(Alvernia et al. 2007) Cluster headache is characterized by a constant unilateral orbital localized pain that radiates into the forehead, temple, and cheek and is associated with ipsilateral autonomic phenomena such as a blocked nostril, rhinorrhea, injected conjunctivum, lacrimation, ptosis, miosis, forehead or facial sweating, lid edema, and a flush and edema of the cheek. Symptomatic cluster headaches have been reported in association with sellar (hypophyseal tumors) and parasellar (meningioma arteriovenous fistula or malformations) lesions, as well as internal carotid artery dissection.(Halker et al. 2010) They can have the similar causal mechanism of the cluster headache. The pathophysiology related to autonomic system imbalance has been proposed as following: 1) swelling of the internal carotid wall compromises the pericarotid sympathetic plexus and causes Horner syndrome, 2) the sympathicoplegia may cause dilatation of the ophthalmic artery and lead to pain, and 3) paroxysmal parasympathetic discharge mediated through the greater petrosal nerve and pterygopalatine ganglion.(Francis et al. 2010) The vidian nerve conveys the autonomic fibers to the pterygopalatine ganglion, thus, the vidian nerve may have an important role in the autonomic dysfunction of the cluster headache and could be a target for the treatment. Lesions in the vidian canal can also cause autonomic disturbances. The majority of the branches of the pterygopalatine ganglion are maxillary division sensory fibers to the palate, nasal mucosa, pharynx, and orbit that pass through the ganglion without synapsing and enter the maxillary nerve through its ganglionic branches. Consequently, therapy targeting the ganglion can cause sensory disturbance in these areas.

Relative contraindications to endoscopic vidian neurectomy include absence of sphenoid pneumatization (conchal type) on radiographic examination or the presence of osteomyelitis of the sphenoid bone. Damage to the vidian nerve can lead to a loss of lacrimation with desiccation of the cornea and dry nose caused by damage to the parasympathetic fibers. This neurectomy does not prevent normal mucosal reaction to colds; however, it may reduce lacrimation as measured by Schirmer's test. Patients who have complained preoperatively of a lack of tears under emotional circumstances, associated eye discomfort and redness, should be considered as a relative contraindication. Most patients without preoperative eye dryness can be treated effectively by the use of tear substitutes when postoperative dry eye is encountered. Bilateral neurotrophic keratopathy with miosis and frontal headache has been a very rare occurrence after the VN.(Lin et al. 2001) Some of the side effects related to neural damage are thought to be attributable to the spread of current from electrocoagulation used to obliterate the branches of the maxillary artery near the vidian nerve. Therefore, thorough explanation and informed consent should be completed before any procedure.

4.2 Instrumentation

VN requires instrumentation that provides good visualization and precise nerve transection. As such, necessary endoscopic equipment includes a 0-, 30- or 70-degree telescope as well as bone-punching instruments. Cameras, monitors, and beam splitters may improve surgeon ergonomics and are important for teaching and documentation. Although the 0-degree is used to identify major landmarks (middle turbinate, anterior sphenoid wall), the angled telescopes allow broader visualization of the more lateralized vidian canal and enable a significantly more thorough surgical dissection.

A Freer elevator (Aesculp, Tuttlingen, Germany) is very suitable for lateralizing the middle turbinate and penetrating the anterior sphenoid sinus wall. A monopolar diathermy or bipolar forceps (such as Stammberger bipolar suction forceps) with suction lumen is used to secure the intraoperation bleeding arising from injury of the pterygovaginal branch from internal maxillary in the inferiolateral aspect of the anterior wall of sphenoid sinus. Kerrison rongeur (Aesculp) instruments are necessary for anterior sphenoid wall removal. Suction elevators are also needed to elevate the mucoperiosteal soft tissue from the anterior surface of sphenoid sinus to the lateral part of pterygoid process. Chisel or osteotome with hammer has enhanced our ability to penetrate the thicker anterior wall of the sphenoid sinus. The embedded vidian canal is sometimes difficult to identify and removal of pterygoid process around the canal can be achieved by Kerrison punch, chisel or osteotome. A double-end probe with a suitably shaped ball tip can be helpful in isolating the vidian nerve from its canal.

Image guidance systems have also improved the accuracy of VN. Computer-assisted surgical navigation aids in intraoperative localization, particularly in cases with accompanied chronic rhinosinusitis in which the anatomy has been significantly altered. They are also helpful in resident teaching. However, in a well-trained hand, the image guidance systems may offer a little help and probably the most important role for computer-assisted surgery is in preoperative surgical planning.

4.3 Patient evaluation

Patient evaluation requires a thorough medical history. The onset, frequency, duration, and severity of the patient's rhinitis should be delineated. A list of previous medical treatments should be obtained to assess whether maximal medical therapy has been administered. The use of topical and systemic medications for the treatment of rhinitis remains the backbone of therapy. There are a variety of classes of medications that are used for the treatment of both AR and NAR. These medications are noted in Table 1. Antihistamines, leukotriene inhibitors, and systemic immunotherapy are available options used for patients with significant symptoms. Steroid preparations are effective for all forms of rhinitis, allergic and nonallergic. They are available both in systemic form for oral or parenteral use and as topical intranasal sprays. Corticosteroids work extremely well in reducing the symptoms of rhinitis when used systemically but are limited by the significant adverse event profile that accompanies systemic steroid use. Depot injections have also been used for many years but are not recommended for use under current guidelines for the management of AR. Oral corticosteroids can be used for short periods of time with significant symptoms. Topical corticosteroids have become the primary treatment and in many analyses have been shown to be more efficacious than antihistamines in the management of AR. Topical nasal corticosteroids have been shown to decrease neutrophil and eosinophil chemotaxis in the nose, as well as reducing intracellular edema. They reduce a variety of inflammatory mediators as well, including interleukin (IL)-6, IL-8, granulocyte-macrophage colony-stimulating factor (GM-CSF), and both IL-4 and IL-5.

Previous surgical attempts and postoperative management should be reviewed and documented. Comorbidities such as asthma, chronic rhinosinusitis, granulomatous diseases, and so forth must be identified. In addition, a detailed allergy history, both pharmacological and environmental, should be obtained as well as any therapeutic measures (i.e., immunotherapy) that have been attempted. A family history is also necessary to determine if a genetic predilection may exist. Finally, a social history is important to ascertain potential exposure to noxious substances either at home or in the workplace (i.e., tobacco, mold) that may influence surgical outcome.

Agent	Rhinorrhea	Congestion	Sneezing	Itching	Eye Symptoms
Oral antihistamines	++	-	++	++	++
Nasal antihistamines	+	-	+	+	-
Intranasal corticosteroid	++	+++	++	++	+
Leukotriene modifiers	+	+	+	+	+
Oral decongestants	-	++	-	-	-
Nasal decongestants	-	+++	-	-	-
Nasal mast-cell stabilizers	+	+	+	+	-
Topical anticholinergics	+++	-	-	-	-

+++, marked benefit; ++, substantial benefit; +, some benefit; +/-, minimal benefit; -, no benefit.

Table 1. Pharmacological effects on symptoms of rhinitis:

The diagnosis of rhinitis involves not only an examination of the nose itself but a complete head and neck examination. Chronic serous otitis media is frequently seen in patients with AR. In addition, asthma is a frequent comorbidity and auscultation of the chest with normal and forced expiration may demonstrate wheezing, suggestive of asthma. The examination should begin with an inspection of the face. Signs of facial puffiness, edema, asymmetry, or discoloration should be noted. Conjunctival injection or erythema should be noted. Darkening of the skin under the eyes from venous stasis is a sign of nasal congestion and is seen commonly in patients with chronic rhinitis. In addition, allergic patients, especially children, often have fine creases in the upper eyelids called Dennie lines, caused by spasms of Mueller muscles. Second, both the external and internal anatomy should be examined. The external structure of the nose is examined for obvious deformity or asymmetry. A transverse crease at the superior border of the lower lateral cartilages is characteristic of the stigmata resulting from repeated rubbing of the itchy allergic nose. The anterior septum is inspected for deformity or deflections that compromise the airway. The size of the turbinates and their degree of impingement on the nasal airway are noted, as well as the reversibility of this hypertrophy with topical decongestants. The appearance of the mucosa and the nasal secretions should be characterized. Allergic mucosa is often edematous and congested and frequently has a boggy gray-to-blue appearance on examination. Erythematous, inflamed mucosa is often seen in the turbinates with rhinitis medicamentosa or in cigarette smokers. Although mucosal appearance can be suggestive of pathophysiology, it is not pathognomonic of any specific disease. Nasal secretions may be present or absent and if present may be described as serous, mucoid, or mucopurulent. Presence of septal excoriations or bloodstained mucus should be noted. Lymphoid islands, which form a raised, red, cobblestone appearance in the posterior pharyngeal wall or lateral raised vertical lymphoid bands behind the tonsillar pillars, are frequently seen in allergic patients. Adenoid hypertrophy is common in allergic children. Chronic nasal obstruction can contribute to dental malocclusion because of chronic mouth breathing.

Comprehensive diagnostic nasal endoscopy has become routine in patients with nasal and sinus complaints. The nasal endoscope allows visualization of the more posterior portions of the nasal cavity and nasopharynx that cannot be appreciated on anterior rhinoscopy alone. Both rigid and flexible fiberoptic endoscopes can be used for this purpose. It is evaluated in the office under topical anesthesia. One method is to systematically examine the sinonasal cavity using three passes with a rigid endoscope and deflected angle of view. The first pass is made along the floor of the nasal cavity proceeding posteriorly toward the nasopharynx. During this pass, the inferior turbinate, septum, nasopharynx, and eustachian tube orifice are all examined for mucosal changes and the presence of secretions. The endoscope may also be rolled under the inferior turbinate to visualize the inferior meatus and Hasner valve. The second pass is made between the inferior and middle turbinate, then courses medial to the middle turbinate into the sphenoethmoidal recess. The superior septum, inferior aspect of the middle meatus, superior turbinate, and sphenoid sinus ostia should all be visualized with this pass. Finally, the third pass involves maneuvering the endoscope below the middle turbinate into the middle meatus to examine the lateral nasal wall and ostiomeatal complex. The ethmoid bulla, hiatus semilunaris, and uncinate process should all be examined with this pass. Not all structures may be visualized on endoscopy if narrowed anatomy is present.

If AR is suspected, specific testing for allergic sensitivities can be conducted both to confirm the diagnosis of AR and to aid in treatment planning. Both in vivo and in vitro methods are available for the testing of allergic sensitivities in adults and children.(Knipping et al. 2009) The most commonly used methods for allergic assessment involve one of several skin testing approaches. Skin testing can be either epicutaneous, as in prick testing, or can be percutaneous, as with intradermal testing. In vitro tests involve the use of laboratory studies to assess both the presence of allergic sensitivity and the specific antigens to which the patient is allergic. Simple screens for allergy include both the calculation of total eosinophilia and the level of total IgE in the serum. Although both of these studies can be useful when levels are markedly elevated, the interpretation of marginal elevations can be difficult and can be influenced by a variety of confounding factors. An additional method for testing allergic sensitivity among patients with rhinitis involves direct provocation of symptoms through introducing allergen directly into the nose. Observations have noted that results obtained through nasal challenge do not necessarily correlate directly with results noted on skin testing. There appear to be differential responses to nasal challenge with various antigens. The use of nasal provocation testing for the diagnosis of AR is not currently used for clinical practice but may offer promise as a technique for future use in the diagnosis of AR versus nonallergic rhinitis.

VN is performed only after aggressive attempts to eliminate symptoms with medical treatment have failed. The surgery is best considered an adjunct to medical therapy in the management of chronic rhinitis rather than being a primary treatment modality. Once the patient is deemed to have completed appropriate medical options and to be a surgical candidate, preoperative CT should be performed to evaluate the anatomy. Because dry eye is emphasized as a possible complication in the preoperative consent procedure it is important to preoperatively assess eye tearing with a Schirmer's test and compare this with the postoperative findings because this symptom may be overreported by patients. Anterior rhinomanometry with a face mask can be used to assess the change of nasal airflow and resistance in patients undergoing VN. However, the value of this exam need to be explored in future studies.

4.4 Preoperative computed tomography evaluation

CT images should be thinly sliced (3 mm or less) and directed in the coronal, sagittal and axial planes using a bony algorithm. Presurgical CT evaluation involves analysis of six specific anatomic areas to avoid possible complications during surgery. First, the sphenoid sinus should be analyzed throughout its length. The pattern of pneumatization and presence of intrasinus septum should be assessed. The degree of pneumatization of the sphenoid is the prime preoperative concern for type I antigrade VN approach.(Liu 2010) Type of sphenoid sinus pneumatization depends on the position of the sinus in relation to the sella turcica, and includes conchal, presellar, sellar, and postsellar type (Fig. 1). This is best seen in the sagittal slices. High-resolution CT scan may show pneumatization of the sphenoid sinuses as early as 2 years of age. Pneumatization progresses in an inferior and posterolateral direction. The pneumatized basisphenoid plate often extends to, but not past, the spheno-occipital synchondrosis in the mature sphenoid sinus. The sinus attains its mature size by the age of 14 years. The degree of pneumatization of the sphenoid sinus varies considerably. The sella turcica is seen as a prominence in the roof of a wellpneumatized sphenoid sinus and is known as the sellar bulge. This is considered one of the most important surgical landmarks to the sellar floor. In the previous study, the most common type of pneumatization of the sphenoid sinus is the sellar type (54.7%). The conchal pneumatization is the least frequent (2%),(Hamid et al. 2008) The conchal nonpneumatized sphenoid is considered to be a relative contraindication to the trans-sphenoid approach. It will make type I approach unavailable and type II approach less favourable. However, with the surgeon informed in advance, different tools can make such an approach feasible. The availability of intraoperative navigational devices can be used to confirm surgical landmarks, making it possible to access the vidian canal even in these poorly pneumatized cases. The operative time is, of course, longer. On the other hand, a highly pneumatized sphenoid sinus may distort the anatomic configuration and may attenuate the bone over the lateral wall, placing the optic nerve and carotid artery at greater risk. The postsellar pneumatization of the sphenoid and that of the dorsum sella may result in penetrating the posterior wall of the sphenoid, with resultant CSF leak. This can result from excessive dissection along the nasal floor, as the speculum will tend to slide downward, directing the surgeon to the posteriorly pneumatized recess. Therefore, type I approach should be performed carefully to avoid morbid consequences during surgery since it bear the risk of intracranial complications. There is usually an intra-sphenoid septum (Fig. 2). Presence of the septum between the canal and the natural ostium would block visualization and hinder surgery. This septum sometimes needs to be removed to access the vidian canal. Removal of the septum is usually time-consuming and may be associated with greater intraoperative bleeding and unintentional skull base penetration. The septum usually deviates to one side. Care should be taken in removing the lateral attachment of these septa, especially when the preoperative imaging showed that it ends on the carotid prominence. In 41 to 89% of patients the septum deviates quite laterally and terminates on the carotid artery.(Fernandez-Miranda et al. 2009) In this situation it is wise to use extreme caution while removing the terminal septum in order to prevent accidental and disastrous injury to the carotid artery. The terminal septa are usually inserted lateral to the sinus floor and may not require complete removal for adequate exposure.

Second, the pterygoid process should also be identified. The anterior opening of the vidian canal is positioned on the superomedial part of the anterior surface of the pterygoid process, at the level of the floor of the sphenoid sinus and inferomedial to the foramen rotundum.

The pterygoid process forms the posterior wall of the PPF. Through the sphenopalatine notch, which is bounded inferiorly by the upper part of the perpendicular plate of the palatine bone, the vidian nerve runs into the PPF. In the anterior opening of the vidian canal, it is located in the line of fusion between the pterygoid process and the body of the sphenoid bone. The gap between the pterygoid process of the sphenoid bone and the sphenoid process of the palatine bone (SPP) determines the feasibility of type II approach (Fig. 3). If the gap allows the passing through of a curved probe, the vidian nerve will be hooked out by the probe or sickle knife. If the gap is too narrow to allow this procedure, the pterygoid process or the SPP need to be partially removed and sometimes the canal opening is not easily accessible due to the severe obscuration of pterygoid process. An image guidance system may be necessary in this situation.

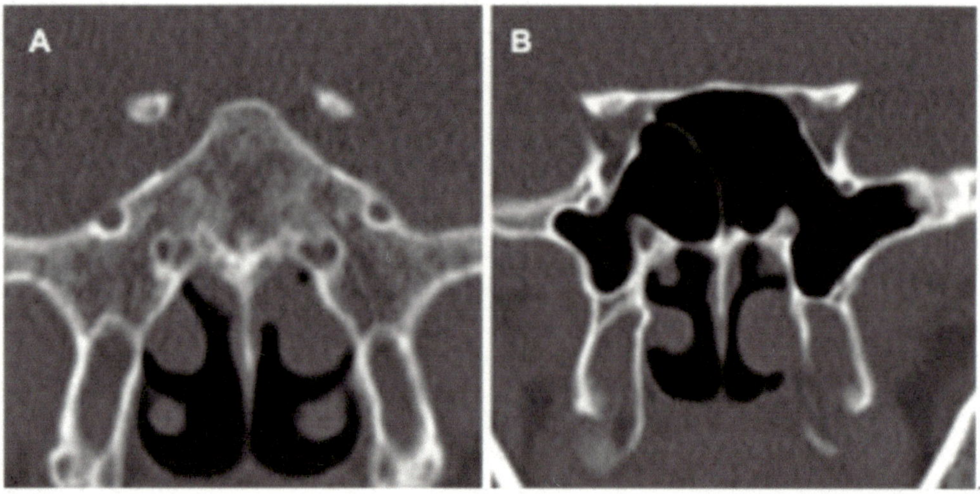

Fig. 1. Coronal CT slices showing the different type of sphenoid sinus pneumatization. A: conchal type. B: sellar type.

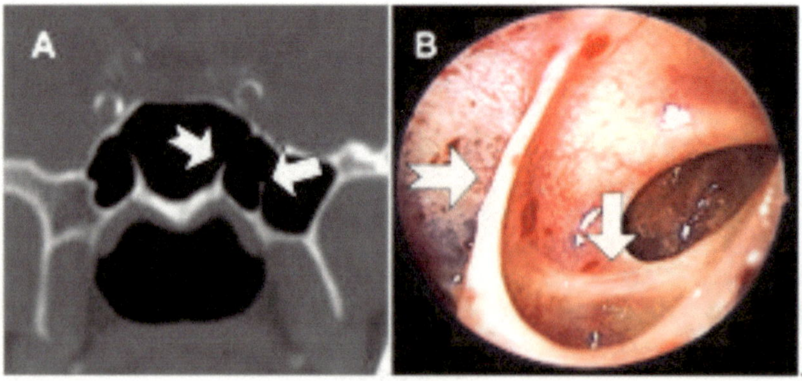

Fig. 2. The intra-sphenoid septum is demonstrated on A: Coronal CT slice; B: intraoperative endoscopic view. Arrows indicate vidian canal; the bifid tail arrow indicates the intra-sphenoid septum

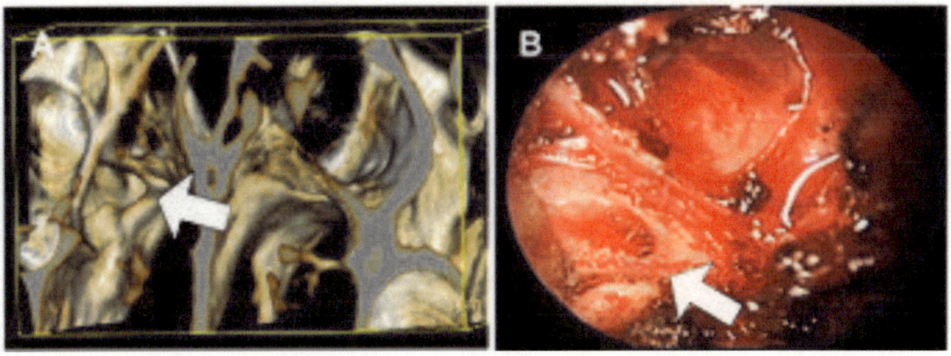

Fig. 3. The gap (arrow) between the sphenoid sinus anterior wall and the pterygoid process or the SPP is demonstrated on A: pre-operative 3D reconstruction CT image; B: intraoperative endoscopic view.

Third, the continuation of the vidian canal bony structure should be identified and its position relative to the sphenoid determined. The relationship between the canal and the sphenoid bone (canal corpus type) can be categorized as follows: (1) embedded inside the sphenoid corpus, (2) partially protruding, or (3) connected to the bone with a stalk inside the sinus. The relationship between the canal and the sphenoid sinus floor (canal floor type) is categorized as follows: (1) the floor is flat, and the canal is at the same level as the floor; (2) the floor is upsloping, and the canal is superior to it; (3) the floor is downsloping; or (4) the canal is inferior to it, and the floor is an inverted V shape (Fig. 4).(Liu 2010) Extrapolation to clinical application has been explored in our previous study. We have shown that it is impossible to precisely identify the vidian canal in the sphenoid sinus floor when it is embedded inside the sphenoid corpus. All patients with this anatomy (canal corpus type 1) should receive VN by type II approach. In patients with the remaining 2 canal corpus types, protrusion of the canal into the floor of the sphenoid sinus can aid in locating the vidian canal, but not all of these patients are candidates for the type I approach. The canal floor relationship influences the choice of surgical approach. The type I approach can be considered only in patients with a canal floor relationship type 1 or type 2. In patients with type 3 or type 4, visualization of the vidian canal and instrument blockage are observed in our study, limiting application of the transsphenoidal approach. In contrast, patients with dehiscence of the bony roof of the canal in the floor of the sphenoid sinus are good candidates for the type I approach. This anatomy is observed in 30.4% (207 of 682 canals) of CT images reviewed in our study and in 4.4% to 32% of canals in other radiologic investigations. In this situation, the nerve can be easily intra-sphenoid transected by a probe
Fourth, the relationship between the anterior opening of the vidian canal and the posterior part of middle turbinate need to be explored. The first step in performing endoscopic VN is to lateralize the prominent middle turbinate in order to access the anterior wall of the sphenoid sinus. Therefore, one of the key points in determining a successful operation is the relationship between the posterior end of the middle turbinate and the lateralization degree of the vidian canal. The anterior opening of the vidian canal is usually positioned at the superiolateral aspect of the posterior end of the middle turbinate. The included angle representing the relationship of those two anatomies can be measured from coronal and axial CT slices (Fig. 5). The results of our study establish the value in both successful and failed cases.(Liu 2011) We found a statistical significance that the greater angle led to a

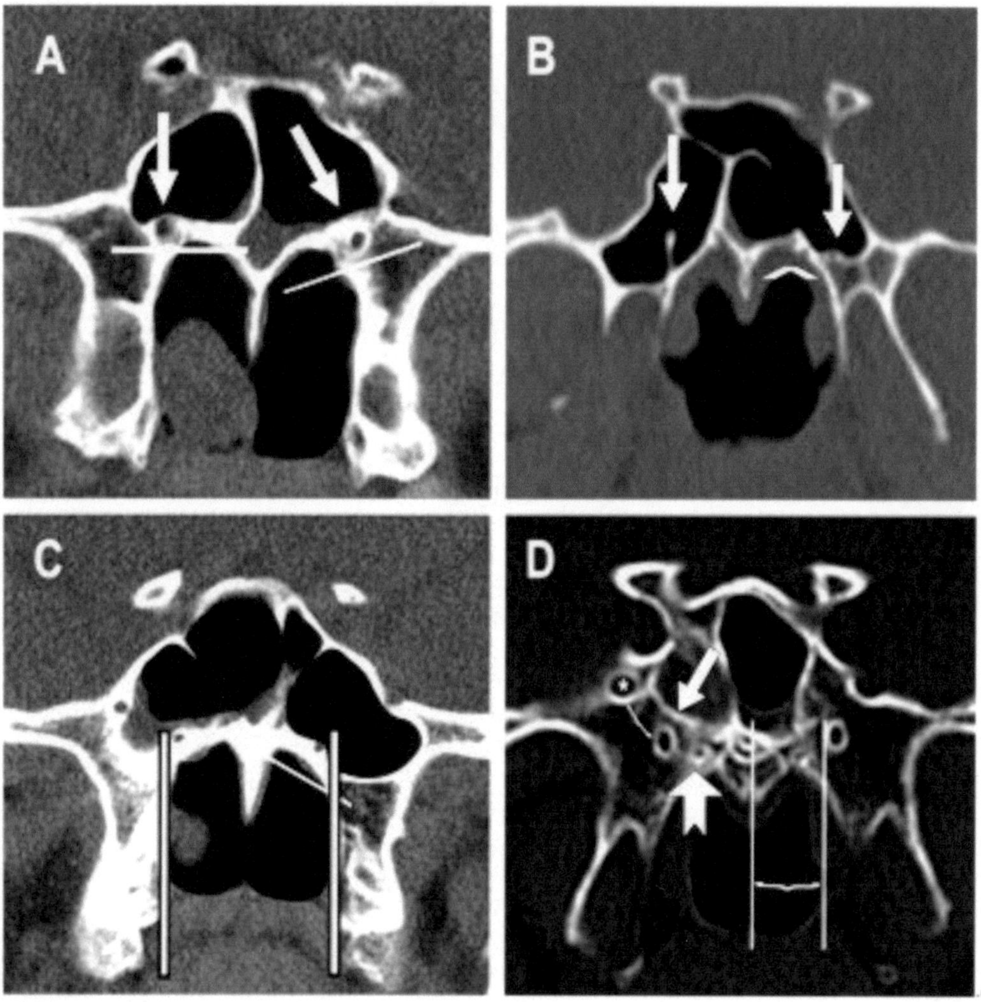

Fig. 4. Coronal computed tomography sections showing the vidian canal and its different positions. A, The vidian canal is embedded in the bone (left). Canal floor type 1 (right) and type 2 (left) are shown. B, Complete (right) and partial protrusion (left) into the sinus. Canal floor type 4 with canal wall dehiscence (left) is shown. C, The vidian canal is medially located close to the medial lamina of the pterygoid process (bilateral). Canal floor type 3 (left) is shown. D, Caliper measurement of the distance between the vidian canal and the vomerine crest (left) and between the vidian canal and the foramen rotundum (right; asterisk). Arrows indicate vidian canal; straight lines in A, C, and D and the caret in B indicate the canal-floor relationships. The bifid tail arrow in D indicates the palatovaginal canal.

higher failure rate. No negative angle value, which represented the anterior opening is medial to the middle turbinate, was recognized. In those difficult cases with a greater angle, a larger area of mucosal destruction and appropriate partial removal of pterygoid process is required. Doing so will bear the risk of brisk bleeding, resulting from injury of the SPA or its major branches. Sometimes, the retrograde nerve resection fashion is employed to handle this situation. Since a unilateral vidian neurectomy already shows acceptable outcomes, choosing an easy-to-approach side is comprehensive. Therefore, the included angle should be assessed and the decision to intervene the surgical side with a smaller angle can be made.

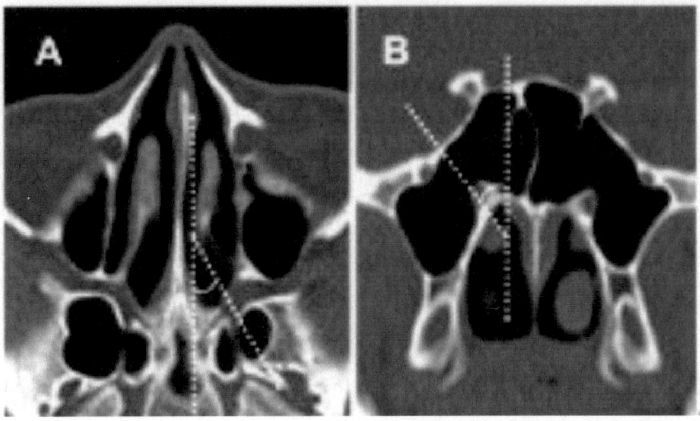

Fig. 5. The included angle between the posterior end of the middle turbinate and the most lateral part of the vidian canal anterior opening was measured (white dotted line). A. Axial view. B. Coronal view.

Fifth, the foramen rotundum on the lateral side and the palatovaginal canal on the medial side should be identified, to prevent it from being mistaken for the vidian canal. In our review of CT images from 341 patients, the foramen rotundum is located 1.7 to 15.5 mm superolateral to the vidian canal. The palatovaginal canal is recognized bilaterally in 37.0% (126 patients) and unilaterally in 19.4% (66 patients). Similar results are obtained by Rumboldt et al, with bilateral and unilateral incidence rates of 38% and 20.7%, respectively.(Rumboldt et al. 2002) The palatovaginal canal is located between the upper edge of the sphenoid process of the palatine bone and the vaginal process of the sphenoid bone, which projects medially from the upper end of the medial pterygoid plate (Fig. 6). This canal opens anteriorly through the posterior wall of the pterygopalatine fossa and transmits the minute pharyngeal branch that arises from the third part of the maxillary artery and the pharyngeal branch of the pterygopalatine ganglion to the pharyngeal orifice of the eustachian tube. Although mistaken transection of this nerve does not lead to any pronounced complication, nasal discomfort will persist, and the patient may require another procedure. Therefore, surgeons should keep this anatomic structure in mind when performing vidian neurectomy transnasally.

Finally, the nasal septum and turbinate should be reviewed. The presence of extreme septum deviation and the relative size of middle and inferior turbinate will effect the surgical feasibility. Choosing an easy side to approach is recommended and sometimes we may need to perform a combined septoplasty, inferior turbinate lateralization or partial inferior turbinectomy in order to access the vidian canal. Overall, preoperative CT images provide objective data for choosing a surgical approach. Interactive coronal, axial, and sagittal reconstructions of the sinuses assist the surgeon in understanding the anatomy in three dimensions. Optimally, the surgeon has a complete mental image of this anatomy prior to the surgical procedure

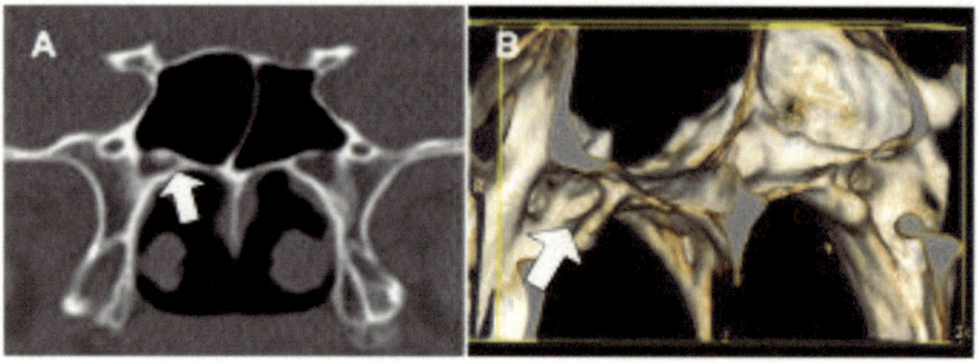

Fig. 6. The presence of palatovaginal canal (arrow) can be demonstrated on A: coronal CT slic and more clearly on B: 3D reconstruction image.

4.5 Anesthesia

VN are now all done under general anesthesia because as the surgery has been performed near the skull base and meticulous management is warrant. However, even with the administration of general anesthesia, topical vasoconstrictors and anesthetics are typically applied prior to surgery to minimize bleeding. It is advantageous to spray oxymetazoline into the nasal cavity 1 hour prior to the procedure. This allows for decongestion prior to introducing applicators or pledgets. A sphenopalatine block is performed transorally or transnasally to augment anesthesia and vasoconstriction as well as reduce bleeding. The transnasal route is usually selected when the nose is widely patent and the inferior part of the basal lamella can be visualized. It is carefully identified by passing the needle posteriorly and laterally through the horizontal part of the basal lamella. Intranasal injection of the nasal wall is performed under direct endoscopic vision into the superior attachment of the middle turbinate, medial surface of the middle turbinate and anterior wall of sphenoid sinus with 1% lidocaine with 1:100,000 epinephrine. As with topical anesthesia, these injections are performed one side at a time; the second side is not injected until surgery on the first side has been completed. Maintenance of an intraoperative heart rate under 60 beats per minute has been found to result in a clearer surgical field.

4.6 Technique

The keys to successful endoscopic VN are to minimize bleeding and how to precisely identify the vidian nerve via the interaction between the CT image guidance and nasal endoscopic visualization. It is particularly important not to traumatize the anterior part of the nose where the endoscope lens will rest or pass during the procedure. This requires using very gentle technique. Nasal mucosal stimulation has been demonstrated to cause vasodilatation and thus may cause bleeding, even at a site some distance from the primary site of stimulation. Additionally, the anterior part of the nose should be carefully suctioned from time to time during the procedure to ensure that the tip of the endoscope does not become contaminated with blood.

VN is begun with the patient placed in the semi-Fowler's position. Cottonoids soaked with diluted epinephrine (1:100 000) and cocaine, 10% (benzoylmethylecgonine), are positioned between the middle turbinate and the nasal septum to enlarge the space between them and to obtain decongestion of the nasal mucosa. The head of the middle turbinate is delicately dislocated laterally to further widen the virtual space between the middle turbinate and the nasal septum. After an adequate space between the middle turbinate and the nasal septum is created, the endoscope is angled upward along the roof of the choana until it reaches the anterior wall of sphenoid sinus. An ostium is created on the anterior wall of sphenoid sinus using a freer, usually located approximately 1.0 cm above the roof of the choana and between the superior turbinate and the nasal septum. Coagulation of the mucosa around the created ostium and inferiolaterally the mucosa on pterygoid process is performed. This serves to avoid arterial bleeding originating from septal branches of the SPA and facilitates the subsequent ostium enlargement. Kerrison's punch is used to enlarge the ostium inferiolaterally in an attempt to enhance the visualization of intrasphenoid cavity. Care must be taken in the inferolateral direction, where the SPA or its major branches lie. To avoid these vessels, it is sufficient to cut away the nasal mucosa slightly in an inferolateral direction and to coagulate it with monopolar diathermy or bipolar forceps, completely exposing the sphenoid rostrum (Fig. 7). The sphenoid rostrum is removed in fragments. Once the anterior sphenoidotomy is completed, small amounts of bleeding originating from the edges of the sphenoidotomy must always be checked to avoid occluding the lens of the endoscope. A 30° or 70° endoscope is used to try to identify the vidian canal, usually at the sphenoid sinus floor. Transection of the nerve is performed using an angle probe when direct vision can be obtained (Fig. 8). Caution must be taken if an intrasinus septum is removed. The incidence of clinical dehiscence of the carotid artery has been demonstrated to be 23%. In addition, the presence of a sphenoethmoid (Onodi) cell, a posterior ethmoid air cell that pneumatizes lateral and superior to the sphenoid sinus, places the optic nerve and occasionally the carotid artery at risk because of the nerve's intimate association with the lateral wall at the apex of the cell.

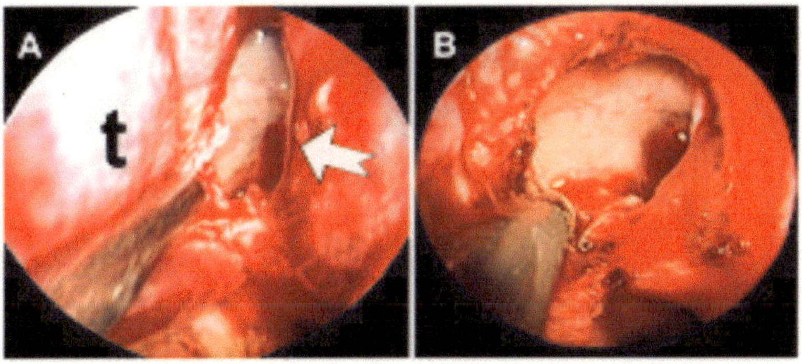

Fig. 7. Intraoperative endoscopic view: A: an ostium (bifid tail arrow) medial to the posterior end of middle turbinate (t) is created on the anterior wall of sphenoid sinus. B: monopolar diathermy is used before further dissection in the inferolateral direction to avoid brisk bleeding.

If there is no bony protrusion inside the sphenoid sinus floor as a visual guidance or the access to the vidian canal with or without protrusion is hampered by the pterygoid process, the approach is extended laterally by removing the pterygoid process around the vidian canal opening using a Kerrison's punch or chisel. The mucoperiosteal soft tissue can be elevated from the anterior surface of sphenoid sinus and then laterally the pterygoid process meticulously by a suction elevator, followed by the bone removal of sphenoid wall, or

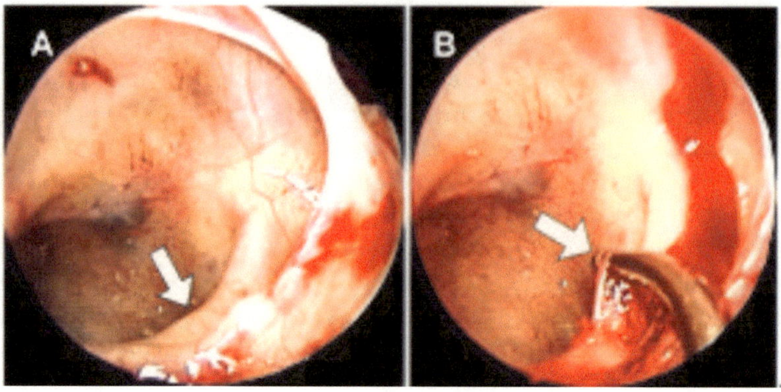

Fig. 8. Intraoperative endoscopic views of type I approach. A: The vidian canal (arrow) can be visualized at the floor of the sphenoid sinus. B: A probe is used to transect the nerve.

SPP. If the gap between sphenoid sinus wall and pterygoid process allows the passing through of a curved probe, the vidian nerve will be hooked out by the probe or sickle knife (Fig. 9). If the gap is too narrow to allow this procedure, the pterygoid process or the SPP will be partially removed by chisel or kerrison's punch based on the anatomical variation to discover the anterior opening of the vidian canal. The nerve hooking by probe can be repeated under this better visualization of canal opening. The vidian nerve can be usually stretched out of the canal opening as long as 2 centimetres and even more. Resection (precise nerve cut) plus cauterization of the nerve ends will follow it. The precise nerve hooking may be occasionally unable to be achieved on account of unintentional cauterization of the nerve during the dissection procedure or an uncertain nerve break

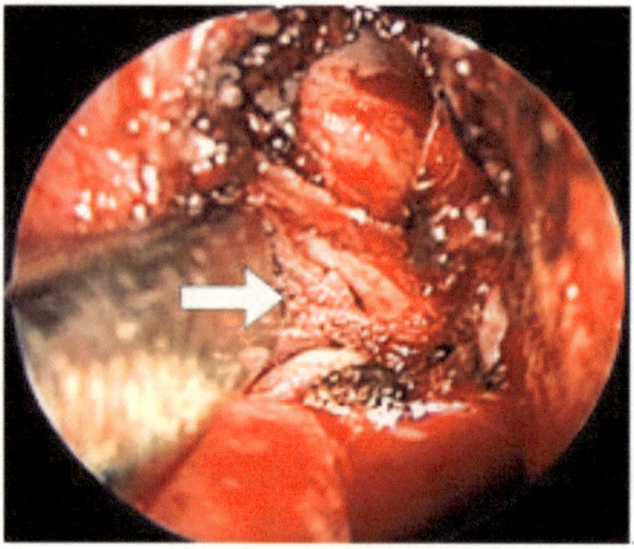

Fig. 9. Intraoperative endoscopic views of type II approach. The vidian canal (arrow) can be visualized at the gap between the anterior sphenoid sinus wall and SPP.

during nerve hooking procedure. Under this situation, the whole edge of the canal opening will be identified and the whole contents will be resected (semiprecise nerve cut). If the canal opening is not easily accessible or not fully exposed due to the severe obscuration of pterygoid process or SPP, a monopolar cauterization can be used to dysfunction the vidian nerve (cauterization) under visual guidance of vidian canal in the sphenoid sinus floor or image guidance of pterygoid process, sphenoid sinus floor, and even the sinus lateral wall.

Concurrent endoscopic septoplasty or partial resection of the inferior turbinate may also be performed once endoscopic VN has been completed on the side opposite from the septal deviation. The incision is made on the wider side. Endoscopic surgery can then proceed on the narrower side after the septoplasty has been completed. The fragment of the nerve is removed whenever possible to avoid nerve regeneration leading to symptom recurrence. Pathologic examination confirms the nerve tissue will help in adding surgeon confidence. At the end of the procedure, hemostasis is obtained, and the middle turbinate is gently restored in a medial direction. Packing of the nasal cavity is not always necessary except in the event of diffuse intraoperative bleeding from the nasal mucosa or in patients with poorly controlled hypertension, in which case packing is usually removed on the second day. Most patients are discharged 2 days after surgery.

4.7 Postoperative care

Meticulous postoperative care is just as critical in producing a successful outcome as the surgery itself. Any sponges placed can be removed the day following surgery and the nose can be suctioned of blood clots. During the initial postoperative period, inflammation and edema is heightened and mucociliary clearance disrupted, thereby increasing the risk of scar formation and development of postoperative sinusitis.

Avoidance of the offending antigens can be very useful in decreasing the burden of exposure, leading to reduced symptoms and improved quality of life. Although avoidance of perennial antigens such as animal dander can be reasonably well accomplished, the avoidance of seasonal pollens and molds can be more challenging due to their widespread airborne distribution. Measures to reduce exposure to dust mite antigen in the home include the use of covers for mattresses and pillows. The use of high-efficiency filtration can also be useful. In more extreme cases the removal of carpeting and curtains can be of benefit. In the case of mold allergy, the home should be kept at a low humidity and any plant material should be removed from the home. In the case of animal allergy, animals should be eliminated from the home, although the clearance of animal dander from the home can take many months.

Continued medical therapy in the postoperative period is still beneficial. In our opinion, topical nasal steroids and antihistamines may be reinitiated in the early postoperative period.

4.8 Outcomes

Multiple retrospective studies have documented the efficacy of VN in treating chronic rhinitis using both subjective and objective outcomes measures. Surgical outcomes of VN are generally good. Published Success rates range from 50% to 90%, with significant improvements in both symptomatology and general health status. Robinson and Wormald performed 14 retrograde VN among 9 patients with vasomotor rhinitis.(Robinson and Wormald 2006) All patients had negative screening for allergies on their serum or on skin-prick tests. A mean follow-up of 25 months of surgical results was analyzed. A significant

improvement in the symptoms of rhinorrhea (p = 0.018) and nasal obstruction (p = 0.011) can be obtained by VAS score analysis. However, there was no significant difference between the pre- to post-operative symptoms for postnasal drip or sneezing. The most common minor adverse effect was dry eyes (35.7%) and nasal crusting (28.6%). One patient complained of a temporary mild numbness of the cheek/gums or palate after surgery. There were no changes to visual acuity after vidian neurectomy. Seven of the 14 (50%) vidian neurectomies were deemed to be successful by the patients. In terms of overall satisfaction, poor satisfaction was encountered in one patient (7.1%) and the rest 92.9% exhibit at least good satisfaction. There was one recurrence case with an initial improvement in their nasal symptoms, which returned to their preoperative state 6 months after the vidian neurectomy.
Jang et al. had performed retrograde VN in 6 intractable rhinitis patients.(Jang et al. 2011) The nasal obstruction and rhinorrhea had the best improvement with significant lower postoperative VAS scores. However, although lower, changes of VAS scores in sneezing and itching were not statistically significant. All patients complained of mild dry eyes in the immediate postoperative period. The results of Schirmer's test performed immediately after surgery were significantly decreased compared to preoperative values (4.6±2.2 mm vs. 14.5±3.7 mm, $P<0.01$). Complaints of mild dry eyes persisted for 1 month after vidian neurectomy, but after 2 months, 5 of 6 patients reported marked improvement of xerophthalmia. The amount of tears by the Schirmer's test was also increased. There were no serious complications, aside from mild crusting of the nasal cavity and mild postoperative pain, which all subsided within 2 weeks. During the follow up period, no patient needed additional treatment, such as antihistamines or corticosteroids. All 6 patients were satisfied with the results of the surgery, although 1 patient reported mild deterioration of symptoms compared to the immediate postoperative period. Improvements persisted for up to 7 years after the primary surgery can be achieved.
In our un-published data, a total of 317 patients who underwent 414 endoscopic vidian neurectomies were reviewed. The change of VAS scores were analyzed in 236 antegrade VN among 163 cases with the mean follow up of 23 months (range, 6-58 months). One hundred and twelve patients underwent unilateral VN and 51 underwent bilateral procedures. The VAS score shows significant improvement in respective item of allergic symptoms, including rhinorrhea, obstruction, sneezing, nasal itchiness, rye itchiness and post-nasal dripping (Fig. 10). The dry eye developed in 172 of 236 sides (72.88%). They felt restored in average of 23 days (from 7 to 60 days). Long term use of eye drop substitute (more than 6 months) was required in 6 sides (2.54%). Palatal numbness occurred in 7 of 236 sides (2.97%) and disappeared in average of 13 days (from one to 21 days). Six postoperative bleeding (2.54%) occurred and stopped spontaneously without any assistance of nasal packing. All except 3 patients felt satisfied with their improvement of symptoms. Three recurrences (1.27%) were detected within one year follow-up and one of them received a successful reoperation.
Seldom reports explore the precise nerve cut rate in retrograde VN. Even in Robinson and Wormald report, we can't see the definite case number that how many of them had precise nerve severance or just function block by cauterization. In our preliminary report with 106 antegrade VN among 67 patients, we found that type I VN was performed successfully in 42 sides (39.6%) while the type II approach achieved 85.8% (91 of 106 sides) operating success rate. The operating success rate largely depended on anatomy variance, which can be pre-operatively recognized by CT images. In type I surgery, the precise nerve cut rates corresponding to the CT canal-corpus type including type 1, 2 and 3 were 0%, 72.1% (31 of 43 sides) and 84.6% (11 of 13 sides), respectively. In view of the CT canal-floor relationship,

the operating success rates for the type I approach were 50% (28 of 56 sides), 51.9% (14 of 27 sides), 0% (0 of 9 sides) and 0% (0 of 14 sides) for type 1, 2, 3 and 4, respectively. Either the embedded canal or the type 3 or 4 canal-floor relationship would fail the type I approach. The presence of the septum made the type I approach more difficult and time-consuming. This anatomic variation failed the type I approach in 6 patients that were viewed as candidates preoperatively. On the other hand, patients with the dehiscence of the canal bony structure were viewed as good candidates for the type I approach. There were 15 canals with more lateral situated anatomy which failed the type II approach. Although the anterior opening of the canals could still be identified, the direct views of nerve transection were not achieved. Further emptying the canal followed by cauterization (semi-precise) was used as a remedy for the 15 canals. With experience growing up with 414 antegrade VN in our un-published data, the precise cut rate of vidian nerve reaches 70.53% and a 19.81%of the semiprecise cut rate can be achieved. Only 9.66% had their nerve function blocked by cauterization. We also found the relationship between the anterior opening of the vidian canal and the posterior end of the middle turbinate had a determining role in antegrade VN. The included angle between the two structures can be measured from CT imaging, both in axial and coronal slices. A more hypertrophied middle turbinate, which represents a larger angle, was associated with a significantly higher surgical failure rate. The findings support the decision to intervene the surgical side with a smaller angle. This result again emphasized the value of pre-operation CT images analysis. As for surgeon's handedness, there was no statistical significance can be observed.

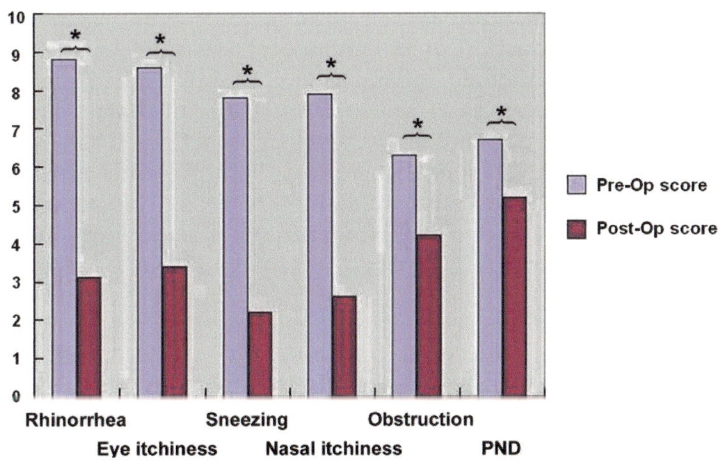

Fig. 10. Mean score for each symptom. *: significant difference. Test applied: paired t test, PND: Post-nasal dripping

The histological difference of the nasal mucosa before and after VN had been seldom discussed. Krajina compared the histological change in 16 VN cases and a very pronounced difference was found.(Krajina 1973) During the operation and 10 days after it, the nasal mucosa was examined. While the mucous membrane of the nose before cutting of the nerve showed very numerous mucous glands in the hyperactive state, after cutting the glands were decreasing in number and also contained some sympathetic branches from stage of normal and stabilized secretion. Moreover, eosinophils in the mucous sympathetic part which had its interruption in the membrane of the nose disappeared after VN. Therefore, the author recommended VN in all cases refractory to all conservative treatment bases on this pathophysiological finding. Ogawa et al. had once employed ELISA to examine local production of cytokines in nasal lavage samples.(Ogawa et al. 2007) A comparison of the cytokine levels (IL-5, eotaxin, and normal T cell expressed and secreted proteins, RANTES) before and 6 month after denervation was performed. The mean levels of both IL-5 and eotaxin significantly decreased after surgery (from 1094.8 to 183.8 pg/mg protein, from 540.6 to 165.0 pg/mg protein, respectively), while the mean levels of RANTES did not (from 385.8 to 331.0 pg/mg protein). The inferior turbinate mucosa was checked and the number of inflammatory cells and nasal glands was markedly reduced in the lamina propria after surgery. Further, the superficial epithelial layer of the turbinate mucosa became covered with stratified columnar cells, and the number of secretory goblet cells decreased. Recent study conducted by Ikeda et al. demonstrated the denervation effect of nasal mucosa.(Ikeda et al. 2008) Morphological analysis of the inferior turbinate mucosa before and after nerve resection showed an apparent decrease in nasal gland acinar cells after surgery, but the vascular structure of the mucosa seemed to be unchanged. Morphometric analysis of the density of the nasal gland showed a significant reduction, whereas no significant change was recognized in the density of the vessels. These findings suggest that denervation results in a decrease in nasal secretion but does not affect the congestion of the nasal mucosa. The reduction in glandular cells may be explained by decreased secretion of the nerve growth factor or epidermal growth factor regulated by acetylcholine, a major neurotransmitter of parasympathetic systems. On the other hand, no change in vascular structures implies that the vascular proliferation cannot be regulated by neural interaction. The infiltration of inflammatory cells in the nasal mucosa was also observed before and after operation. A significant reduction in the number of infiltrating neutrophils, eosinophils, and lymphocytes was recognized. The reduction of inflammatory cells may be explained by inhibition of nerve activities via neurogenic inflammation. In both allergic and idiopathic rhinitis, pathophysiological features such as fluid secretion mediated by orothrodromic reflex involving efferent nerve predominantly parasympathetic and release of neurotransmitters and neuropeptides from the sensory neurons via antidromic reflex are characterized by interaction of nerve activities with inflammatory cells. This report support the VN did improve the symptom of rhinorrhea. However, other underlying mechanisms still need to be evaluated in further work.

5. Conclusion

AR and NAR are significant, burdensome disorders that affect a large number of adults and children around the world. Rhinitis is associated with several important comorbid conditions, including asthma, rhinosinusitis, and otitis media with effusion. The use of appropriate therapeutic options will improve the outcome of patients with both AR and NAR. Medical treatment remains the backbone in treating chronic rhinitis.

VN can have some adjuvant benefit in patients who showed poor response to medical approaches. However the availability of nerve resection is largely determined by a favourable anatomy. The course of the vidian canal may vary from person to person, and it may also vary from one side to the other side in the same person. Therefore, a careful preoperative planning is warrant. CT imaging can offer good delineation of it and its relationship with the neighboring structures. Surgeons dealing with disease in this area must be familiar with the classic imaging characterization before initiation.

The transsphenoid approach is a simple method to accomplish a vidian neurectomy, able to spare SPA ligation and even duplicable in an occasional endoscopist. However, the recurrence of disease needs further investigation in the long term follow-up although the outcome is comparable with other reports in the 6 months follow-up. In view of anatomical variation, there is still no a completely satisfactory and consistent procedure to handle this entity. More powerful instrumentation is expected to facilitate this procedure.

6. References

Alvernia, J. E.; Spomar, D. G.; Olivero, W. C. (2007). A computed tomography scan and anatomical cadaveric study of the pterygopalatine ganglion for use in Gamma Knife treatment of cluster headache. *J Neurosurg*, Vol.107, No.4, (October 2007), pp. 805-8, ISSN 0022-3085

Bernstein, J. A. (2010). Allergic and mixed rhinitis: Epidemiology and natural history. *Allergy Asthma Proc*, Vol.31, No.5, (October 2010), pp. 365-9, ISSN 1539-6304

Broide, D. H. (2010). Allergic rhinitis: Pathophysiology. *Allergy Asthma Proc*, Vol.31, No.5, (October 2010), pp. 370-4, ISSN 1539-6304

Brozek, J. L.; Bousquet, J.; Baena-Cagnani, C. E.; Bonini, S.; Canonica, G. W.; Casale, T. B.; van Wijk, R. G.; Ohta, K.; Zuberbier, T.; Schunemann, H. J. (2010). Allergic Rhinitis and its Impact on Asthma (ARIA) guidelines: 2010 revision. *J Allergy Clin Immunol*, Vol.126, No.3, (September 2010), pp. 466-76, ISSN 1097-6825

Chandra, R. (1969). Transpalatal approach for vidian neurectomy. *Arch Otolaryngol*, Vol.89, No.3, (March 1969), pp. 542-5, ISSN 0003-9977

el Shazly, M. A. (1991). Endoscopic surgery of the vidian nerve. Preliminary report. *Ann Otol Rhinol Laryngol*, Vol.100, No.7, (July 1991), pp. 536-9, ISSN 0003-4894

Fernandez-Miranda, J. C.; Prevedello, D. M.; Madhok, R.; Morera, V.; Barges-Coll, J.; Reineman, K.; Snyderman, C. H.; Gardner, P.; Carrau, R.; Kassam, A. B. (2009). Sphenoid septations and their relationship with internal carotid arteries: anatomical and radiological study. *Laryngoscope*, Vol.119, No.10, (October 2009), pp. 1893-6, ISSN 1531-4995

Francis, G. J.; Becker, W. J.; Pringsheim, T. M. (2010). Acute and preventive pharmacologic treatment of cluster headache. *Neurology*, Vol.75, No.5, (August 2010), pp. 463-73, ISSN 1526-632X

Golding-Wood, P. H. (1961). Observations on petrosal and vidian neurectomy in chronic vasomotor rhinitis. *J Laryngol Otol.*, Vol.75, (March 1961), pp. 232-47, ISSN 0022-2151

Gregson, A. E. (1969). Relief of chronic epiphora by transantral vidian neurectomy. *Br J Ophthalmol*, Vol.53, No.12, (December 1969), pp. 858-9, ISSN 0007-1161

Halker, R.; Vargas, B.; Dodick, D. W. (2010). Cluster headache: diagnosis and treatment. *Semin Neurol*, Vol.20, No.2, (April 2010), pp. 175-85, ISSN 1098-9021

Hamid, O.; El Fiky, L.; Hassan, O.; Kotb, A.; El Fiky, S. (2008). Anatomic Variations of the Sphenoid Sinus and Their Impact on Trans-sphenoid Pituitary Surgery. *Skull Base*, Vol.18, No.1, (January 2008), pp. 9-15, ISSN 1531-5010

Ikeda, K.; Yokoi, H.; Saito, T.; Kawano, K.; Yao, T.; Furukawa, M. (2008). Effect of resection of the posterior nasal nerve on functional and morphological changes in the inferior turbinate mucosa. *Acta Otolaryngol*, Vol.128, No.12, (July 2008), pp. 1337-41, ISSN 1651-2251

Jang, T. Y.; Kim, Y. H.; Shin, S. H. (2011). Long-term effectiveness and safety of endoscopic vidian neurectomy for the treatment of intractable rhinitis. Clin Exp Otorhinolaryngol, Vol.3, No.4, (January 2011), pp. 212-6, ISSN 2005-0720

Kamel, R. and S. Zaher (1991). Endoscopic transnasal vidian neurectomy. *Laryngoscope*, Vol.101, No.3, (March 1991), pp. 316-9, ISSN 1531-4995

Knipping, S.; Holzhausen, H. J.; Riederer, A.; Schrom, T. (2009). Allergic and idiopathic rhinitis: an ultrastructural study. *Eur Arch Otorhinolaryngol*, Vol.266, No.8, (August 2009), pp. 1249-56, ISSN 1434-4726

Konno, A. (2010). Historical, pathophysiological, and therapeutic aspects of vidian neurectomy. *Curr Allergy Asthma Rep*, Vol.10, No.2, (March 2010), pp. 105-12, ISSN 1534-6315

Krajina, Z. (1973). Vidian neurectomy in vasomotor rhinitis. *Acta Otolaryngol*, Vol.76, No.5, (November 1973), pp. 366-71, ISSN 0001-6489

Krajina, Z. (1989). Critical review of Vidian neurectomy. *Rhinology*, Vol.27, No.4, (December 1989), pp. 271-6, ISSN 0300-0729

Lin, P. Y.; Cheng, C. Y.; Wu, C. C.; Yen, M. Y.; Wang, S. J.; Liao, K. K.; Lee, S. M. (2001). Bilateral neurotrophic keratopathy complicating Vidian neurectomy. *Am J Ophthalmol*, Vol.132, No.1, (July 2001), pp. 106-8, ISSN 0002-9394

Liu, S. C. and W. F. Su (2011). Evaluation of the feasibility of the vidian neurectomy using computed tomography. *Eur Arch Otorhinolaryngol.*, Vol., No., (February 2011), pp. , ISSN 1434-4726

Liu, S. C.; Wang, H. W.; Su, W. F. (2010). Endoscopic vidian neurectomy: the value of preoperative computed tomographic guidance. *Arch Otolaryngol Head Neck Surg*, Vol.136, No.6, (June 2010), pp. 595-602, ISSN 1538-361X

Minnis, N. L. and A. W. Morrison (1971). Trans-septal approach for Vidian neurectomy. *J Laryngol Otol.*, Vol.85, No.3, (March 1971), pp. 255-60, ISSN 0022-2151

Mora, F.; Cassano, M.; Mora, R.; Gallina, A. M.; Ciprandi, G. (2009). V.A.S. in the follow-up of turbinectomy. *Rhinology*, Vol.47, No.4, (December 2009), pp. 450-3, ISSN 0300-0729

Nomura, Y. (1974). Vidian neurectomy-some technical remarks. *Laryngoscope*, Vol.84, No.4, (April 1974), pp. 578-85, ISSN 0023-852X

Nomura, Y.; Terao, H.; Matsuura, T. (1971). Method in the vidian neurectomy. *Nippon Jibiinkoka Gakkai Kaiho*, Vol.74, No.2, (February 1971), pp. 504-5, ISSN 0030-6622

Ogawa, T.; Takeno, S.; Ishino, T.; Hirakawa, K. (2007). Submucous turbinectomy combined with posterior nasal neurectomy in the management of severe allergic rhinitis: clinical outcomes and local cytokine changes. *Auris Nasus Larynx*, Vol.34, No.3, (September 2007), pp. 319-26, ISSN 0385-8146

Osawa, S.; Rhoton, A. L., Jr.; Seker, A.; Shimizu, S.; Fujii, K.; Kassam, A. B. (2009). Microsurgical and endoscopic anatomy of the vidian canal. *Neurosurgery*, Vol.64, No.5 Suppl 2, (May 2009), pp. 385-411, discussion 411-2, ISSN 1524-4040

Robinson, S. R. and P. J. Wormald (2006). Endoscopic vidian neurectomy. *Am J Rhinol*, Vol.20, No.2, (May 2006), pp. 197-202, ISSN 1050-6586

Rumboldt, Z.; Castillo, M.; Smith, J. K. (2002). The palatovaginal canal: can it be identified on routine CT and MR imaging? *AJR Am J Roentgenol*, Vol.179, No.1, (July 2002), pp. 267-72, ISSN 0361-803X

Salib, R. J.; Harries, P. G.; Nair, S. B.; Howarth, P. H. (2008). Mechanisms and mediators of nasal symptoms in non-allergic rhinitis. *Clin Exp Allergy*, Vol.38, No.3, (March 2008), pp. 393-404, ISSN 1365-2222

Scadding, G. K.; Durham, S. R.; Mirakian, R.; Jones, N. S.; Leech, S. C.; Farooque, S.; Ryan, D.; Walker, S. M.; Clark, A. T.; Dixon, T. A.; Jolles, S. R.; Siddique, N.; Cullinan, P.; Howarth, P. H.; Nasser, S. M. (2008). BSACI guidelines for the management of allergic and non-allergic rhinitis. *Clin Exp Allergy*, Vol.38, No.1, (January 2008), pp. 19-42, ISSN 1365-2222

van Rijswijk, J. B.; Blom, H. M.; Fokkens, W. J. (2005). Idiopathic rhinitis, the ongoing quest. *Allergy*, Vol.60, No.12, (December 2005), pp. 1471-81, ISSN 0105-4538

6

Phase Contrast Computed Tomography

Fu Jian
Beijing University of Aeronautics and Astronautics
China

1. Introduction

Absorption-based X-ray imaging has been used for medical and industrial applications and become an invaluable tool since German scientist Röntgen's discovery more than a hundred years ago. By the development of computed tomography (CT), absorption-based X-ray imaging could be further improved and non-destructive three-dimensional (3D) views of internal structures became possible. In particular, for medical diagnostics applications, X-ray CT became an invaluable tool during the last 30 years. However, this kind of techniques provides poor contrast and spatial resolution for weakly absorption materials and structures with low atomic number. For example, since the absorption coefficients of soft tissue are very close to that of water, it is very difficult to distinguish internal features in the soft material.

In the quest of better contrast in X-ray imaging, a number of different phase contrast imaging (PCI) techniques have been explored during the last few decades. The phase shift cross section is three orders of magnitude larger than the absorption cross section for materials with low atomic number, which is an indication that PCI is more sensitive to density variation than absorption-based X-ray imaging. As one of the important research topics in the field of PCI, phase contrast CT (PC-CT) has consequently been developed to get the phase shift cross section tomography image of the samples. Unlike absorption-based CT, PC-CT uses the phase shift rather than the absorption as the imaging signal and may provide better image quality in soft tissue and low atomic number samples.

In this chapter, an overview of PCI and PC-CT methods was presented. Some of contents are directly adapted from the literatures. We will firstly introduce the concept of X-ray refraction, the complex refractive index and the phase signal. Then we will discuss the imaging principles of several kinds of PCI methods including crystal interferometer, analyzer based imaging, propagation based imaging and grating based imaging. Followed is the description of several PC-CT methods. PC-CT based on gratings and ordinary X-ray source will be the focus of discussion. Finally a description about the future of PC-CT will be presented.

2. X-ray refraction

It is well-known that refraction will be observed when light wave passes from one medium to another medium at any angle other than 90° or 0°. Refraction is the change in direction of a wave due to a change in its speed. It is described by Snell's law, which states that the angle of incidence is related to the angle of refraction. The index of refraction represents the refraction property of one media, which is relative to the propagation speed of light in this media.

As a form of electromagnetic wave, X-ray also has refraction phenomenon when it interacts with matter. Meanwhile, X-ray is shorter in the wavelength than visible light and easier to penetrate matter. It has a wavelength in the range of 0.01 to 10nm, corresponding to frequencies in the range 30 petahertz to 30 exahertz (3×10^{16} Hz to 3×10^{19} Hz) and energies in the range 120 eV to 120 keV. Due to refraction, both the amplitude and the phase of the electromagnetic wave describing the X-ray beam are affected when X-rays penetrate matter. The amplitude gets attenuated and the phase gets shifted.

When calculating refraction effects of X-rays penetrating matter, one can calculate both absorption and phase shift of the X-ray wave from the complex index of refraction n. In homogeneous media with a nonzero electron density, the refractive index is usually written as $n = 1 - \delta + i\beta$. Where δ and β are given by equations (1) and (2). λ is the wavelength, $r_0 = 2.82 \times 10^{-15}$ m is the Thomson scattering length (classical electron radius), Z is the atomic number, and ρ_A is the atomic number density. σ_p and σ_α are phase shift cross section and the absorption cross section respectively (Jensen 2010).

$$\delta = (\lambda / 2 / \pi)\rho_A(\lambda r_0 Z) = (\lambda / 2 / \pi)\rho_A\sigma_p \tag{1}$$

$$\beta = (\lambda / 4 / \pi)\rho_A\sigma_\alpha \tag{2}$$

To see the effect of the refractive index, we consider a wave propagating through a medium. The propagation of an electromagnetic wave through a medium with index of refraction n is described by equation (3). $\bar{k}$ is the wave vector, $\bar{r}$ is the position vector, and E_0 is the amplitude of the electric field.

$$\Psi(\bar{r}) = E_0 e^{in\bar{k}\cdot\bar{r}} = E_0 e^{i(1-\delta)\bar{k}\cdot\bar{r}} e^{-\beta\bar{k}\cdot\bar{r}} \tag{3}$$

In vacuum, the index of refraction n is unity, and hence the propagation of a plane wave in vacuum can be described by equation (4).

$$\Psi(\bar{r}) = E_0 e^{i\bar{k}\cdot\bar{r}} \tag{4}$$

In Figure 1 an example of how a plane wave changes as it interacts with a block of material is displayed. A wave travelling through a medium with refractive index n is both attenuated and phase shifted relative to a ray travelling through vacuum. The imaginary part of the refractive index describes the attenuation, here illustrated by the loss in amplitude and indicated by green lines in figure 1. The change in amplitude and intensity are given by equations (5) and (6) respectively. $\mu = 2k\beta$ is the linear absorption coefficient for absorption imaging. r is the length of the block of material.

$$\Delta E = E_0(1 - e^{-\beta kr}) \tag{5}$$

$$\Delta I = |E_0|^2 - |E_0 e^{-\beta kr}|^2 = I_0 - I_0 e^{-2\beta kr} = I_0(1 - e^{-\mu r}) \tag{6}$$

The second part of the refractive index is the real part δ. The real part describes the change in wavelength of the X-rays inside the material. The change in wavelength causes a phase difference between the X-rays that pass through the material and the X-rays that do not. This change in phase is,

$$\Delta\Phi = \delta\bar{k}\cdot\bar{r} \tag{7}$$

In general this can be rewritten as,

$$\Delta\Phi = \bar{k}\int\delta(x,y)\cdot d\bar{r} = \bar{k}\int\delta(x,y)\cdot dy \tag{8}$$

The change in phase also results in a change in direction of the X-rays as seen in Figure 1. The angular change in the direction is given as,

$$\alpha = \partial(\int\delta(x,y)dy)/\partial x \tag{9}$$

From the derivations above we now see how the real and the imaginary parts of the refractive index describe the behavior of X-rays as they pass through the material. These descriptions can be used to determine how to measure the real and imaginary parts of the refractive index, which are corresponding to phase contrast imaging and the conventional attenuation-based imaging (Jensen 2010).

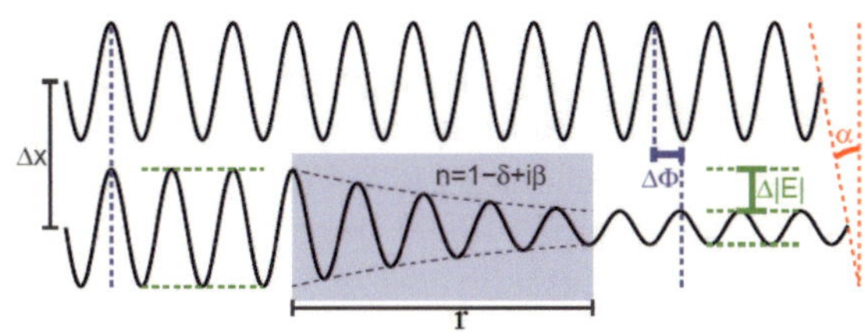

Fig. 1. Phase shift and attenuation of a wave in a medium. Inside the medium with refractive index $n = 1 - \delta + i\beta$ the wave get phase shifted with respect to the wave propagating in free space, as indicated by red lines, and attenuated, as indicated by green lines. Figure adapted from (Jensen 2010).

3. Why is phase contrast imaging?

The complex refractive index of the sample implies the features of phase contrast imaging and the conventional attenuation-based imaging.

From equations (1) and (2), we see that the ratio between the two cross sections σ_p and σ_α is given as

$$\sigma_p/\sigma_\alpha = (2\delta)/\beta \tag{10}$$

In Figure 2(a) the refractive index per mass unit is plotted for elements with atomic number lower than or equal to 20 for a number of different x-ray energies (data from Henke et al. , 1993). For water at 23.0keV, $\delta = 4.36\times10^{-7}$ and $\beta = 2.20\times10^{-10}$. In Figure 2(b) the ratio between the phase shift cross sections and the absorption cross sections is plotted. We see that the ratio is in the range $10^2 - 10^4$ (for water at 23.0 keV, $\sigma_\alpha/\sigma_p = 3.97\times10^3$). The cross section for the phase shift is thus 2-4 orders of magnitude greater than the cross section for the absorption.

It is this large difference that is one of the motivations for performing phase contrast imaging, as phase contrast imaging has the potential to deliver contrast that is orders of magnitude better than standard absorption images. Phase contrast imaging is especially beneficial for soft tissue as it mainly consists of materials of low atomic number (C, O and H). From Figure 2(b) we also see that except for the lowest atomic numbers the cross section ratio increases with energy (Jensen 2010).

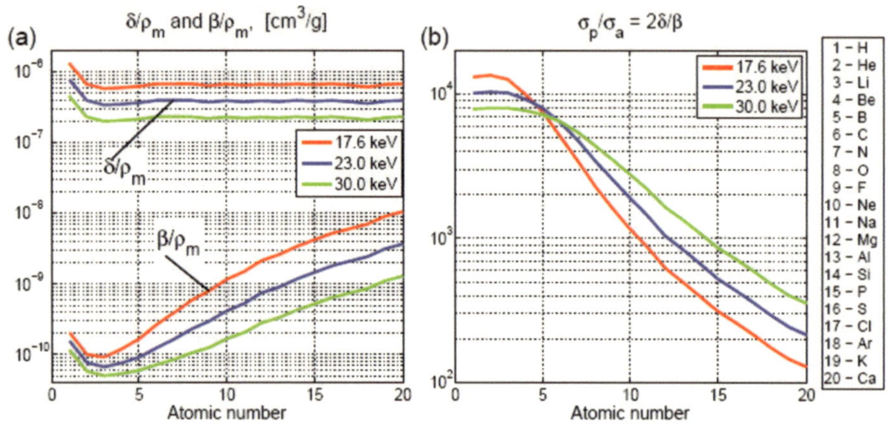

Fig. 2. Refractive index. (a) The real part (δ) and the imaginary (β) part of the refractive index per mass unit are plotted for various elements at various energies. (b) The ratio between the phase-shift and the absorption cross sections is plotted for various elements at various energies. Note that the ratio is between $10^2 - 10^4$ for these low Z elements, and except for the lowest atomic number this ratio increases with energy. Figure adapted from (Jensen 2010).

4. Several phase contrast imaging methods

Above we see how the derivative of the phase could be determined by measuring the change in direction of the X-rays. To determine the phase shift one method is thus to measure the change in direction of the X-rays. There currently exist several ways to probe this change, depicted in figure 3. In the following we will introduce them briefly.

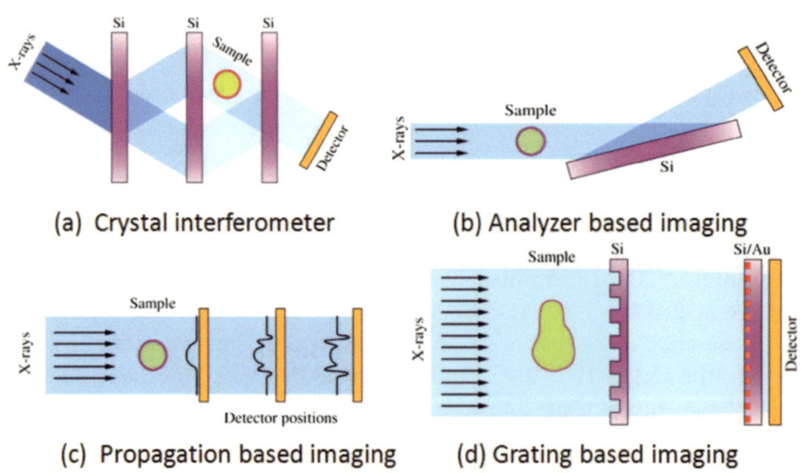

Fig. 3. Schematic drawing of several phase contrast imaging methods. Figure adapted from (Bech 2009).

4.1 Crystal interferometer

Crystal interferometers were first used for imaging by Bonse & Hart (1965). The method uses a number of crystal reflections to split an X-ray beam in two and let one part of the beam pass through the sample before the two beams are recombined. A sketch of a crystal interferometer set-up is shown in Figure 3(a). The method has later been extended to cover tomography (Momose 1995, Momose et al. 1996). As the method is based on the optical path length difference between the two beams, there are very stringent requirements to the stability of the interferometer. The interferometer has to be stable to better than a part of the X-ray wavelength (Momose 2003b). Resolving the stability issue can be aided through the use of monolithic crystal optics. Using Bragg reflections from crystals the method is limited to a temporal coherence of $\Delta\lambda / \lambda \rightarrow 10^{-4}$. A high degree of spatial coherence is also needed (Momose 2003b).

The method is very good for synchrotron use and high resolution studies. It was originally demonstrated with a laboratory X-ray source (Bonse & Hart1965), but the temporal coherence limits the available flux. The method is limited in the field of view by the size of the crystal optics. The widespread use is also limited by the need for stability where small vibrations can change the optical path length enough to disturb the measurements.

4.2 Analyzer based imaging

As a well collimated X-ray beam passes through a sample, the beam is slightly refracted. In analyzer based imaging (ABI) the refraction is imaged using the Bragg reflection of one or multiple analyzer crystals. A sketch of an ABI setup is shown in Figure 3(b). The method measures the derivative of the phase. The method was first introduced by Goetz et al. (1979), Ingal & Beliaevskaya (1995), Davis et al. (1995), Chapman et al. (1997). Chapman et al. (1997) demonstrated that it is possible to determine the phase quantitatively for pure phase objects. Later the same was shown in general (Pagot et al. 2003, Wernick et al. 2003, Rigon et al. 2003). The method is difficult to extend to tomography as the crystals are normally aligned such that the derivative of the refractive index is measured in the direction parallel to the tomographic axis. The tomographic reconstruction thus provides the out-of-plane derivative of the phase $\partial\delta(x,y) / \partial z$ and the apparent absorption reconstruction.

If the method is to be used with a laboratory source the main limitations are the need for temporal coherence, which limits the available flux. Due to the diffraction angles and sizes of the analyzer crystals the field of view will normally also be limited.

4.3 Propagation based imaging

A different approach to phase imaging is propagation based phase contrast (Snigirev et al. 1995). The propagation based imaging (PBI) is in many senses the simplest kind of phase contrast imaging, as no optical elements are required in the beam and the constraint on spectral width is relaxed (Wilkins et al. 1996, Cloetens et al. 1999a). PBI rely on interference fringes arising in the free space propagation in the Fresnel regime, as illustrated in figure 3(c). The measured intensity fringes are thus not a direct measure of the phase like the crystal interferometer, but rather the Laplacian of the phase front (Cloetens et al. 1997).

In order to achieve interference of the propagating beam, a very high degree of spatial coherence is required, and a high resolution detector is needed to observe the fringes. A series of images is then recorded at different propagation distances in order to unambiguously determine the phase of the wave front.

This method is particularly good at edge enhancement, and is hence well suited for e.g. fiber samples, foam or localization of non-homogeneity in metals (Cloetens et al. 1999b) also in tomography setup. But for imaging of soft tissue and small density variations this method is not optimal (Nesterets & Wilkins 2008).

4.4 Grating based imaging

Grating based imaging (GBI) or shearing interferometer is a fourth approach to phase contrast imaging (Clauser 1998). It is related to the crystal interferometer in the sense that it consists of a beam splitter and a beam analyzer, and GBI is related to ABI by the fact that the first derivative of the phase front is measured. GBI has previously been applied to visible light phase contrast (Lohmann & Silva 1971), and has recently been applied to X-ray imaging as well (David et al. 2002, Momose et al. 2003a, Pfeiffer et al. 2006).

The beam splitter grating splits the beam by diffraction, but the diffraction orders are separated by less than a milli-radian, and the diffracted beams are hence not spatially separated, but will interfere to create an intensity pattern downstream of the beam-splitter at a distance defined by the Talbot effect (Talbot 1836, Weitkamp et al. 2005), see figure 3(d). Refraction in a sample is measured by detecting the transverse shift of the interference pattern with a high resolution detector or an analyzer grating.

Tomographic reconstruction of the differential phase is possible even without initial integration to retrieve the quantitative phase shift (Pfeiffer et al. 2007), and this kind of tomographic reconstruction has turned out to be an advantage to local tomography (Pfeiffer et al. (2008)).

5. Phase contrast computed tomography

The quantity that serves as imaging information is not the distribution function of the real part δ of the refractive index, but its projection along the propagation direction of X-ray beam. In order to implement the quantitative analysis, δ should be reconstructed from the measured projections. Phase contrast computed tomography consequently appears as the result of the efforts to combine phase contrast imaging with computed tomography. There are mainly three kinds of PC-CT which are based on ABI, PBI and GBI. In the following we will present them.

5.1 PC-CT based on ABI

This kind of PC-CT adopts two scanning configurations to acquire phase projection data, depicted in figure 4. In the case of figure 4(a), the incidence direction of X-ray is parallel to lattice plane. The angular change in the direction is given as,

$$\alpha = \int (\partial \delta(x,y,z) / \partial z) dl \tag{11}$$

In this case, the value $\partial \delta / \partial z$ keeps invariant under all the projection view angle. It is similar to the conventional absorption-based CT. So the classical CT algorithms could be adopted to reconstruct the distribution of $\partial \delta / \partial z$, such as filtered back-projection algorithm (FBP) and algebraic reconstruction technique (ART).

In the case of figure 4(b), the incidence direction of X-ray is perpendicular to lattice plane. The angular change in the direction is given as,

$$\alpha = \int (\partial \delta / \partial x_r) dl \tag{12}$$

$$x_r = x\cos\varphi + y\sin\varphi \tag{13}$$

In this case, the value $\partial\delta / \partial x_r$ always changes under different projection view angle φ. This is against the principle of Radon transform and the classical CT algorithm can not be adopted to reconstruct the phase CT images.

There exist two methods to resolve this question. The first one applies the cubic spline integral to retrieve the value $\int \delta dl$ from the measured angular change α and the classical CT algorithm to reconstruct δ (Huang 2006).

The second one is based on an assumption which is expressed as,

$$\alpha\cos\varphi = \int (\partial\delta(x,y,z) / \partial x) dl \tag{14}$$

Under this assumption, the value $\partial\delta / \partial x$ keeps invariant under all the projection view angle φ. It is similar to the conventional absorption-based CT. So the classical CT algorithms could be adopted to reconstruct the first-order partial differential $\partial\delta / \partial x$.

5.2 PC-CT based on PBI

Figure 5 gives the scanning configuration adopted by this kind of PC-CT. In this case, no optical device is used except the coherent X-ray source.

According to the Transport of Intensity Equation (TIE), the intensity distribution $I_{\varphi,z}(x,y)$ at a distance z from the sample and angle of rotation φ can, for weakly absorbing samples and distance d in the near Fresnel region, be expressed as (Nugent 1996, Xu & Liu 2003),

$$I_{\varphi,d}(x,y) = I_{\varphi,0}(1 - (\lambda d / 2 / \pi) \cdot \nabla^2 \Phi(x,y)) \tag{15}$$

where $I_{\varphi,0}(x,y)$ is the absorption contrast intensity measured at $z = 0$.

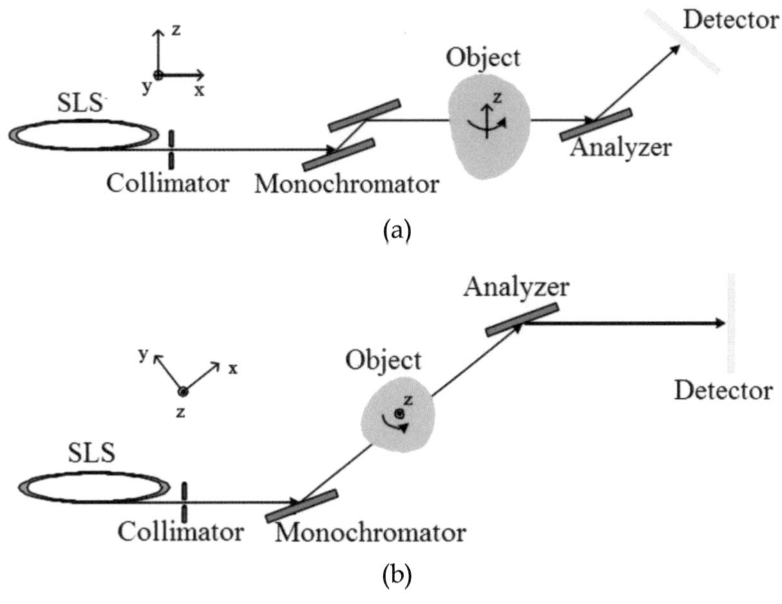

Fig. 4. Two scanning configurations adopted by PCT-CT based on ABI.

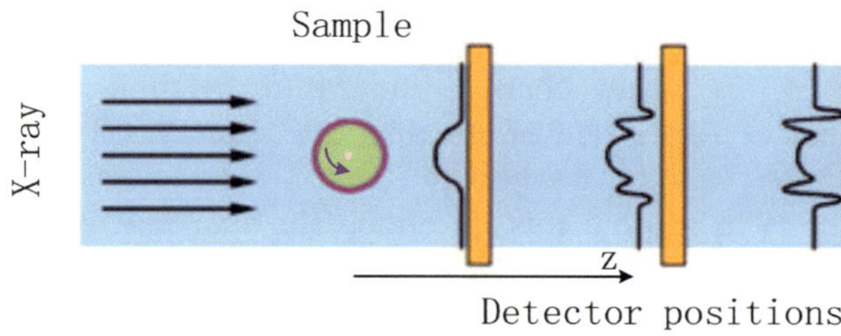

Fig. 5. The scanning configuration for PBI PC-CT.

Based on this equation, a reconstruction algorithm is deduced, which is similar to the conventional FBP, and expressed as (Bronnikov 2002),

$$\delta = \frac{1}{4\pi^2 d}\int_0^{\pi} q ** g_{\varphi} d\varphi \tag{16}$$

$$g_{\varphi} = I_{\varphi,d} / I_{\varphi,0} - 1 \tag{17}$$

$$q = |y| / (x^2 + y^2) \tag{18}$$

Where the filter function q is convolved with the data g_{φ}. This convolution can easily be implemented in the Fourier domain where the filter has the following form:

$$Q = |\xi| / (\xi^2 + \eta^2) \tag{19}$$

In the numerator of this filter, one can recognize the ramp filter $|\xi|$ of standard FBP. For easy implementation, the filtering is done separately where only the denominator is retained, because the ramp filter is implemented in the FBP reconstruction software. This reduces the algorithm to one extra filtering step in the reconstruction progress (Boone 2009).

In this algorithm, it was assumed that g_{φ} is known. For a cone beam scanning configuration, g_{φ} can not be calculated because of the changing magnification, except for objects with no absorption, i.e. pure phase objects. For weakly absorbing objects, this problem can be partially corrected by adding a correction parameter to the filter

$$Q_{cor} = |\xi| / (\xi^2 + \eta^2 + \tau) \tag{20}$$

as suggested by Groso et al. (2006), who named this algorithm the Modified Bronnikov Algorithm (MBA). A similar algorithm, the TIE phase retrieval, was derived by Paganin et al. (2002) and successfully applied by Mayo et al. (2003). When the assumption of a homogeneous object is made, the presence of the parameter τ can be derived directly from the TIE. The value of this parameter is determined using a semi-empirical approach. A too small constant leads to blurry results, where a too large constant eliminates the filter. Based on a single filtered projection, a good compromise can easily be chosen for the best results.

5.3 PC-CT based on GBI

Figure 6 gives the typical scanning configuration adopted by this kind of PC-CT. It usually uses a two-grating interferometer to retrieve the phase shift signal. When an incoherent X-ray source is adopted, a three-grating interferometer can be adopted to provide the retrieval of the phase shift signal. It permits the use of ordinary incoherent X-ray sources and has a much better potential to clinical applications and industrial non-destructive testing than other methods. In the following we will present this method in detail.

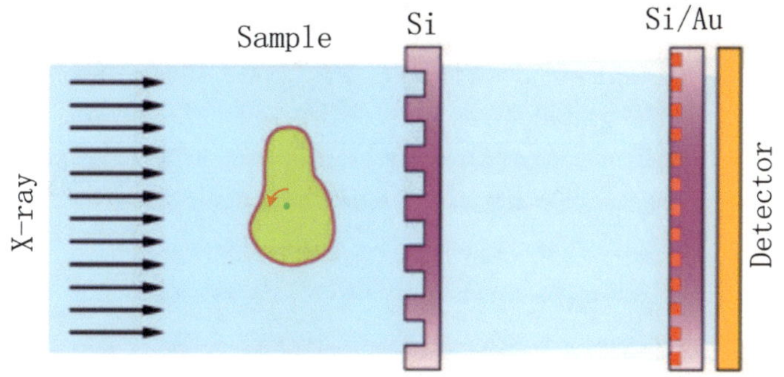

Fig. 6. The PC-CT scanning configuration with a two-grating interferometer.

5.3.1 Grating interferometer

Here we focus on the grating interferometer consisted of two x-ray gratings. A sketch of the grating interferometer can be seen in figure 7. The first grating is a beam splitting phase grating, G1. The grating is designed with a 0.5 duty cycle, such that the width of the phase shifting part of the grating is half of the period, g1 of the grating. The grating is designed so that the phase shift part of the grating introduces a π phase shift at the selected energy. Using these parameters it can be shown that the grating produces a box shaped interference pattern of alternating high and low intensity at uneven fractional Talbot distances, $d_T^{(n)}$, behind the grating (Jensen 2010). The fractional Talbot distance is given as,

$$d_T^{(n)} = n\frac{g1^2}{8\lambda} \tag{21}$$

Figure 7 shows an example of how the interference behind such a phase grating will be if the incoming beam is a plane wave. We note that the maximum intensity variation takes place at the uneven fractional Talbot distances. We also note that the period of the interference pattern is half the period of the phase grating. In Figure 7 the 5th, 9th and 11th fractional Talbot distances are marked with red dashed lines. These three distances are often selected as the experimental parameters.

5.3.2 Phase retrieval

If an object is placed in front of the phase grating it will change the intensity and the direction of the x-rays as described by the refractive index and explained above. As the direction of the x-rays changes, the vertical position of the interference pattern will also change. The principle idea of the grating interferometer imaging method is thus to determine the refraction of the x-rays through the sample, by performing measurements with and without sample and determine the change in position of the interference pattern caused by the sample.

One way to measure the position of the interference pattern is to use an analyzer grating. This grating, G2, has a duty cycle of 0.5 and a period that is matched to the period of the interference pattern g2 (see Figure 7). The idea is then to scan G2 in small increments perpendicular to the grating lines to detect the position of the interference pattern. An

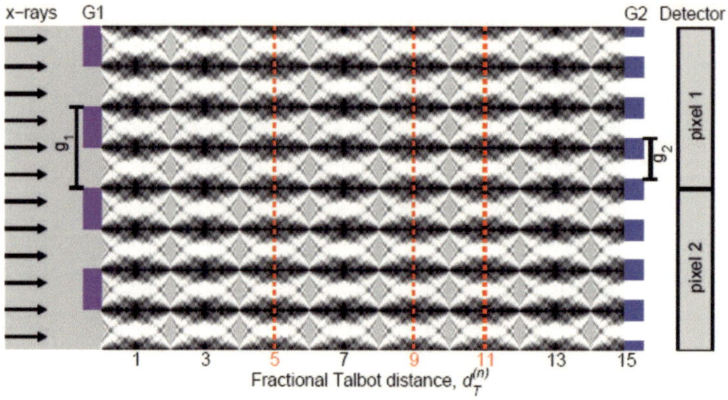

Fig. 7. The two-grating interferometer. On the left a phase grating, G1,of period, g1, splits the incoming plane wave. As a result an interference pattern is produced behind the grating. At uneven fractional Talbot distances, the interference pattern produces lines of alternating high and low intensity. The intensity pattern can be analyzed using an absorption grating, G2, of period g2 = g1/2. Depending on the alignment of the second grating it will either block or transmit the x-rays. A detector is placed behind the second grating. By scanning the second grating the position of the interference pattern can be determined. Figure adapted from (Jensen 2010).

example of the result of scanning G2 is shown in Figure 8. When G2 is aligned with the interference pattern all the x-rays will pass through the grating and high intensity will be recorded in the detector (Figure 8(a)). When G2 is moved half a period most of the x-rays will be absorbed, and low intensity will be recorded in the detector (Figure 8(c)). It can be shown that for real life set-ups the intensity variations when scanning one of the gratings will be well approximated by a first order Fourier expansion (Pfeiffer et al. 2008),

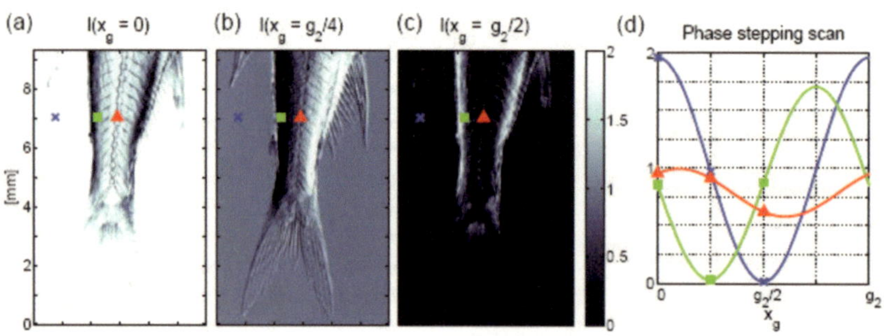

Fig. 8. Stepping the grating. (a)-(c) Projections of a fish for the grating positioned at x_g = [0; g2/4; g2/2] respectively. (d) Plot of the intensity in three pixels as a function of the grating position. The three points are marked in panels (a)-(c). Note how the phase and amplitude of the oscillation varies. Figure adapted from (Jensen 2010).

$$I(j,k,x_g)=\sum_{n=0}^{\infty}a_n(j,k)\cos(\frac{2n\pi}{g_2}x_g-\phi_n(j,k))\approx a_0(j,k)+a_1(j,k)\cos(\frac{2n\pi}{g_2}x_g-\phi_1(j,k)) \quad (22)$$

where (j,k) refers to the pixel numbers, a_n are the amplitude coefficients, ϕ_n the corresponding phase coefficients. An example of such an intensity variation is seen in Figure 9. The parameter a_0 describes the average intensity, a_1 the oscillation amplitude and ϕ_1 the position of the interference pattern.

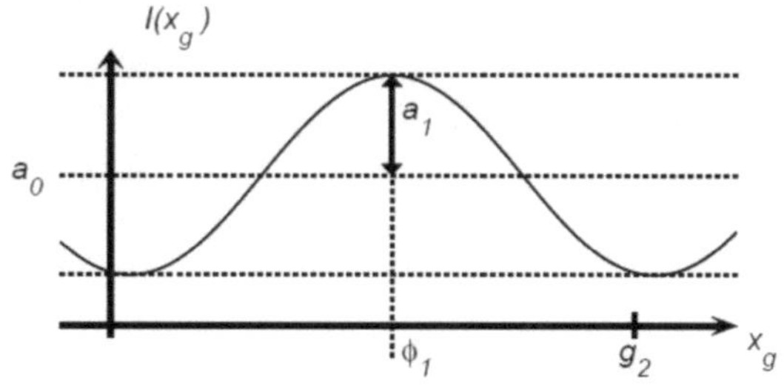

Fig. 9. Intensity variation in a single pixel. Figure adapted from (Jensen 2010).

In order to determine the refraction caused by the sample, it is necessary to include in the image processing a set of reference images recorded with an empty beam. The reference images are recorded during a phase stepping scan as described above under conditions identical to those recorded of the sample. From the reference images and the sample images, we get a set of parameters a_0, a_n and ϕ_n. If we denote the parameters obtained from the reference beam with a superscript r and those from the sample with a superscript s, we can retrieve the relative absorption, phase shift and visibility images as (Bech 2009),

$$a_0 = a_0^{\ s} \ / \ a_0^{\ r} \quad (23)$$

$$\phi 1 = \phi_1^{\ s} \ / \ \phi_1^{\ r} \quad (24)$$

$$V = \frac{a_0^{\ r}}{\phi_0^{\ s}} \sum_{n\ odd} \frac{a_n^{\ s}}{a_n^{\ r}} \quad (25)$$

In figure 10 an example of the three types of images produced with a grating interferometer is presented. The imaged specimen is a small fish. We can now see the individual strengths of the three different imaging modalities. The absorption image (Figure 10(a)) is the classical x-ray image, showing both the tissue and the bone of the fish. Figure 10(b) shows the differential phase contrast image. These images illustrate how the phase contrast can provide added contrast especially for soft tissue as described in the beginning of this chapter. Finally the dark field image (Figure 10(c)) shows that the micro-structure of the bones produces a lot of scattering. The dark field signal thus delineates the bones even more clearly than the standard absorption image.

5.3.3 Tomographic reconstruction from phase data

In this kind of PC-CT, the experiment configuration provides the line projections of the partial derivative of the object function. In this case tomographic reconstruction based on the conventional FBP using the standard Ramp linear filter function will not result in a correct reconstruction of the original object function.

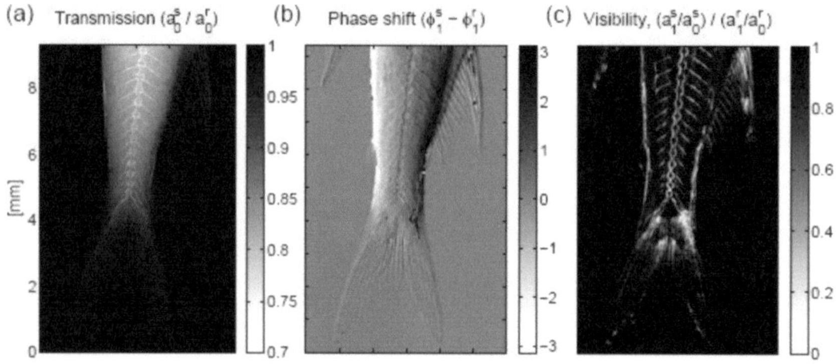

Fig. 10. Three types of images are recorded with the grating interferometer. (a) The transmission, which is the standard x-ray absorption contrast image. (b) The differential phase contrast image, which is very sensitive to e.g. soft tissue. (c) The dark field image, which shows the scattering structures of the sample. Figure adapted from (Jensen 2010).

Franz Pfeiffer et al(2007) proposed a reconstruction resolution for this question, expressed in the following equations. The procedure is the same as that to reconstruct absorption data, except for the imaginary filter $\tilde{h}(v)$ replacing the Ram-Lak filter $|r|$.

$$\delta(x,y) = \int_0^{\pi} FT^{-1}(FT(a_\varphi(r)) \cdot \tilde{h}(v))d\varphi \tag{26}$$

$$\tilde{h}(v) = |v| \frac{1}{2\pi i v} \tag{27}$$

This reconstruction resolution can be extend to three dimensional imaging by replacing the Ram-Lak filter $|r|$ in the standard Feldkamp algorithm with the imaginary filter $\tilde{h}(v)$. After this replacement we can obtain the three dimensional distribution of the real part of the object's refractive index.

6. Discussion

PC-CT uses the phase shift as the imaging signal and may provide better contrast in soft tissue and low atomic number samples. In this chapter, an overview of PCI and PC-CT methods was presented. The approach using grating interferometer permits the use of ordinary X-ray sources and has brought a break-through for various applications, such as clinical diagnosis, material evaluation and non-destructive testing. The practical application of X-ray PC-CT is becoming a reality with this technique.

To push the application of PC-CT based on ordinary X-ray source and grating interferometer, many questions still need to be resolved. For example, a common and matured theoretical basis, including three aspects of physics, mathematics and engineering techniques, should be created. A high-speed phase signal retrieval method should be found to reduce the exposure time and improve the efficiency. The fabrication technique of gratings should be developed to decrease the cost and improve the manufacture capability.

Additionally, PC-CT should be also combined with other visible light imaging methods to improve further the imaging resolution and contrast. We believe that nanometre resolution PC-CT will appear in several years.

7. Acknowledgment

Special thanks to Prof. Franz Pfeiffer and Dr. Martin Bech at the department of physics in Technische Universität München (TUM), Munich, German, for introducing me to the field and for the many shared valuable discussion, and experiments. I acknowledge support from National Natural Science Foundation of China (50875013), China Beijing municipal natural science foundation (4102036), Beijing NOVA program (2009A09) and Beijing University of Aeronautics and Astronautics young scholar cultivation program (YWF-11-03-Q-043).

8. References

Bech, M. (2009). PhD thesis, *X-ray imaging with a grating interferometer*, University of Copenhagen.

Bonse, U. & Hart, M. (1965). An x-ray interferometer, *Applied Physics Letters*, Vol. 6, No.8, (April 1965), pp.155-156, ISSN 0003-6951.

Boone, M., Witte, Y. De, Dierick, M., Bulcke, J. Van den, Vlassenbroeck, J. & Hoorebeke, L. Van. (2009). Practical use of the Modi_ed Bronnikov Algorithm in micro-CT, *Nuclear Instruments and Methods in Physics Research Section B*, Vol.267, No.7, (April 2009), pp.1182-1186, ISSN 0168-583X.

Bronnikov, A. V. (2002). Theory of quantitative phase-contrast computed tomography, *Journal of the Optical Society of America A*, Vol.19, No.3, (March 2002), pp.472-480, ISSN 1084-7529.

Clauser, J. F. (1998). Us patent No. 5,812,629: Ultrahigh resolution interferometric x-ray imaging.

Chapman, D., Thomlinson, W., Johnston, R. E., Washburn, D., Pisano, E., Gmur, N., Zhong, Z., Menk, R., Arfelli, F. & Sayers, D. (1997). Diffraction enhanced x-ray imaging, *Physics in Medicine and Biology*, Vol.42, No.11, (May 1997), pp.2015-2025, ISSN 0031-9155.

Cloetens, P., Ludwig, W., Baruchel, J., Dyck, D. V., Landuyt, J. V., Guigay, J.-P. & Schlenker, M. (1999a). Holotomography: Quantitative phase tomography with micrometer resolution using hard synchrotron radiation xrays, *Applied Physics Letters*, Vol. 75, No.19, (September 1999), pp.2912-2914, ISSN 0003-6951.

Cloetens, P., Ludwig, W., Baruchel, J., Guigay, J.-P., Pernot-Rejmankova, P., Salome-Pateyron, M., Schlenker, M., Buffierec, J.-Y., Maire, E. & Peix, G. (1999b). Hard x-ray phase imaging using simple propagation of a coherent synchrotron radiation beam, *Journal of Physics D: Applied Physics*, Vol.32, No. 10A, (January 1999), pp.A145-A151, ISSN 0022-3727.

Cloetens, P., Pateyron-Salome, M., Buffiere, J.Y., Peix, G., Baruchel, J., Peyrin, F. & Schlenker, M. (1997). Observation of microstructure and damage in materials by phase sensitive radiography and tomography, *Journal of Applied Physics,* Vol. 81, No.9, (May 1997), pp.5878-5886, ISSN 0021-8979.

Davis, T. J., Gao, D., Gureyev, T. E., Stevenson, A. W. & Wilkins, S. W. (1995). Phase-contrast imaging of weakly absorbing materials using hard x-rays, *Nature,* Vol.373, (February 1995), pp.595-598, ISSN 0028-0836.

David, C., Nohammer, B., Solak, H. H. & Ziegler, E. (2002). Differential x-ray phase contrast imaging using a shearing interferometer, *Applied Physics Letters,* Vol.81, No.17, (October 2002), pp.3287-3289, ISSN 0003-6951.

Goetz, K., Kalashnikov, M. P., Mikhailov, Y. A., Sklizkov, G. V., Fedotov,S. I., Foerster, E. & Zaumseil, P. (1979). Measurements of the parameters of shell targets for laser thermonuclear fusion using an x-ray schlieren method, *Soviet Journal of Quantum Electronics,* Vol.9, No.5, (May 1979), pp.607-610, ISSN 0049-1748.

Groso, A., Abela, R. & Stampanoni, M. (2006). Implementation of a fast method for high resolution phase contrast tomography, *Optics Express,* Vol.14, No.18, (September 2006), pp.8103-8110, ISSN 1094-4087.

Henke, B. L., Gullikson, E. M. & Davis, J. C. (1993). X-ray interactions: photoabsorption, scattering, transmission, and reflection at E=50-30000eV, Z=1-92, *Atomic Data and Nuclear Data Tables,* Vol. 54, No.2, (July 1993), pp.181-342, ISSN 0092-640X.

Huang Z. F. (2006). PhD thesis, *Research on extraction methods of phase information and CT reconstruction algorithms in diffraction enhanced imaging,* Tsinghua University.

Ingal, V. & Beliaevskaya, E. (1995). X-ray plane-wave topography observation of the phase contrast from a non-crystalline object, *Journal of Physics D: Applied Physics,* Vol.28, No.11, (May 1995), pp.2314-2317, ISSN 0022-3727.

Jensen, T. H. (2010). PhD thesis, *Refraction and scattering based x-ray imaging,* University of Copenhagen.

Lohmann, A. W. & Silva, D. E. (1971). An interferometer based on the talbot effect, *Optics Communications,* Vol.2, No.9, (1971), pp.413-415, ISSN 0030-4018.

Mayo, S. C., Davis, T., Gureyev, T. E., Miller, P. R., Paganin, D., Pogany, A., Stevenson, A. &Wilkins, S.(2003). X-ray phase-contrast microscopy and microtomography, Optics Express, Vo.11, No.19, (September 2003), pp.2289-2302, ISSN 1094-4087.

Momose, A. (1995). Demonstration of phase-contrast x-ray computed tomography using an x-ray interferometer, *Nuclear Instruments and Methods in Physics Research Section A,* No.352, No.3, (January 1995), pp.622-628, ISSN 0168-9002.

Momose, A. (2003b). Phase-sensitive imaging and phase tomography using x-ray interferometers, *Optics Express,* Vol.11, No. 19, (September 2003), pp.2303 - 2314, ISSN 1094-4087.

Momose, A., Kawamoto, S., Koyama, I., Hamaishi, Y., Takai, K. & Suzuki, Y. (2003a). Demonstration of x-ray talbot interferometry, *Japanese Journal of Applied Physics,* Vol.42, No.7B, (Seven 2003), pp.L866-L868, ISSN 0021-4922.

Momose, A., Takeda, T., Itai, Y. & Hirano, K. (1996). Phase-contrast x-ray computed tomography for observing biological soft tissues, *Nature Medicine*, No.2, No.4, (April 1996), pp.473-475, ISSN 1078-8956.

Nesterets, Y. I. & Wilkins, S. W. (2008). Phase-contrast imaging using a scanning-double-grating configuration, *Optics Express*, Vol.16, No.8, (April 2008), pp.5849-5867, ISSN 1094-4087.

Nugent, K. A., Gureyev, T. E., Cookson, D. F., Paganin, D. & Barnea, Z. (1996). Quantitative Phase Imaging Using Hard X Rays, *Physical Review Letters*, Vol.77, (September 1996), pp.2961-2964, ISSN 0031-9007.

Paganin, D., Mayo, S. C., Gureyev, T. E., Miller, P. R. &Wilkins, S. W. (2002). Simultaneous phase and amplitude extraction from a single defocused image of a homogeneous object, *Journal of Microscopy*, Vol.206, (April 2002), pp.33-40, ISSN 0022-2720 .

Pagot, E., Cloetens, P., Fiedler, S., Bravin, A., Coan, P., Baruchel, J., Hartwig, J. & Thomlinson, W. (2003). A method to extract quantitative information in analyzer-based x-ray phase contrast imaging, Applied Physics Letter, Vol.82, No.20, (October 2003), pp.3421-3423, ISSN 0003-6951.

Pfeiffer, F., David, C., Bunk, O., Donath, T., Bech, M., Duc, G. L., Bravin, A. & Cloetens, P. (2008). Region-of-interest tomography for gratingbased x-ray differential phase-contrast imaging, *Physical Review Letters*, Vol.101, (October 2008), pp.168101, ISSN 0031-9007.

Pfeiffer, F., Kottler, C., Bunk, O. & David, C. (2007). Hard x-ray phase tomography with low-brilliance sources, *Physical Review Letters*, Vol.98, (March 2007), pp.108105, ISSN 0031-9007.

Pfeiffer, F., Weitkamp, T., Bunk, O. & David, C. (2006). Phase retrieval and diffrential phase-contrast imaging with low-brilliance x-ray sources, *Nature Physics*, Vol.2, No.4, (March 2006), pp.258-261, ISSN 1745-2473.

Rigon, L., Besch, H. J., Arfelli, F., Menk, R. H., Heitner, G. & Plothow-Besch, H. (2003). A new DEI algorithm capable of investigating sub-pixel structures, *Journal of Physics D: Applied Physics*, Vol.36, No.10A, (May 2003), pp.A107-A112, ISSN 0022-3727.

Snigirev, A., Snigireva, I., Kohn, V., Kuznetsov, S. & Schelokov, I. (1995). On the possibilities of x-ray phase contrast microimaging by coherent high energy synchrotron radiation, *Review of Scientific Instruments*, Vol.66, No.12, (November 1995), pp.5486-5492, ISSN 0034-6748.

Talbot, H. F. (1836). Facts relating to optical science, *Philosophical Magazine*, Vol.9, No.56, pp.401-407, ISSN 19415966.

Weitkamp, T., Diaz, A., David, C., Pfeiffer, F., Stampanoni, M., Cloetens, P. & Ziegler, E. (2005). X-ray phase imaging with a grating interferometer, *Optics Express*, Vol.13, No.16, (August 2005), pp.6296-6304, ISSN 1094-4087.

Wernick, M. N., Wirjadi, O., Chapman, D., Zhong, Z., Galatsanos, N. P., Yang, Y., Brankov, J. G., Oltulu, O., Anastasio, M. A. & Muehleman, C. (2003). Multiple-image radiography, *Physics in Medicine and Biology*, Vol.48, No.23, (December 2003), pp.3875-3895, ISSN 0031-9155.

Wilkins, S. W., Gureyev, T. E., Gao, D., Pogany, A. & Stevenson, A. W. (1996). Phase-contrast imaging using polychromatic hard x-rays, Nature, Vol.384, (November 1996), pp.335-337, ISSN 0028-0836.

Wu, X. & Liu, H. (2003). A general theoretical formalism for X-ray phase contrast imaging, *Journal of X-Ray Science and Technology*, Vol.11, No.1, (January 2003), pp.33-42, ISSN 0895-3996.

7

Bone Density Measurement Using Computed Tomography

Cetin Celenk[1] and Peruze Celenk[2]
[1]*Department of Radiology, Faculty of Medicine, Ondokuzmayis University, Samsun*
[2]*Department of Oral and Maxillofacial Radiology, Faculty of Dentistry*
Ondokuzmayis University, Samsun
Turkey

1. Introduction

Osteoporosis is a major medical, social, and economic problem. Osteoporosis and low bone mass affect an estimated 44 million Americans (National Osteoporosis Foundation, 2008). The lifetime risk of hip, spine, or forearm fractures is estimated to be 40% in white women and 13% in white men above 50 years of age. Considerable attention is therefore focused on assessing bone mass and the ability to identify people at risk of fracture. Determining bone density (BD) helps a doctor determine those at increased risk for osteoporosis-related fracture.

Bone density (or bone mineral density) is a medical term that refers to the amount of matter per square centimeter of bone. Bone density is used in clinical medicine as an indirect indicator of osteoporosis and fracture risk. BD measurements are most commonly made over the lumbar spine and over the upper part of the hip. In recent literature, several approaches have been introduced to measure mandibular and skeletal BD, and then compare these measurements with BD in other parts of the skeleton. The measurement is painless, non-invasive, and involves minimal radiation exposure. In this chapter, bone density using computed the tomography technique will be introduced and discussed.

CT is an imaging technique that shows human anatomy in cross sections and provides a three-dimensional dataset that can be used for image reconstruction and analysis in several planes or three-dimensional settings. CT is used to study bone pathology, from traumatic lesions to bone neoplasm. In addition to morphologic information, CT also provides information about tissue attenuation. Direct Hounsfield unit measurements for BD may be used to examine bone quality. Attenuation values can be extracted from raw CT data and used to reconstruct images. These values can also be used to estimate the density of tissues. CT accurately measures bone density. CT density measurement methods can be used as to separate the trabecular bone from the cortical shell and the posterior elements of vertebrae.

CT density measurements have shown superiority to other modalities Using CT for take density measurements is discussed, including several of its challenges, in the current clinic. The foundations of CT density, classification, and registration are discussed in detail.

2. Osteoporosis

2.1 What is osteoporosis?

Osteoporosis is a multifactorial pathologic condition that affects the entire skeleton and is characterized by low bone mass in combination with microarchitectural changes, particularly in cancellous and cortical bone. Osteoporosis is the end result of bone loss. Osteoporosis is the most common type of the metabolic disorders of bone. The condition is characterized by reduced bone mass and increased risk of fracture (fragility). Osteoporosis occurs when bones lose minerals, such as calcium, more quickly than the body can replace them, leading to a loss of bone thickness (bone mass or density). As a result, bones become thinner and less dense so that, eventually, even a minor bump or accident can cause serious fractures. These are known as fragility or minimal trauma fractures.

Osteoporosis, which literally means "porous bone," is a disease that reduces the density and quality of bones. As the bones become more porous and fragile, the risk of fracture is greatly increased. The loss of bone occurs "silently" and progressively. Often, there are no symptoms until the first fracture occurs.

Based on the World Health Organization's (WHO) definition of osteoporosis, Melton (1995) estimated that 30% of postmenopausal white women in the United States have osteoporosis. Asthmatics, other lung patients, or rheumatoid arthritis patients treated with high-dose corticosteroids lose trabecular bone and experience fractures, as do patients with Cushing's syndrome. Other disorders including renal failure and certain types of cancer cause bone loss, along with chronic use of drugs such as anticonvulsants, anticoagulants, excess alcohol, and too much thyroid medication. Young women who experience amenorrhea due to athletic activity, weight loss, stress, nutritional deficiency, bulimia, anorexia nervosa, or those who have early natural or surgical menopause and do not take estrogen replacement therapy lose bone. Not all of the patients in these groups will develop osteoporosis. However, most of them will lose some bone and thus increase their long-term risk for fractures.

2.2 The clinical indication for bone mass measurement

- Estrogen deficient women at clinical risk for osteoporosis
- Individuals planning to dental implant therapy
- Individuals with vertebral abnormalities
- Individuals receiving, or planning to receive, long-term glucocorticoids
- Individuals with primary hyperparathyroidism
- Individuals being monitored to assess the efficacy of an approved osteoporosis drug therapy
- Medicare will only reimburse when BD tests are ordered by the treating health care provider
- Frequency of BD testing is once per two years
- Benefit applies to all Medicare patients including managed care programs
- Non-Medicare payers may have different guidelines (Christopher&Cann, 1989)

2.3 Why we measure bone density?

Bone density (or bone mineral density) is a medical term referring to the amount of matter per square centimeter of bone. Bone density is used in clinical medicine as an indirect indicator of osteoporosis and fracture risk.

Simple measurement of bone mineral density using SXA, DXA, QCT, or ultrasound does not predict which patient will develop osteoporosis. However, low bone density, as measured by any of the above techniques, is a strong risk factor for the occurrence of non-traumatic bone fractures that are characteristic of osteoporosis.
Slightly more than half of the overall risk for the development of osteoporosis is associated with low bone density, as measured quantitatively. The other factors contributing to fractures are varied, including the internal structure of bone, level of physical activity, neuromuscular coordination, and lifestyle factors that are difficult to quantify. Because of this, bone density is the most useful measurement in estimating an individual patient's relative risk for osteoporosis.
Osteoporosis is a major public health concern, with up to half of all women and even 20% of men having a lifetime risk for osteoporosis-related fracture. Bone mineral density increases until around age 35 and then levels off until menopause. There is an increase in the amount of fat within the trabecular field with age. During the first six to eight years of menopause, there is a sharp decline in bone mineral density. An estimated 1% to 5% of bone density is lost at this time. The higher a woman's overall bone density, the less she will be affected when she loses bone density at menopause. Persons have limited or no estrogen replacement therapies at menopause are the major high-risk group (Reinbold et al., 1988).
Also, one impetus behind this new research is that desire to examine jaw bone quality before osseo-integrated implant treatment has begun. It is hoped, with further research, the success rates of implant therapy will increase (Celenk&Celenk, 2008, 2010)

2.4 How we measure bone density?

Bone density (BD) is the amount of bone tissue in a certain volume of bone. In recent literature, several approaches have been introduced to measure skeletal BD.
All commercially-available methods for bone density measurement pass a low-intensity beam of x-rays or gamma-rays through a patient, and a radiation detector on the other side measures how much of the beam is absorbed. Part of the beam is absorbed by the bone and part by the surrounding soft tissue, and each technique measures these differently. But, quantitative computed tomography provides a cross-sectional or 3-dimensional image from which the bone is measured directly, independent of the surrounding soft tissue.

3. Types of bone mineral density tests

- Ultrasound
- DEXA (Dual Energy X-ray Absorptiometry)
- SXA (single Energy X-ray Absorptiometry)
- PDXA (Peripheral Dual Energy X-ray Absorptiometry)
- RA (Radiographic Absorptiometry)
- DPA (Dual Photon Absorptiometry)
- SPA (Single Photon Absorptiometry)
- MRI (Magnetic Resonance Imaging)
- QCT (Quantitative Computed Tomography)
- Laboratory tests

3.1 Ultrasound

Measuring area is the heel. New methods of measuring osteoporosis using ultrasound have also been developed. One such ultrasound system measures BMD at the patient's heel and takes about a minute. Non absorptiometric methods such as ultrasound of bone do not directly measure bone density, but give alternative information about properties of bone, such as the speed of sound, that are related to bone density and structure. The ultrasound systems for testing osteoporosis are smaller and less expensive than traditional methods. Further, density changes in the heel occur much slower than in the hip or spine. Therefore, ultrasound densitometry should not be used to monitor a patient's response to the therapy (Njeh et al., 1997 & Rang et al., 1998).

Ultrasound densitometry may not be as sensitive as other techniques, such as DEXA or QCT, that measure the spine or hip, since the heel may be normal in bone density even when central sites such as the hip or spine are already significantly abnormal.

However, the new ultrasound densitometry systems will allow many more people access to bone densitometry and potentially diagnose osteoporosis before a traumatic fracture occurs (Njeh et al., 1997 & Rang&Speller., 1998).

3.2 DEXA (dual energy X-ray absorptiometry)

The measuring area is spine, hip, or total body. DEXA (dual energy X-ray absorptiometry) is the most widely available method of bone densitometry, and most insurance plans will cover the cost for the test, given that certain medical indicators are present. Bone mineral density measurement with DEXA is painless and requires no injections, invasive procedures, sedation, special diet, or any other advance preparation. During a DEXA exam, the patient lies fully clothed on a padded table while the system scans one or more areas of bone (usually the lower spine or hip). The entire exam typically takes just a few minutes to complete.

Dual energy x-ray absorptiometry (DXA) measures the bone by computing the difference in absorption of low-energy photons and high energy photons by the mixture of soft tissue and bone in the path of the beam and can generate a 2-dimensional image for localization of the bone.

While DEXA uses x-rays, the radiation dose is less than during a chest x-ray. Each patient's bone density is plotted against the "norm" for a healthy young adult or against age-matched control data. A radiologist or other physician then interprets the data and creates a concise report on the status of the patient's bone density.

DEXA systems have recently received US Food and Drug Administration (FDA) clearance. The accuracy of bone mineral density testing is high, ranging from 85% to 99%. DEXA is the most accurate and widely available BMD test (Mazess et al., 1992).

The interpretation of individual DXA studies is not difficult. However, the responsibility of a physician overseeing a densitometry service lies more in familiarity with the conceptual context as it relates to the role of densitometry in and the management of osteoporosis (Lentle&Prior, 2003).

3.3 SXA (single energy X-ray absorptiometry)

Measuring area is the wrist or heel. This is a method of assessing bone mineral density using a single energy X-ray beam. Single energy x-ray absorptiometry (SXA) computes bone mineral from the increased absorption of the beam as it passes from a constant thickness of soft tissue or water bag into the bone. Localization for SXA is normally done using external landmarks without an image. It is now widely considered inferior to dual-energy X-ray absorptiometry, which uses a second energy beam to correct for absorption of X-ray energy by non-calcium containing tissues (Adams, 1997).

3.4 PDXA (peripheral dual energy X-ray absorptiometry)

Measuring area is the wrist, heel, or finger. The acronym pDXA (peripheral dual-energy X-ray absorptiometry) is used to describe dedicated devices that are specifically designed to measure the BMD of peripheral skeletal sites using DXA. There is no fundamental difference in technology between peripheral and central DXA. pDXA (Hans et al., 2008),

3.5 RA (radiographic absorptiometry)

The measuring area is the hand. RA, or radiographic absorptiometry, uses an X-ray of the hand and a small metal wedge to calculate bone density in the middle phalanges. Radiographic absorptiometry (RA) measures bone density in the fingers relative to an aluminum calibration wedge on the film. RA is one of the most preferred bone mass measurements because it can calculate bone loss quickly and it is a relatively inexpensive option for any medical specialist and medical office (Yang et al., 1994),

3.6 DPA (dual photon absorptiometry)

The measuring area is the spine, hip, or total body. Measurement of the BMC of spine and proximal femur (or any part or the entire skeleton) requires measurement of the relative attenuation of two differing photon energies to permit a correction for soft-tissue attenuation. This allows an assay of the calcium content in deeper structures, although the technique only provides an real density of calcium (in grams per square centimeter) not true volumetric density such as may be achieved with quantitative CT (Blake &Fogelman 1997, Genant & Boyd 1977).

3.7 SPA (single photon absorptiometry)

The measuring area is the wrist. The method overcame the problems for radiographic photodensitometric techniques, caused by polychromatic X-rays and nonuniformity of film sensitivity and development, by using a single energy g-ray source (125I, photon energy 27.3 KeV) and a scintillation detector to measure transmitted photons (Adams 1997). SPA was used to advance bone measurement from the early days of measurement of bone size on radiographs of the hand or crude determinations of optical density from similar images. It is an effective technique for measurements of bone in the distal radius and ulna (Duppe et al., 1997).

3.8 MRI (magnetic resonance imaging)

The measuring area is the spine, hip, or total body. MRI might be used effectively, as it is noninvasive and radiation-free, and it is a reliable in vivo method for assessing features of the trabecular bone structure (Wehrli et al. 2000; Majumdar 2002; Strolka et al 2005, Celenk&Celenk 2010). Trabecular bone is highly responsive to metabolic stimuli and has a turnover rate approximately three to 10 times higher than cortical bone, and so it is a prime site for detecting early bone loss and monitoring response to therapeutic intervention.

3.9 Laboratory tests

Laboratory tests that measure the amount of collagen in urine samples can indicate bone loss. Lab tests may also be used in conjunction with DEXA or other methods of bone densitometry to diagnose osteoporosis.

4. QCT (quantitative computed tomography) and osteoporosis

4.1 The foundations of the CT density

Measuring area is the entire body

QCT refers to a class of techniques in which the CT numbers, or x-ray attenuation, of a tissue is properly referenced to a calibration standard and then used to quantify some property of the tissue. Techniques were developed and published from 1978 to 1982 for bone density, lung nodule calcification, liver and brain tumor volumes, body fat measurement, muscle mass, liver iron measurement, kidney stone composition, and tissue blood flow. Of these, bone mineral density, lung nodule calcification, and tissue blood flow have been commercialized.

4.2 Why quantitative computed tomography?

CT numbers (i.e., Hounsfield units, HU) are strongly related to biological tissues density (Ciarelli et al., 1991; McB- room et al., 1985). The directly measured Hounsfield number for bone density may be used to examine bone quality. This method is recommended by some authors (Nilsson et al 1988, Shapurian et al 2006, Norton et al 2001). The mean number of HU within each ROI measures and uses the BD as the marker of metabolic alterations within the trabecular field.

QCT was one of the earliest ways of measuring bone density its use has largely been superseded by the use of dual energy x-ray absorptiometry (DXA) (Adams et al. 1997). QCT has several advantages over DXA, providing true volumetric density (so being size independent) separately in trabecular and cortical bone and being free of the inaccuracies caused by spinal DXA by extra-osseous calcification and hyperostosis. Quantitative CT and simple trabecular ROI attenuation approaches bone density measurement simply and accurately. QCT also shows promise as effective tools in measuring BD. However, QCT is not widely available and delivers more radiation to the patient than DEXA.

DEXA T-scores are the standard used by "all the major national and international societies, including the World Health Organization."

Gugliemi et al (1994) said we believe that considerations should be given to the use of QCT as the gold standard against which other measurements of spinal BD are judged. Development in QCT technology (spiral acquisition) and software has enabled rapid acquisition of 3D volume images and application to other relevant sites. We have therefore reassessed QCT in the assessment of patients with osteoporosis. The analysis showed similar results across the board—with no significant differences for any of the measurements versus DEXA.

Given the poor agreement between the two methods for the diagnosis of osteoporosis and the much better fracture discrimination with QCT, we believe that consideration should be given to the use of QCT as the "gold standard" against which other measurements of spinal BMD are judged.

Investigators often diagnose osteoporosis by measuring a patient's bone mineral density (BMD). Bone mineral density measures the amount of calcium in regions of the bones. Bone density is a good measurement for bone quality but it is not sufficient in itself. However, BD might be used to imply bone quality when the density alterations represent changes in trabecular structure (Celenk&Celenk, 2008).

Most methods for measuring BD (also called bone densitometry) are fast, non-invasive, painless, and available on an outpatient basis. Bone densitometry can also be used to estimate a patient's risk of fracture. These methods compare the numerical density of the bone (calculated from the image), with empirical (historical) databases of bone density to determine whether a patient has osteoporosis, and often, to what degree.

The accuracy of the results remained high whether BD was measured by using QCT or by means of a simple region of interest (ROI) CT density assessment. The "simple ROI" technique can perform without angulations or precise measurements

This information at CT is currently being wasted. ROI measurement of vertebral body trabecular attenuation takes a matter of seconds" and adds value to any routine BD measurement that can be performed with the same CT data. This means that any CT examination that covers any bone alone can effectively rule out osteoporosis and osteopeni without need of a second test.

Reinbold et al. (1986) said that trabecular bone is approximately eight times more metabolically active than cortical bone. Quantitative computed tomography (QCT), which measures trabecular bone density, is therefore highly sensitive to changes in skeletal density.

We can use QCT as the reference standard and any CT examination covers vertebra. The investigators are also looking to detect suspected lumbar compression factors with QCT, which DEXA can miss this condition.

QCT is the only commercially available 3-dimensional technique, meaning it can be used to measure 100% isolated trabecular bone. All other techniques measure the mixture of trabecular bone and the overlying compact bone. In the spine, trabecular bone is 30-35% of the total, in the distal radius it is 35-50%, and 60-75% in the calcaneus. Trabecular bone is important to measure because it is more metabolically active than compact bone and is the first to change in response to a stimulus such as estrogen deficiency. Trabecular bone in the spine is a more reliable indicator of overall skeletal response than the heavily weight-bearing bone in the calcaneus. However, it is also important to consider that any measurement must be done precisely; otherwise, the measurement will be insensitive.

DEXA can produce false-negative results for osteoporosis in the setting of unsuspected lumbar compression fractures that CT can potentially detect. While DEXA uses x-rays, the radiation dose is less than during a chest x-ray.

Baran et al. (1997) said that the QCT examination, when performed correctly, gives relatively low radiation exposure compared with conventional radiographs or standard CT studies, typically equivalent to a transcontinental airline trip.

Summers et al. (2001) said that ''we can record the actual bone mineral density value in grams per cubic centimeter instead of using the T-scores or Z-scores produced by the DEXA phantomless QCT software "because they don't really have a reference standard that's accepted".

Both lumbar QCT and simple ROI measurements are effective at assessing bone mineral density relative to DEXA, which is a reference standard we have to use. We can set a certain level and be at 100% sensitivity for osteoporosis and also exclude osteoporosis in a large fraction of people—over half of people depending on the level—and actually preclude the possible need for DEXA in those cases (Summers et al.,2001).

For the same precision, QCT is 2-3 times more sensitive than DXA and 5 times more than SXA for detecting a change in bone mineral density in early postmenopausal women (Reinbold et al 1988).

4.3 How is bone density measured by QCT?

Trabecular bone is approximately eight times more metabolically active than cortical bone (Reinbold 1986. Quantitative computed tomography, which measures trabecular bone, is therefore highly sensitive to changes in skeletal density.

For this purpose we can use both single energy quantitative computed tomography (SEQCT) and dual energy (DEQCT). One disadvantage of single-energy QCT (SEQCT) is that bone mineral measurements are affected by varying quantities of intraosseous fat. It has been calculated. For example, that a 10% increase in intraosseous fat results in underestimation of actual bone mineral content by **7** mg/ml. (Reinbold et al., 1986)

QC T scanning done with dual energy has the advantage of eliminating the effect of marrow fat, resulting in increased accuracy. However, the reproducibility is decreased and there is increased radiation dosage (Genant&Boyd, 1977). The use of dual energy QCT using preprocessing or post processing techniques can reduce this fat induced error in the elderly to 2% to 4%, but it is considered unnecessary for most clinical applications because the inaccuracy is small relative to the normal biological range (Cann&Genant, 1983).

DEQCT correlates well with SEQCT for estimation of bone density and alterations in marrow fat are therefore not a significant problem (Rosenthal et al., 1989).

As a result we are using single energy quantitative computed tomography for measurement bone density.

4.4 What is Hounsfield unit?

The Hounsfield unit (HU) scale is a linear transformation of the original linear attenuation coefficient measurement in one in which the radio density of distilled water at standard pressure and temperature (STP) is defined as zero, while the radio density of air at STP is defined as -1000 HU. Hounsfield unit are used in medical imaging to describe the amount of x-ray attenuation of each "voxel" in the 3D image. Voxels are normally represented as 12-bit binary numbers and therefore have $2^{12} = 4096$ possible values. These values are arranged on a scale from -1024 HU to +3071 HU, calibrated so that -1024 HU is the attenuation produced by air and 0 HU is the attenuation produced by water.

For a material X with linear attenuation coefficient μ_X, the corresponding HU value is therefore given by

$$HU = \frac{\mu_x - \mu_{water}}{\mu_{water} - \mu_{air}} \times 1000$$

where μ_{water} and μ_{air} are the linear attenuation coefficients of water and air, respectively. Thus, a change of one Hounsfield unit (HU) represents a change of 0.1% of the attenuation coefficient of water since the attenuation coefficient of air is nearly zero. CT scanners are calibrated with reference to water (Brooks &Chiro 1976**)**. The CT number is directly related to the linear attenuation coefficient for the x-ray and is usually calibrated to 0 for water and to −1000 for air, -120 for fat, +40 for muscle, and +400 or more for bone.

The Hounsfield number of a tissue varies according to the density of the tissue; the higher the number, the denser the tissue. Consequently, the mean Hounsfield number is a ratio in proportion to the atomic weights of the whole particles and particle numbers within the evaluation site. It has been discovered that when there is an increase in the fat amount of ROI volume, there is a corresponding decrease in the amount of minerals and in the Hounsfield number. The reverse has also been observed. The mean Hounsfield number

decreases when the amount of fat increases or the amount of mineral decreases. The Hounsfield number can be used directly to determine bone quality alterations.
CT is another extension of photon absorptiometry, but for a much more general purpose. Rather than a simple measurement of the photon attenuation along a fixed line through an object, as in SPA, a series of measurements are made at any point along that line by (in effect) rotating the source and detector about that point. Thus, a point on the line is "viewed" from up to a thousand different directions. Through the mathematical process known as projection reconstruction, these points along the line are separated from one another, as are points along other lines that make up the two-dimensional axial image plane. This process of reconstructing the CT image produces a map of the x-ray attenuation coefficients in a cross-sectional "slice" of the body, and these coefficients can be used to determine tissue density at any point in the image. The size and number of points along a line in current CT scanners is variable depending on the object being scanned, but ranges from points 0.25 mm up to 1.5 mm in size, and typically 256–512 elements lie along the line. Each "slice" of a patient scanned can also have variable thickness (the portion exposed to the x-ray beam), ranging from 1 mm up to 10 mm thick. Each point, or element, in a given reconstructed image is the same size, but this size can vary from 0.25 x 0.25 x 1 mm (0.0625 mm^3) to 1.5 x 1.5 x 10 mm (22.5 mm^3). When viewed on a display monitor, these points are called picture elements or "pixels"; when stored in the computer and used for quantitative purposes, they represent volume elements because of the finite slice thickness and are termed "voxels" (Christopher et al 1989,. Cann&Genant 1980).

4.5 Phantom and calibration

Determination of a linear correlation between HU and density is called calibrating the CT dataset and is obtained with a standard protocol-based procedure scanning a calibration phantom with known densities.
Recent commercial modifications of this design, including both liquid and solid bone-equivalent materials, provide slightly different scanning geometries and require scanner-specific cross-calibration to this standard reference using patient data or development of their own normative databases.
Since commercially available CT scanners use kilovoltage x-rays, where the photoelectric effect and coherent scattering play substantial roles, the x-ray attenuation depends not only on the electron density but also on atomic composition of the material. In addition, the CT number also depends on photon energy spectrum, geometrical configuration of the phantom system, detector sensitivity, and, possibly, reconstruction algorithm.
Therefore, the relationship between CT number and effective density for body tissues should be calibrated specifically for each scanning condition of each CT system. However, the involved theoretical calculations may be too complicated to practice without complete understanding of the underlying physics.
All the techniques provide a result for trabecular bone mineral density in terms of mg/cm^3 relative to the K_2HPO_4 or calcium hydroxyapatite mineral equivalent standard.
The calibration materials are air, water, and ethanol. The polybinary calibration requires only a CT scan of a fat substitute (ethanol) and a bone substitute (40%K2HPO4) besides water and air. Simplicity and specificity should be mandatory for a standard that has to be routinely practiced by the relevant facilities with the same quality. Furthermore, the simplicity will possibly enable the self-calibration of planning CT images if the patient is scanned with the calibration materials appropriately placed in the scanning field.

The detector response profile of the CT machines restores the use air or water calibration. The HU curves for the CT scanner are seen to be extremely stable by the use of a phantom in a weekly quality control program.
Also, Reinbold et al. (1988) and Cann&Genant (1980) said that in an effort to improve accuracy and reproducibility, a number of phantoms have been developed to offer reference standards and/or methodologies for QCT studies.
Boden et al. (1989) said that "the early thrust of research in phantom development was directed at correction for CT instability or scan-to- scan variations." Although early third-generation scanners may have shown considerable scanto-scan variation, it is no longer the case that functional CT scanners show such variations. Over the last decade, one of the authors, has measured hundreds of CT scanners in the public and private sectors; the variation of intra-scanner CT numbers is within 1 to 2 Hounsfield units (HU) and is systematic and reproducible.
At the same time, Zhao and colleagues (2009) also claim that spine BMD can be automatically calculated without phantom. By accurately segmenting cortical bone and trabecular bone, determining ROI and removing inappropriate data, it is proved that the BMD measurement result by this method is highly consistent with that by with-phantom method.
As a result, BMD calculations with and without phantom are highly correlated.

4.6 Examination procedures

4.6.1 Spine

The following protocols can be used to calculate density in addition to routine CT, specially by taking CT crossections to evaluate osteoporosis.
The patient place supine on the CT table and a cushion places under the knees to reduce the lumbar lordosis. CT sections are usually taken from lumbar vertebrae. The calibration standard is placed under the lumbar vertebrae. A lateral scanogram (topogram) is made from approximately T12 to S1. This use positions the axial slices through the mid vertebral levels of three to four consecutive lumbar vertebral bodies. Scans are made perpendicular to the axis of the vertebrae. Usually, a low-dose technique is used (120 kVp, 140 mAs) with the table increment and scan thickness, which were both set at 5 mm- 10 mm. Also it can be use **a** low radiation dose technique (80 kVp, 140 mAs**;** 140 kVp, 80 mAs) for DEQCT, which results in a skin exposure of 313 mR for each 80- 140 kVp pair (Rosenthal et al., 1989).
We simply lay an ovoid ROI and measure the mean attenuation in Hounsfield units. Reconstructions can perform any thicknesses (at both 1.5-mm and 5-mm) but the 5-mm thicknesses are more compatible with any routine CT study. Regions of interest (ROIs) are manually defined in every axial CT slice. When the ROI is defined, every image may be enlarged to increase accuracy. At the same time, BD values for all patients are determined in the trabecular field of the vertebral corpus by removal of the vertebral cortex (approximately 2-3.5 cm^2).

4.6.2 Mandible

The mandibular trabecular field (including incisor, molar, and premolar areas) is largely determined by leaving out nontrabecular fields such as teeth, bony cortex, mental symphysis and mandibular canal (approximately 1–1.5cm^2), and BD measures. In order to show a more accurate measured density value of the tissue characteristic under study, the measurement sites must be done as large as possible.

4.7 How do we comment QCT results?

QCT, like any bone density measurement, is used to compare a patient with normal control data or an absolute reference value, and to measure the change in bone density with time in a given patient. Researchers have established a "fracture threshold" level for all bone density methods; patients with bone density above this level are rarely seen with osteoporotic fractures, while below it, the prevalence of patients with fractures rises. This level is about 100-110 mg/cm^3 for QCT. As the value decreases below this, the fracture prevalence increases, so below 50 mg/cm^3 most patients already have spinal fractures. At quantitative CT, a BMD threshold of 90 mg/cm^3 yielded 100% sensitivity for osteoporosis or at the L3 level, a trabecular attenuation threshold of 130 HU was 100% sensitive for osteoporosis (Shapurian et al., 2006).

Figures show measurement values on different persons with different Hounsfield Unit to determine bone density (Fig 1-3).

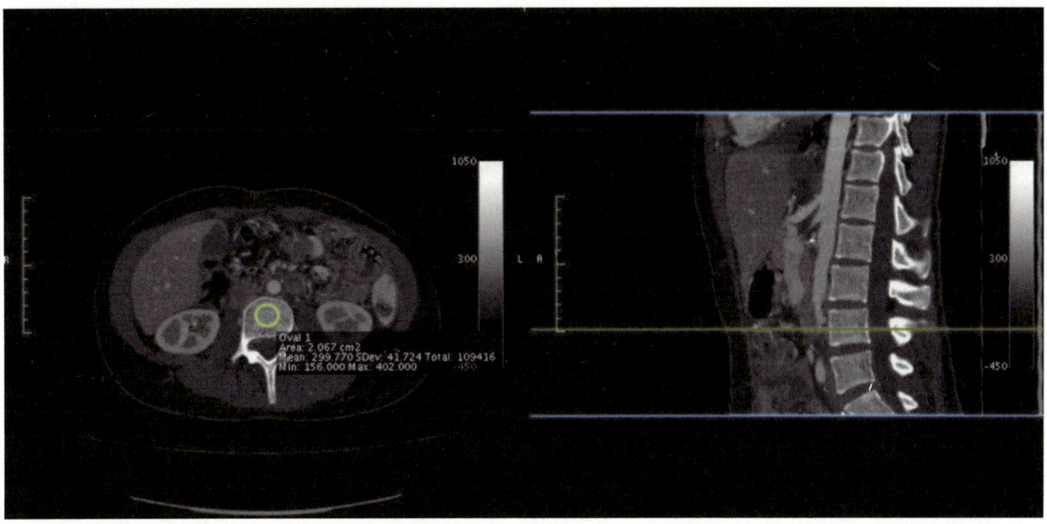

Fig. 1. Axial L3 vertebral CT slice of 20-year old woman shows nonosteoporotic L3 vertebral bone density measurement in Hounsfield Unit (mean: 299 HU).

The QCT value for a patient, when added to other diagnostic information, can be helpful in deciding an approach to treatment. Serial QCT measurements can establish the rate of change of bone mineral density in both treated and untreated patients, but the sensitivity of the method depends on how well the technique is done at a given hospital. In most cases, a change of 8-10 mg/cm^3 can be significant or at least indicate a trend, and several serial measurements all changing the same way improve confidence in the result. Women who are 1-3 years post menopause average 7 mg/cm^3/yr loss, so yearly measurements can be helpful. Bone loss may be slower in older individuals. The frequency for each patient will depend on other diagnostic and treatment factors, and it is important to interpret the bone density results within the context of each individual's clinical status.

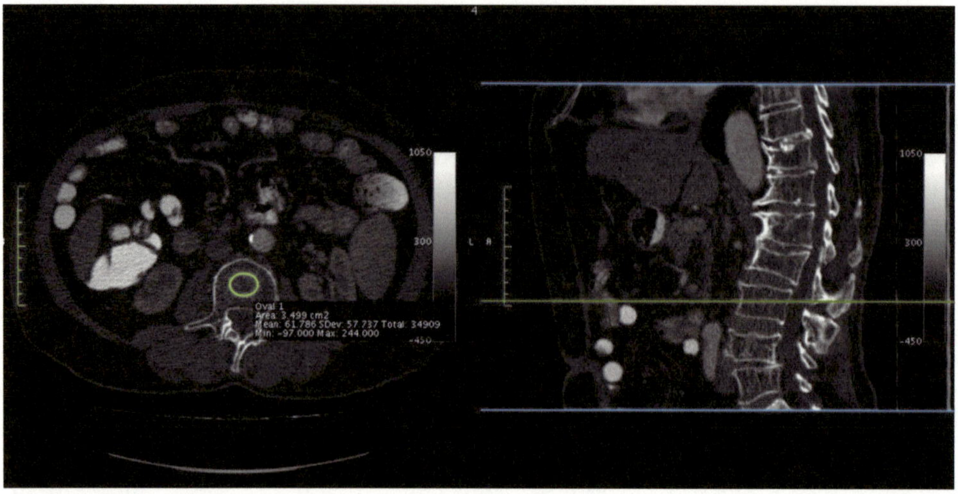

Fig. 2. Axial L3 vertebral CT slice of 61-year old man shows osteoporotic L3 vertebral bone density measurement in Hounsfield Unit (mean: 63 HU).

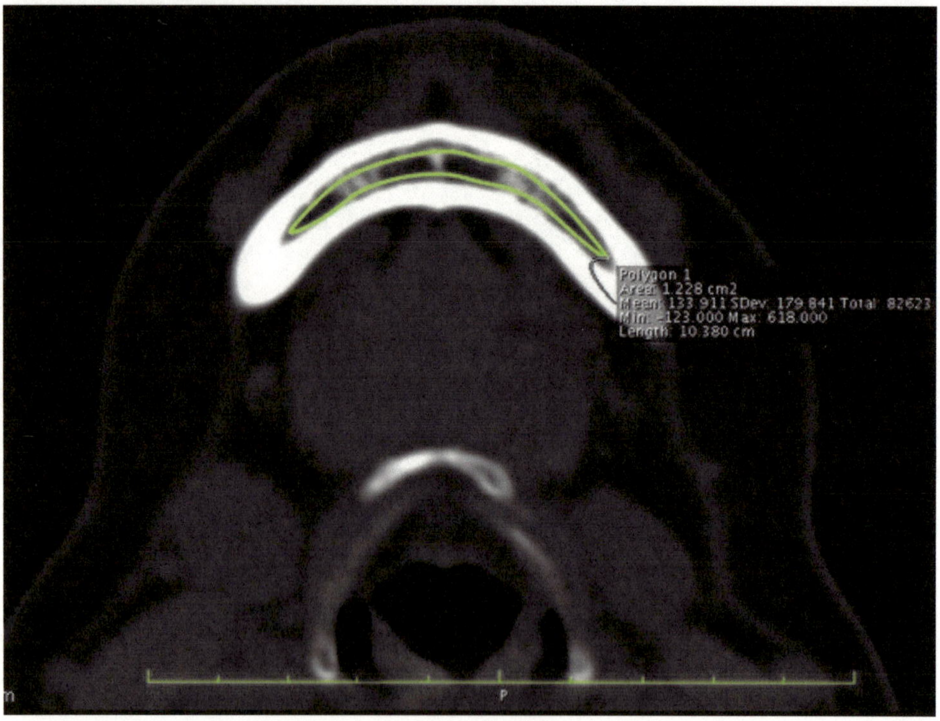

Fig. 3. Axial mandible CT slice of 36-year old woman shows nonosteoporotic mandible bone density measurement in Hounsfield Unit (mean: 133 HU).

4.8 Conclusion

1. The density of trabecular areas where QCT and bones metabolic changes are highest can be calculated in addition to their cortexes, specially, at vertebra.

2. There is no need to use fantom if routine calibrations are made during measurements on the latest generation devices.
3. We can obtain accurate and precise osteoporosis results with QCT bone density measurement as a HU.

5. References

Adams J.E. (1997). Single and dual energy X-ray absorptiometry. Eur. Radiol. 7 (Suppl. 2), S20–S31

Adams J.E., Alsop C., Harrison E.J., Lernbass I., Davies M., et al. (2000). Quantitative Computed Tomograpy (QCT): The Forgotten Gold Standard? Journal of Bone Mineral Research 15:S169

Baran D.T., Faulkner K.G., Genant H.K., Miller P.D., Pacifici R. (1997). Diagnosis and management of osteoporosis: guidelines for the utilization of bone densitometry. Calcif Tissue Int. Dec;61(6):433-40.

Blake G.M., Fogelman I. (1997) Technical principles of dual energy x-ray absorptiometry. Semin Nucl Med ; 27:210–228.

Boden S.D., Goodenough D.J., Stockham C.D., Jacobs E., Dina T., et al. (1989)Precise measurement of vertebral bone density using computed tomography without the use of an external reference phantom. J Digit Imaging.;2(1):31-38.

Brooks R.A., Di Chiro G. (1976). Principles of computer assisted tomography (CAT) in radiographic and radioisotropic imaging. Phys Med Biol ;21:689–732.

Cann C.E., Genant H.K. (1980).Precise measurement of vertebral mineral content using computed tomography. J Comput Assist Tomogr 4:493-500

Cann C.E., Genant H.K. (1983) Single versus dual energy CT for vertebral mineral quantification (abst). J Comput Assist Tomogr ; 7: 551-552

Celenk C., Celenk P. (2008) Relationship of mandibular and cervical vertebral bone density using computed tomography. Dentomaxillofac Radiol ;37(1):47-518.

Celenk P., Celenk C. (2010) Evaluation by quantitative magnetic resonance imaging of trabecular bone quality in mandible and cervical vertebrae. Clin Oral Implants Res. Apr 1;21(4):409-13

Christopher E. C,. (1989). Why, When and How to Measure Bone Mass: A Guide for the Beginning User. AIP Publishing, Woodbury NY, pp 250-285.

Ciarelli M.J., Goldstein S.A., Kuhn J.L., Cody D.D., Brown M.B. (1991). Evaluation of orthogonal mechanical properties and density of human trabecular bone from the major mrtaphyseal regions with materials testing and computed tomography. J Orthop Res, vol. 9, is. 5, pp. 674-82

Duppe H.R., Gardsell P, Nilsson B., Johnell O. (1997) A single bone density measurement can predict fractures over 25 years. Calcif Tissue Int ; 60:171–174.

Genant H.K., Boyd D. (1977). Quantitative bone mineral analysis using dual energy computed tomography. Invest Radiol 12:545 -551.

Genant H.K., Engelke K., Fuerst T., et al. (1996). Noninvasive assessment of bone mineral and structure: state of the art. J Bone Miner Res ; 11:707–730.

Guglielmi G., Grimston S.K., Fischer K.C., Pacifici R. (1994). Osteoporosis: diagnosis with lateral and posteroanterior dual x-ray absorptiometry compared with quantitative CT. Radiology;192(3):845-50.

Hans D.B., Shepherd J.A., Schwartz E.N., Reid D.M., Blake G.M., et al. (2007). Peripheral dual-energy X-ray absorptiometry in the management of osteoporosis: the 2007 ISCD Official Positions. J Clin Densitom. 2008 Jan-Mar;11(1):188-206.

Khosla S., Melton L.J.III. (1995) Secondary osteoporosis. In: Riggs BL, Melton LJ III, eds. Osteoporosis: etiology, diagnosis, and management. 2nd ed. Philadelphia, Pa: Lippincott- Raven ; 183–204.

Lentle B.C., Prior J.C. (2003). Osteoporosis: What a clinician expects to learn from a patient's bone density examination. Radiology ;228(3):620-8.

Majumdar S. (2002). Magnetic resonance imaging of trabecular bone structure. Topics in Magnetic Resonance Imaging 13: 323–334.

Melton R.D. III (1995). How many women have osteoporosis now? J Bone Miner Res 10:175177.

Nilsson M., Johnell O., Jonsson K., Redlund-Johnell I.(1988). Quantitative computed tomography in measurement of vertebral trabecular bone mass. A modified method. Acta Radiol ; 29: 719–725.

Njeh C.F., Boivin C.M., Langton C.M., (1977).The role of ultrasound in the assessment of osteoporosis: a review. Osteoporos Int ; 7:7–22.

Norton M.R., Gamble C. (2001). Bone classification: an objective scale of bone density using the computerized tomography scan. Clin Oral Implants Res ; 12: 79–84.

Mazess R., Chestnut C. III, McClung M., Genant H. (1992). Enhanced precision with dual-energy x-ray absorptiometry. Calcif Tissue Int ; 51:14– 17.

Nilsson, M., Johnell, O., Jonsson, K. & Redlund- Johnell, I. (1988). Quantitative computed tomography in measurement of vertebral trabecular bone mass. A modified method. Acta Radiologica 29: 719–725.

Rang C., Speller R. (1998). Comparison of ultrasound and dual energy x-ray absorptiometry measurements in the calcaneus. Br J Radiol ; 71:861–867.

Reinbold W.D., Genant H.K., Reiser U.J., Harris S.T., Ettinger B. (1986). Bone mineral content in early postmenopausal and postmenopausal osteoporotic women: Comparison of measurement methods. Radiology 160:469-478.

Rosenthal D.I., Mayo-Smith W., Hayes C.W., Khurana .J.S, Biller BM, et al. (1989). Age and bone mass in premenopausal women. J Bone Miner Res ;4(4):533-8.

Shapurian T., Damoulis P.D., Reiser G.M., Griffin T.J., Rand W.M. (2006). Quantitative evaluation of bone density using the Hounsfield index. Int J Oral Maxillofac Implants ; 21: 290–297.

Strolka I., Toffanin, R., Guglielmi G., & Frollo, I. (2005). Image Registration in the T2n measurements of the calcaneus used to predict osteoporotic fractures. Measurement Science Review 5: 79–81.

Summers R.M., Baecher N., Yao J., Liu J., Pickhardt P.J., et al. (2011). Feasibility of simultaneous computed tomographic colonography and fully automated bone mineral densitometry in a single examination. J Comput asist Tomogr ;35(2):212-6.

Wehrli, F.W., Hopkins, J.A., Hwang, S.N., Song, H.K., Snyder, P.J. Et al. (2000). Crosssectional study of osteopenia with quantitative magnetic resonance imaging and bone densitometry. Radiology 217: 527–538.

World Health Organization. (1994).Assessment of osteoporotic fracture risk and its role inscreening for postmenopausal osteoporosis. WHO Technical Report Series, no. 843. Geneva, Switzerland: World Health Organization ; 5.

Yang S.O., Hagiwara S., Engelke K. et al. Radiographic absorptiometry for bone mineral measurement of the phalanges: precision and accuracy study. Radiology 1994; 192:857–859.

Zhao K., Pan X., Zou Y., Wang Z., Zhang T. et al. (2009). An automatic method for measurement of vertebral bone density based on QCT without an external reference phantom, Proc. SPIE 7497, 74972I ; doi:10.1117/12.830955

8

Extraction of Airway in Computed Tomography

Ken Inohara[1,2], Yuka I. Sumita[3] and Shuichi Ino[4]
[1]*University of Alberta*
[2]*Nihon University School of Dentistry*
[3]*Tokyo Medical and Dental University*
[4]*National Institute of Advanced Industrial Science and Technology*
[1]*Canada*
[2,3,4]*Japan*

1. Introduction

Computed tomography (CT) developed by Hounsfield (Hounsfield, 1973) extended the usefulness of radiography as a diagnostic technique. It enabled users to examine soft tissue in axial images, which previously had been limited mainly to hard tissue, e.g. bone and tooth. This was accomplished by the depiction of air space surrounding the soft tissue. Moreover, the development of high-speed scanning CT enabled three-dimensional observation of the anatomical structure of the human body. Slip-ring CT was developed by Toshiba in 1985 (Mori et. al., 1987) and by Siemens in 1987 (Kalender et. al., 1997), and Helical CT was in the practical application by the both companies in 1990 (Katakura, 1989) (Kalender et. al., 1990) (Kageyama et. al., 1992).

Furthermore, CT imaging in biomedical science has transcended its use as a diagnostic tool only. For example, three-dimensional reconstruction through rapid-prototyping techniques has been accomplished through application of CT imaging for novel use.

In this chapter, a standardized method for airway extraction from CT of the head and neck region is described. This process applies further to simulation of speech and swallowing, and for diagnosis of sleep apnea syndrome (SAS).

2. Airway extraction

2.1 Air as contrast material in general radiography and CT

The main target in general radiography is often hard tissues of the body such as bone and teeth. However, in some cases, air space can be taken as a contrast material when interested in the soft tissues of the body. Air encephalography was a typical example of instrumental assessment using air as contrast material before CT developed. This obsolete radiographic examination of the basal cisterns and ventricles of the brain was performed by filling the intracranial cerebrospinal fluid spaces with air, which was normally introduced through a lumbar puncture while the patient sat in an upright position. In chest radiography, air may be also used as a contrast material. For upper gastrointestinal tract radiography, a double contrast material (barium and air) method was developed by Shirakabe and Ichikawa (Kawai et. al., 1970), and is still widely used for cancer screening of stomach.

In CT examination, some methods using air as contrast material have been reported for exposure of the stomach and large intestine (Nagata et. al., 2004).

2.2 Extraction of airway in CT

In the head and neck region, photographs of air space were taken in early stages of CT development, especially exposure for diagnosis of SAS (Haponik et. al., 1983; Suratt et. al., 1983). However, there was a problem in that the conventional CT machine spent too much time to acquire images. As a solution, a slip-ring CT was developed and applied in the 1990s (Burger et. al., 1993). Additionally, trials for application of Helical CT have been performed (Lowe et. al., 1995).

In the field of phonetics, some studies using CT have been carried out for analysis of resonance characteristics of the vocal tract (airway). Story et al. investigated CT images of an adult woman's airway during vocalization to understand its transmission characteristics (Story et. al., 1998). Sundberg et al. took CT images of an opera singer during singing, followed by three-dimensional reconstruction for analysing the oropharyngeal shape (Sundberg et. al., 2007).

There is an important difference between surgical use and airway extraction in CT. The former is mainly for simulation which assists surgeons at operations by providing biomedical models. In the majority of cases, a main target of extraction from CT for biomedical modeling is hard tissue, mainly bone. In the field of head and neck defects, a prediction of facial change after sagittal splitting ramus osteotomy and a simulation of fibula grafting for resected mandible would be examples of use of such technology. Thus it permits a rough estimate of the outcome. However, the latter is for measurement of area and/or volume, thus it needs accuracy and reproducibility.

2.2.1 Determination of threshold

Determination of threshold is performed when converting CT images into binary values in order to measure volume of air space, followed by analysis of acoustical characteristics and diagnosing SAS (Fig. 1). It may seem that the threshold should be determined reasonably, but actually some difficulties exist.

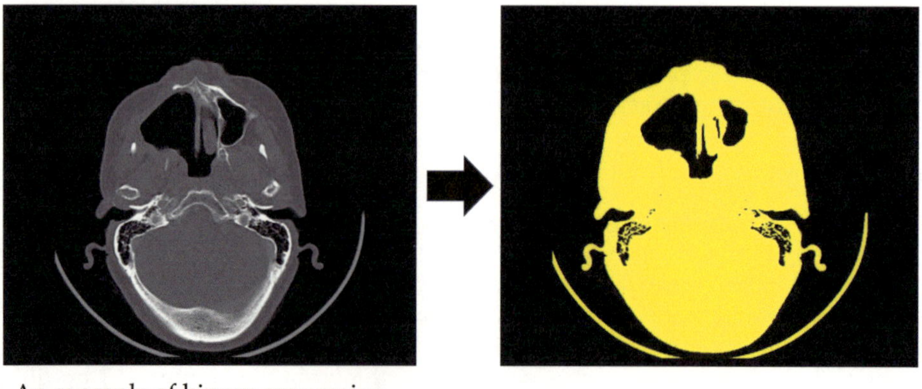

Fig. 1. An example of binary conversion.

2.2.2 Hounsfield number of air

The Hounsfield number (CT number) is a quantitative value for describing radiodensity. According to definition in Wikipedia, "The Hounsfield unit (HU) scale is a linear transformation of the original linear attenuation coefficient measurement into one in which the radiodensity of water is defined as 0 HU, while the radiodensity of air is defined as -1000

HU. For a material X with linear attenuation coefficient μ_x, the corresponding HU value is therefore given as below where μ_{water} and μ_{air} are the linear attenuation coefficients of water and air, respectively." (1)

$$HU = \frac{\mu_x - \mu_{water}}{\mu_{water} - \mu_{air}} \times 1000 \tag{1}$$

In biomedical engineering, 1024 (= 2^{10}) is usually substituted for 1000, thus the Hounsfield number of air should be -1024 HU.

According to the above definition, air space can be extracted when the threshold is set as -1024 HU. However, the area must be smaller than actual air space. Fig. 2 shows an example of vocal tract shape when threshold was set as -1024 HU. In the oropharynx region, the discontinuous form of the vocal tract was presented; this occurred because the air space was too small. This problem is known mainly as the "partial volume effect".

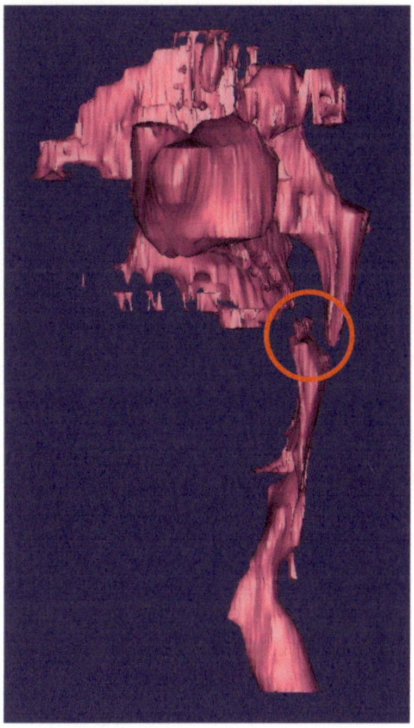

Fig. 2. A discontinuous vocal tract because of too low setting of threshold.

2.2.3 Pixel and voxel

Because one axial plane of the CT image generally consists of 512 x 512 pixels, minuteness of the image depends on the size of field of view (FOV) (Fig. 3).

In the case of 400 mm x 400 mm FOV, which is generally set in truncal imaging, the length of the side of the pixel is calculated as below (2).

$$400 \text{ mm} / 512 \text{ pixels} = 0.78125 \text{ mm} \tag{2}$$

With regard to the Z axis, it depends on the slice thickness/interval of imaging. The latest CT machines can take images in 0.5 mm or smaller intervals, but sometimes radiologists capture in thicker slices in order to reduce radiation to the patient.

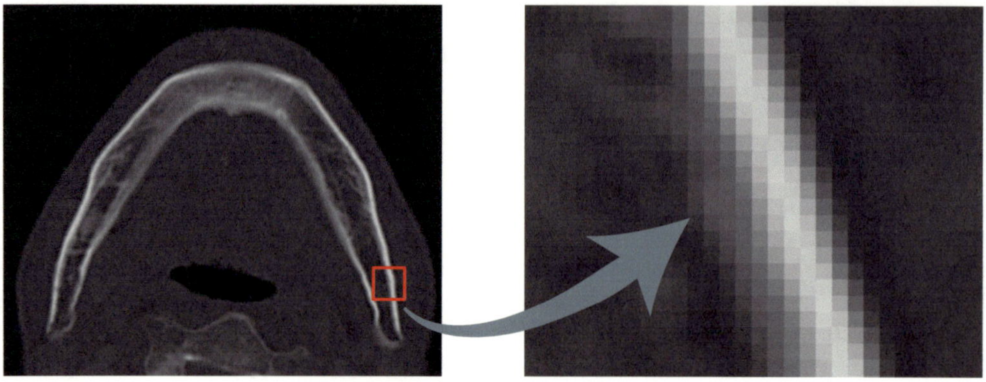

Fig. 3. Enlarged CT image (mandibular bone).

A rectangular prism with a pixel and Z axis slice thickness is named a "voxel" (Fig. 4). Three-dimensional CT data are an aggregate of voxels.

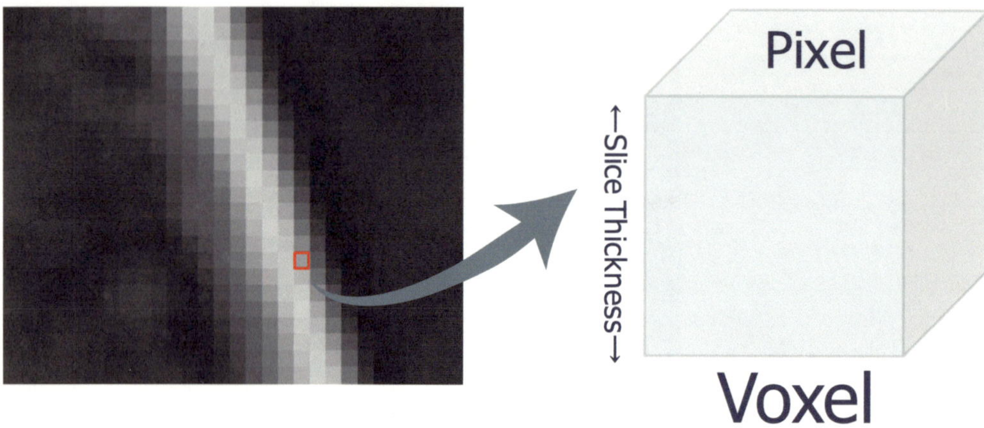

Fig. 4. Voxel is a rectangular prism with a pixel and slice thickness of Z axis.

2.2.4 Partial volume effect

The partial volume effect occurs when a single voxel contains a mixture of multiple tissue values. Each voxel has its own Hounsfield number. The Hounsfield number of the voxel at the boundary area between air and soft tissue is influenced by the both substances. (Fig. 5)
Following the definition of Hounsfield number, those of water and air are 0 HU and 1024 HU, respectively. However, the Hounsfield number of the internal air actually presents a higher value than 1024 HU. This is because of the partial volume effect, mentioned above. Therefore, we have to define precisely the threshold of Hounsfield number between soft tissue and air when images are converted into binary.
It means that setting of threshold influences the size of air space. For instance, when the Hounsfield number of a voxel is -600 HU and the threshold is set as -800 HU, the voxel may be judged as soft tissue. On the other hand, when the threshold is set as -500 HU, it may be as air. Thus, the area of air space can be changed to a couple of millimetres as setting of threshold easily, because the length of the side is approximately 0.5 to 2 mm that is depended on a voxel size (FOV and slice interval).

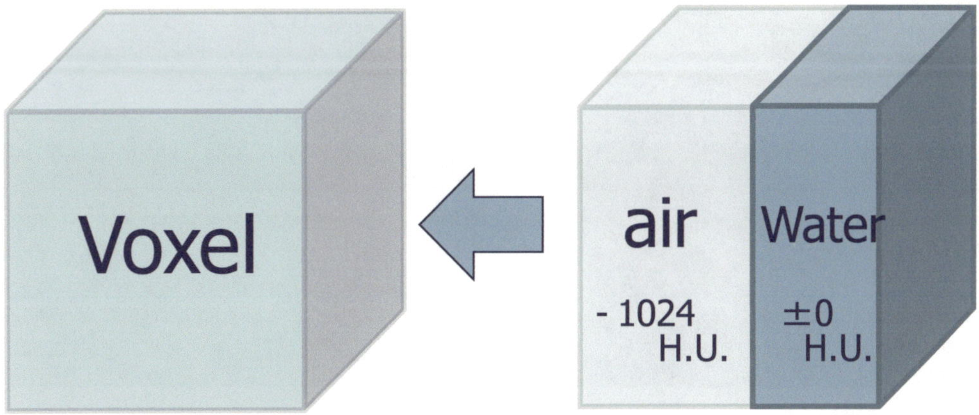

Fig. 5. Voxel contains a mixture of multiple tissue values.

In other research, the threshold generally has been decided by the operators' own subjective judgement, not in an objective way. Hence, the values have varied with different studies. It seems to be a serious problem for measuring size, area and/or volume, followed by transmission functions from data inaccuracy. Unfortunately, few studies have referred to the problem. For these reasons, standardized reconstruction methods have to be established.

3. Standardized airway extraction

In order to convert into binary objectively, standards must be set for thresholding. We noted that fat tissue has a Hounsfield number that is the lowest in human body. The following is a standardized method what we propose (Inohara et. al., 2010).

3.1 Hounsfield number of fat tissue

As described in formula (1), the Hounsfield number is a quantitative value for describing the radiodensity of each tissue of human body, where the radiodensity of water is 0 HU and that of air is -1024 HU. Fat tissue represents the lowest Hounsfield number in human body, which is approximately -80 HU. (Fig. 6)

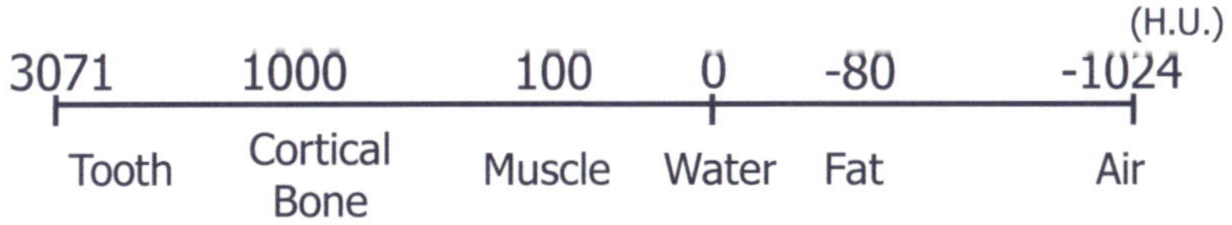

Fig. 6. Hounsfield value of each tissue of human body.

We hypothesized that objective binary conversion would be enabled by identification of the minimum setting of the Hounsfield value of fat tissue in the body. The Hounsfield number of fat tissue is generally said to be approximately -80 HU. However, the value has some spread-width actually. The optimal threshold value cannot exceed the minimum setting of fat tissue.

Fortunately, it is easy to find fat tissue, specifically the "Buccal fat-pad", in head and neck CT images for airway extraction. (Fig. 7)

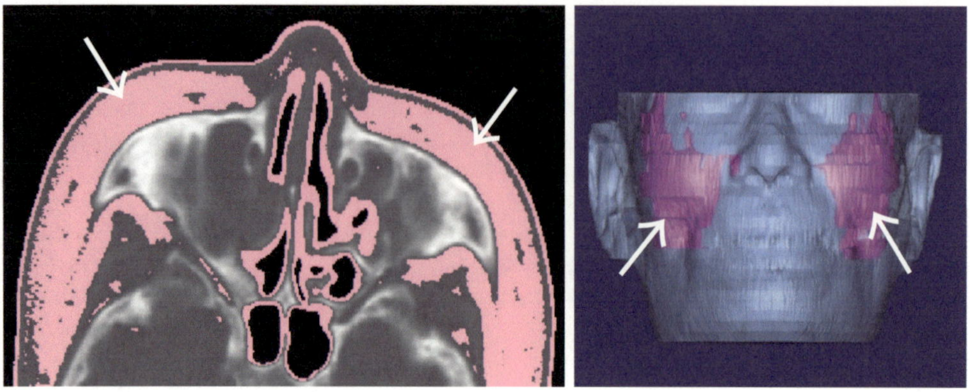

Fig. 7. Buccal fat-pad (arrow).

3.2 Detection of minimum setting of buccal fat-pad

To measure the bottom line of the Hounsfield number for the buccal fat-pad, a number of images that include the buccal fat-pad site should be examined. As the threshold value is down-regulated gradually, the voxels also decrease. The threshold value at which all representing voxels disappear in the images is the minimum setting of the buccal fat-pad. As an example, a process for detecting the minimum setting of Hounsfield value is shown in figure 8. In this subject, the minimum setting is determined as -247 HU. (Fig. 8)

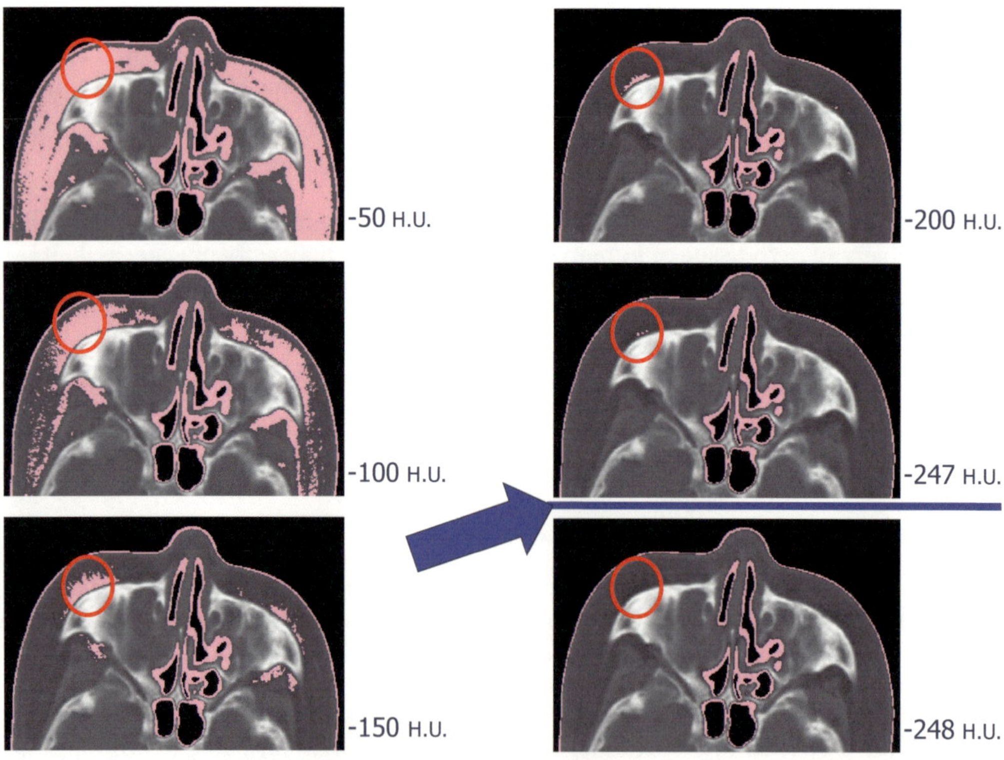

Fig. 8. Process of measuring minimum setting Hounsfield value of buccal fat-pad.

3.3 Evaluation of CT images in three-grade system

We describe the summary of process to determine the suitable threshold value on the following. The thresholds were set as the bottom line of the buccal fat-pad Hounsfield number, and the values of 50, 100, 150, 200, 250, and 300 HU were subtracted from the bottom line. (Fig.9)

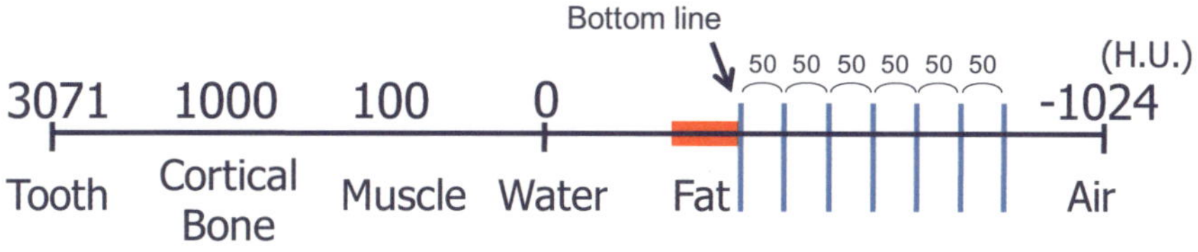

Fig. 9. Setting of threshold to evaluate images.

The regions where the structures were different among the thresholds were found in a series of each subject's images. In our previous study (Inohara et al, 2010) we evaluated the images as follows: G—the regions where the anatomical structure in the original images was revealed to be similar were judged to be good; NG—the regions where the structure was different from the original images were judged to be incorrect; P—the regions which came neither under G nor NG were judged passable. Following figure showed the judgment of nasal area. With regarding to turbinate and the nasal septum, the image that has separate parts is judged to be good (G), because the turbinate is generally separated from the nasal septum, because they should be actually separated in the normal human body. (Fig. 10)

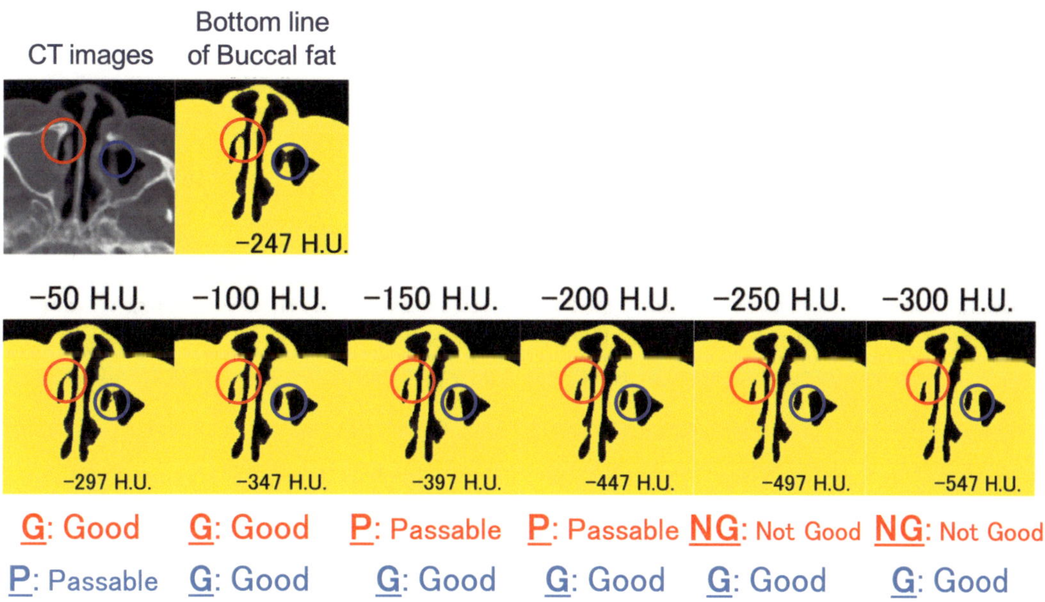

Fig. 10. An example of judgement by three-grade system.

In our study, five patients' CT images who had undergone maxillectomy of malignant tumors and had no resection of the zygomatic arch (because buccal fat pad was expected to be a criterion for thresholding) were employed. Slice distance of these images is 3 mm by

using a single-beam CT scanner. Data processing was performed by Mimics (Materialise NV, Belgium).
Each subject's G, P, and NG position numbers were counted and scored per the aforementioned thresholds as 2, 1, and -1 point respectively. Both positive and negative scores were summed as per the thresholds per subject, followed by being plotted on the graph. Regression analysis was performed, and the minimal Hounsfield value was calculated. (Fig. 11)

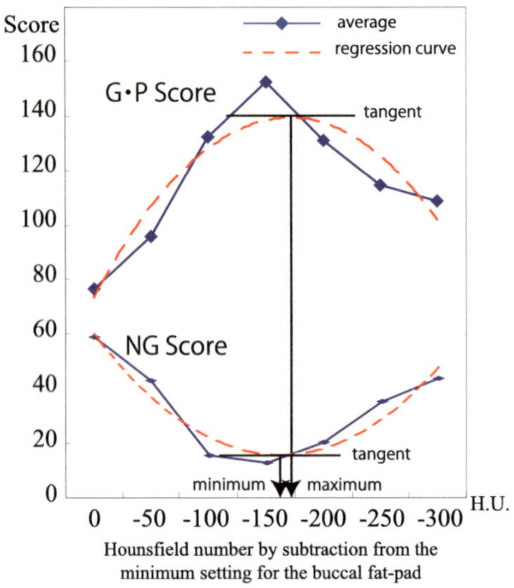

Fig. 11. Plot graphs of average scores, regression curves, tangents, and local maximum and minimum.

For the G and P positions (positive factor), the multiple regression equation (3) is as follows:

$$y = -9.40 \times 10^{-4}x - 2.25 \times 10^{-5}x^2 + 1.38 \qquad (3)$$

As adjusted $R^2 = 0.855$, fitness is good. As significance probability of the binomial term was $p = 0.012$ and the sign was negative, this regression curve was convex upward. The local maximal was the minimum setting of -170 HU.
For the NG positions (negative factor), the multiple regression equation (4) is as follows:

$$y = 4.10 \times 10^{-4}x + 1.72 \times 10^{-5}x^2 + 0.164 \qquad (4)$$

As adjusted $R^2 = 0.866$, fitness is good. As significance probability of the binomial term was $p = 0.004$ and the sign is positive, this regression curve was convex downward. The local minimum was the minimum setting of -161 HU. From these results, the optimal threshold as -165 HU from each patient's minimum values of the buccal fat-pad region was deduced in our previous study.

3.4 Verification of the standardized method

As mentioned above, first, we hypothesized that objective binary conversion would be enabled by identification of the minimum setting of the Hounsfield value of fat tissue in the

body. The minimum setting of the buccal fat-pad could be clearly measured individually, which varied between approximately -200 and -310 HU. This result is explainable because the Hounsfield value of each tissue has some spread-width actually, although the value of fat tissue is generally said to be approximately -80 HU.
Optimal threshold value could be calculated objectively by applying anatomical and statistical analysis. We have built a solid model of the vocal tract by the aforementioned method to confirm accuracy of the method what we proposed. (Fig. 12)
We have already started new research by using these models to disclose transmission characteristics of patients with surgical resection in the head and neck.

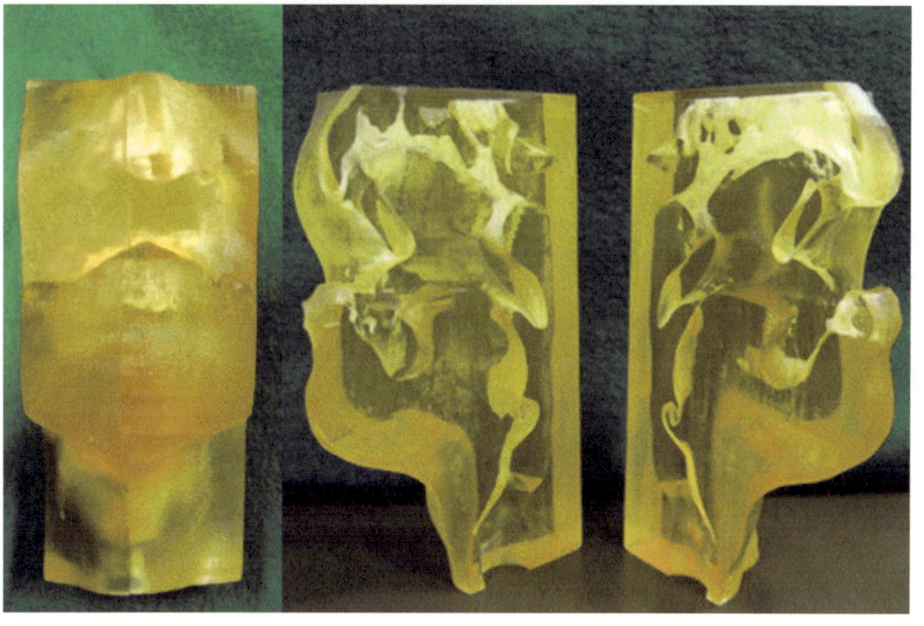

Fig. 12. A model reconstructed by rapid prototyping what applied the standardized method

4. Future of airway extraction

The use of CT imaging in biomedical science has been developing rapidly, transcending its use as a diagnostic tool only. Three-dimensional reconstruction and rapid-prototyping, enabled by CT imaging, are particularly important in the field of biomedical science. The field of air extraction benefits from development of biomedical science.
Our main interest is the shape of the vocal tract during phonation, especially head and neck cancer patients. (Fig. 13) The standardized method of airway extraction that we proposed can contribute to accuracy of measuring and analysis.
Technology of airway extraction in CT is applied in various diagnostic and research scenes, especially for SAS patients. For instance, there is a study to assess the predictive power of an otorhinolaryngological examination of the upper airway to identify risk factors of SAS in the patients (Yagi et. al., 2009). In addition, there is research about airway obstruction in infants with a hypoplastic mandible (Looby et. al., 2009).
Moreover, some recent studies have been performed by using four-dimensional reconstruction in multi detector-row CT (MDCT); this means using dynamic images,

especially in a field of swallowing assessment. Although videofluorography with a modified barium swallowing test (Martin-Harris et. al., 2000) is applied generally in dysphagia assessment, there is risk of aspiration, followed by pneumonia. To avoid this risk, research has been performed where a subject swallowed just air, captured by a 64-row MDCT that is generally used for cardiac cine-CT (Fudeya et. al., 2010). In addition, there is recent research of applying 320-row MDCT, which is the most up-to date facility (Inomoto et. al., 2010).

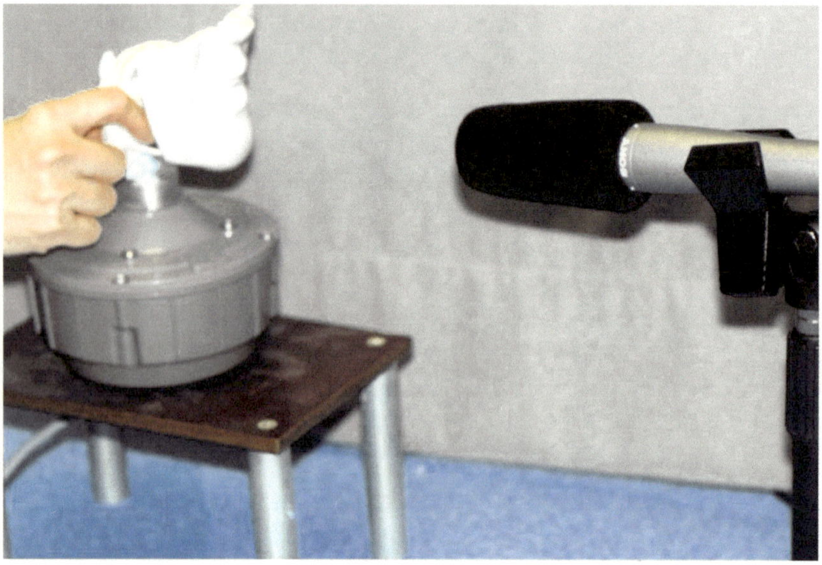

Fig. 13. Examination of analysis of vocal tract transmission characteristics using a model that was rapid-prototyped by our proposed method.

5. Conclusion

In this chapter, the standardized method for airway extraction was described in detail. As the necessity of airway extraction in CT is now increasing, establishment of a standardized method for air extraction is needed. The method that we proposed is simple, objective, and effective.

6. Acknowledgements

This work was partially supported by the Grant-in-Aid for Young Scientist (B), the Ministry of Education, Culture, Sports, Science and Technology, Japan (MEXT Grant). The authors would like to thank for Ms. L. Dunwald in Misericordia Community Hospital, Drs. H. Taniguchi, T. Kurabayashi, N. Ohbayashi in Tokyo Medical and Dental University, T. Ifukube in University of Tokyo, and J. Rieger in University of Alberta.

7. References

Burger, C. D.; Stanson, A. W.; Daniels, B. K.; Sheedy, P. F. & Shepard, J. W. (1993). Fast-computed tomographic evaluation of the effect of route of breathing on upper airway size and function in normal men. *Chest*, Vol. 103, No. 4, pp. 1032-1037

Fudeya, T.; Otake, S.; Watabe, H.; Mitsuoka, T. & Yoshikawa, A. (2010). Visualization of laryngopharynx during swallowing of negative contrast media (air) with cine mode 64-row MDCT. *Nippon Hoshasen Gijutsu Gakkai Zasshi*, Vol. 66, No. 5, pp. 535-539

Haponik, E. F.; Smith, P. L.; Bohlman, M. E.; Allen, R. P. & Goldman, S. M. (1983). Computerized tomography in obstructive sleep apnea. Correlation of airway size with physiology during sleep and wakefulness. *American Review of Respiratory Disease*, Vol. 127, No. 2, pp. 221-226

Hounsfield, G. N. (1973). Computerized transverse axial scanning (tomography) .1. description of system. *British Journal of Radiology*, Vol. 46, No. 552, pp. 1016-1022

Inohara, K,; Sumita, Y. I.; Ohbayashi, N.; Ino, S.; Kurabayashi, T.; Ifukube, T. & Taniguchi, H. (2010). Standardization of thresholding for binary conversion of vocal tract modeling in computed tomography. *Journal of Voice*, Vol. 24, No. 4, pp. 503-509

Inamoto, Y.; Fujii, N.; Saitoh, E.; Baba, M.; Okada, S.; Katada, K.; Ozeki, Y.; Kanamori D. & Palmer, J.B. (2010). Evaluation of swallowing using 320-detector-row multislice 16 CT. Part II: Kinematic analysis of laryngeal closure during normal swallowing. *Dysphagia*, DOI : 10.1007/s00455-010-9276-2

Kageyama, K.; Kimura, K.; Katakura, T.; Suzuki, K.; Aizumi, J. & Seino, O. (1992). Helical volume CT and its clinical significance. *Fukushima Journal of Medical Science*, Vol. 38, No. 2, pp. 67-74

Kalender, W. A.; Engelke, K. & Schaller, S. (1997). Spiral CT: medical use and potential industrial applications. *SPIE*, Vol. 3149, pp. 188-202

Kalender, W. A.; Seissler, W.; Klotz, E. & Vock, P. (1990). Spiral volumetric CT with single-breath-hold technique, continuous transport, and continuous scanner rotation. *Radiology*, Vol. 176, No. 1, pp. 181-183

Katakura, T. (1989). Basic research of Computed Tomography (IX) - Helical CT scanner. *Dansou Eizou Kenkyukai Zasshi*, Vol. 16, pp. 247-250

Kawai, K.; Takada, H.; Takekoshi, T.; Misaki, F.; Murakami, K.; Masada, M.; Nishizawa, M.; Hayakawa, H. & Shirakabe, H. (1970). Double contrast radiograph on routine examination of the stomach. *American Journal of Gastroenterology*, Vol. 53, No. 2, pp. 147-153

Looby, J. F.; Schendel, S. A.; Lorenz, H. P.; Hopkins, E. M. & Aizenbud, D. (2009). Airway analysis: with bilateral distraction of the infant mandible. *Journal of Craniofacial Surgery*, Vol. 20, No. 5, pp. 1341-1346

Lowe, A. A., Fleetham, J. A., Adachi, S. & Ryan, C. F. (1995). Cephalometric and computed tomographic predictors of obstructive sleep apnea severity. *American Journal of Orthodontics and Dentofacial Orthopedics*, Vol. 107, No. 6, pp. 589-595

Martin-Harris, B.; Logemann, J. A.; McMahon, S.; Schleicher, M. & Sandidge, J. (2000). Clinical utility of the modified barium swallow. *Dysphagia*, Vol. 15, No. 3, pp. 136-141

Mori, K.; Saito, K. & Asahina, K. (1987). X-ray CT TCT-900S. *Toshiba review*, Vol. 42, No. 2, pp. 80-82

Nagata, K.; Endo, S.; Kudo, S.; Kitanosono, T. & Kushihashi, T. (2004). CT air-contrast enema as a preoperative examination for colorectal cancer. *Digestive Surgery*, Vol. 21, No. 5-6, pp. 352-358

Story, B. H.; Titze, I. R. & Hoffman, E. A. (1998). Vocal tract area functions for an adult female speaker based on volumetric imaging. *Journal of the Acoustical Society of America*, Vol. 104, No. 1, pp. 471-487

Sundberg, J.; Birch, P.; Gumoes, B.; Stavad, H.; Prytz, S. & Karle, A. (2007). Experimental findings on the nasal tract resonator in singing. *Journal of Voice*. Vol. 21, No. 2, pp. 127-137

Suratt, P. M.; Dee, P.; Atkinson, R. L.; Armstrong, P. & Wilhoit, S. C. (1983). Fluoroscopic and computed tomographic features of the pharyngeal airway in obstructive sleep apnea. *American Review of Respiratory Disease*, Vol. 127, No. 4, pp. 487-492

Yagi, H.; Nakata, S.; Tsuge, H.; Yasuma, F.; Noda, A.; Morinaga, M.; Tagaya, M. & Nakashima, T. (2009). Morphological examination of upper airway in obstructive sleep apnea. *Auris Nasus Larynx*, Vol. 36, No. 4, pp. 444-449

Part 2

CAD and Advanced Imaging Application

9

QCT as a Base of Computer Aided Diagnosis of Osteoporotical Changes

Antoni John and Piotr Wysota
Silesian University of Technology
Department of Strength of Materials and Computational Mechanics
Poland

1. Introduction

The osteoporosis is a systemic disease of bone which leads to progressive decrease of the bone mass and the changes of bone structure. As the years went by these changes became so serious that it can cause the disorders of functioning of bone in organism (bones become weak and more subject on fracture). At people suffering from this disease more often occurred the fractures e.g. in reach of hip joint and vertebral of spine. One of characteristic feature of osteoporosis is asymptomatic progress. The first signs - difficulties during move and appearing pains in the spine and in the hip joint appear when it is the big loss of bone mass and it is the large risk of fractures. Unfortunately it is a serious phase and the fractures are common - after fracture one should stabilization of places of fracture. Differences between correct tissue and tissue with osteoporosis are presented in Fig.1 [1].

a) b)

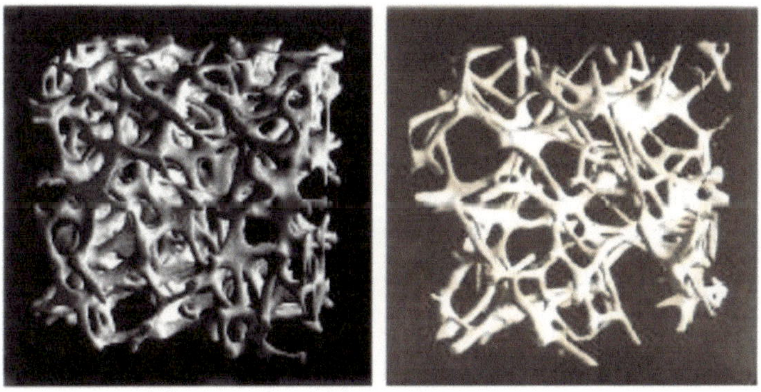

Fig. 1. Microstructure of bone: a) healthy, b) with osteoporotical changes [1]

From mechanical point of view the fracture of bone occurs in two cases:

- the correct structure of bone but the loads are so big that cause the stresses larger than stress limit,
- the disorders of bone structure caused decrease of strength properties of bone when normal activity of organism can results stresses larger than stress limit.

The attention is concentrated on the second situation (when only the physiology loading of organism can cause accidental fracture of bone) because it takes place in osteoporosis.
Very important factor is diagnosis of osteoporosis. It is a serious problem because this disease progress without symptoms. First signs appear when it is the big loss of bone mass (about 30%) and the risk of fracture is high. Comparison of radiological images of hip joint for healthy state and state with osteoporosis is shown in Fig. 2 [11].

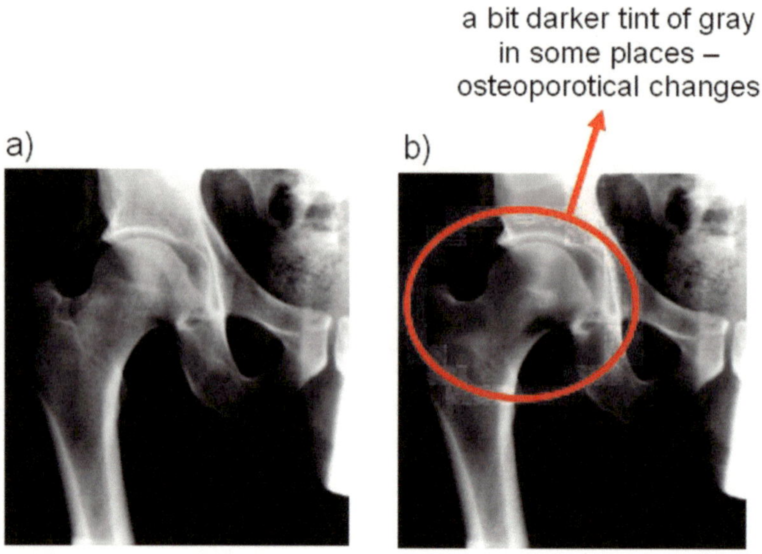

Fig. 2. Hip joint: a) correct, b) with osteoporotical changes [11]

Usually patients come to doctors when have difficulties during move and pains in spine and/or in hip joint. Unfortunately until then osteoporosis is recognized and treatment is begun. The treatment of osteoporosis usually consists of providing analgesic and stabilization of places of fractures. It would be better to prevent this disease because lack of movement is causes of weakness of bones. Knowledge of physical properties of bone tissue is helpful in diagnosing of the diseases of the bone system (especially that properties change during progress of disease).
To diagnose the osteoporosis the following preventive examinations are realized:

a. Radiology Absorptiometry (RA),
b. Roentgen Absorptiometry:
   - Single X-ray Absorptiometry (SXA),
   - Dual-energy X-ray absorptiometry (DXA),
c. Quantitative Ultrasonography (QUS),
d. Quantitative Computed Tomography (QCT).

These methods work on the base of Lambert-Beer's low which describes phenomenon of weakness of the radiation during crossing by through object. In the course of examination the part of radiation is absorbed or distracted. The intensity of radiation depends on thickness as well as the content of minerals in the bone. In result of iterative reading of photos for individual pixels, after transformation, the measurement density of whole object is obtained. In estimate the progress of osteoporosis the largest meaning have DXA and QCT.

These are densitometry methods which risky of osteoporosis estimate on the basis of distributions of density of bone tissue. In literature there are many publications about using both of these methods in aid of diagnosis osteoporosis. Good source of knowledge about computed tomography is paper [3]. Cierniak R. characterized this method in overall way. He presented the algorithms and the principles of creating images. He described also applying measuring techniques as well as CT scanners. Computed tomography is inverse problem - on the base of gathered data the model is created (on the basis of information about absorbed radiation in individual slice of scanning the images are generated). Adams J. E. in [2] described in details QCT. Authoress go into genesis of these method, its development, clinical applying, in particular diagnosis of osteoporosis. She presented different variety of QCT and described density phantoms Adams J. E. compare QCT with other methods and gave example when QCT is more useful: in case when we can obtain more information about researched bone (because images from QCT after conversion are good sources of information). Sawada K. et al. in papers [16] and [17] pay attention that if we want to find physical properties of bones same places are more useful (e.g. spine or hip joint) and same places are less useful (e.g. wrist or limbs). Engelke K. et al. in paper [4] presented the official state the International Densitometry Society about applying of quantitative computed tomography and peripheral quantitative computed tomography in diagnosis of osteoporosis at adults person. Authors pay attention that although the dual energy x-ray absorptiometry is often used in recognition of osteoporotical changes, in some cases better solution is applying the QCT. Engelke K. et al. emphasize that important matter is calibration of density phantom (the more accurate calibration the better results from tomography). Authors put many details about methods of performing QCT examinations, technical parameters of tomographs as well as gave advice to interpreting of results from tomography. On the base of the papers: Adams J. E. [2], Engelke K. et al. [4] and Nayak S., Roberts M.S. & Greenspan S.L. [14] we can say that when we compare both of these methods: DXA and QCT, more precise data of bone density is from QCT (from DXA we obtain "surface density" - in g/cm^2, from QCT "volume density" - in g/cm^3). Besides, in DXA is more difficult to distinction the kind of bone at the densitometry images. Second reason is the fact that data from QCT is more useful to create numerical model. In our case better solution is to use quantitative computed tomography - that's why we applied this method.

2. Quantitative computed tomography

2.1 Description of QCT

In this method the tomograms from CT are used to analyze the mineral density of bone. Through using the composition of projection images from different directions one can get cross-sectional and solid images in all researched structures (Fig. 3) [19]. Tomograms consist of individual voxels. Each voxel is characterized by coordinates x, y, z and color in gray scale. On the base of amount of radiation (absorbed in different places) one can determined density in these places with exact to one voxel.

QCT differs than standard approach occurrence of density phantom which is X-rayed together with patients. The phantom is composed of regions representing specimens of bone density in Hounsfield Units. The density phantom is presented in Fig. 4.

Here, phantom is composed of six specimens. On the base of these standard density the calibration curve is drown. Formula of this curve enables to determinate the density for each voxel of researched bone. The calibration curves for four series were presented on Fig. 5.

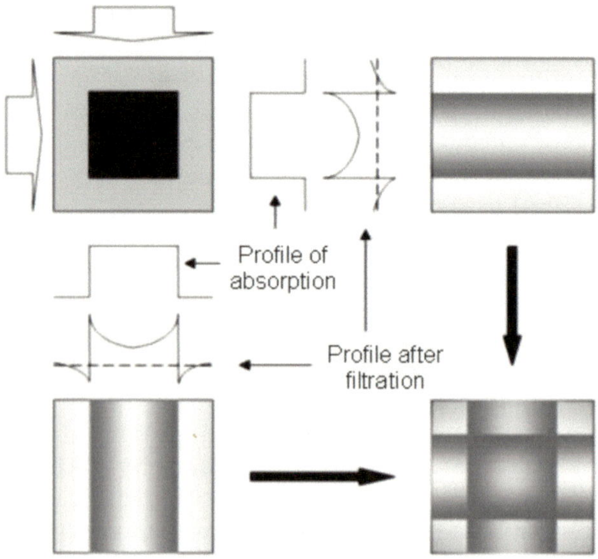

Fig. 3. Reconstruction images by analytical method with filtration [19]

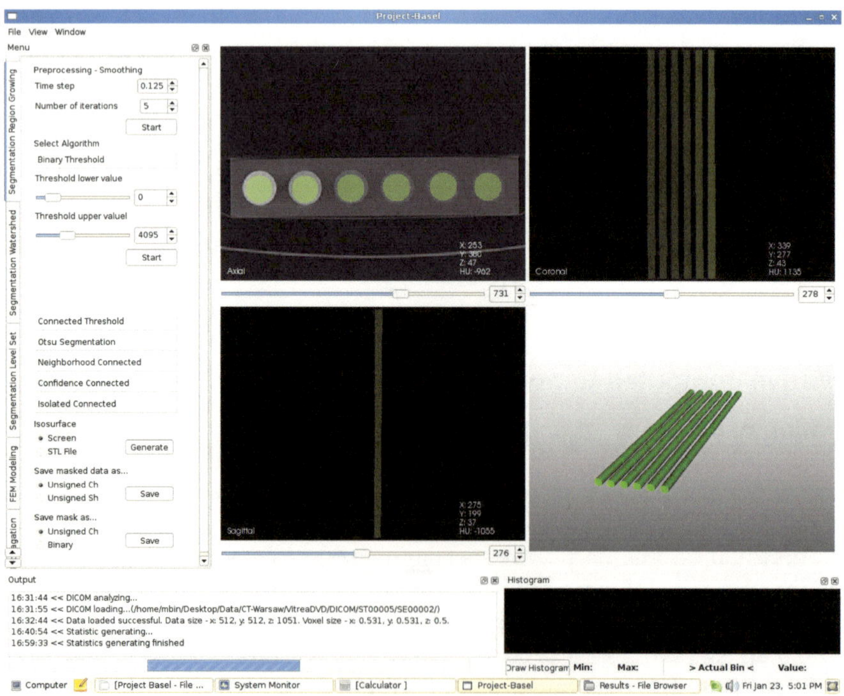

Fig. 4. The density phantom in different views

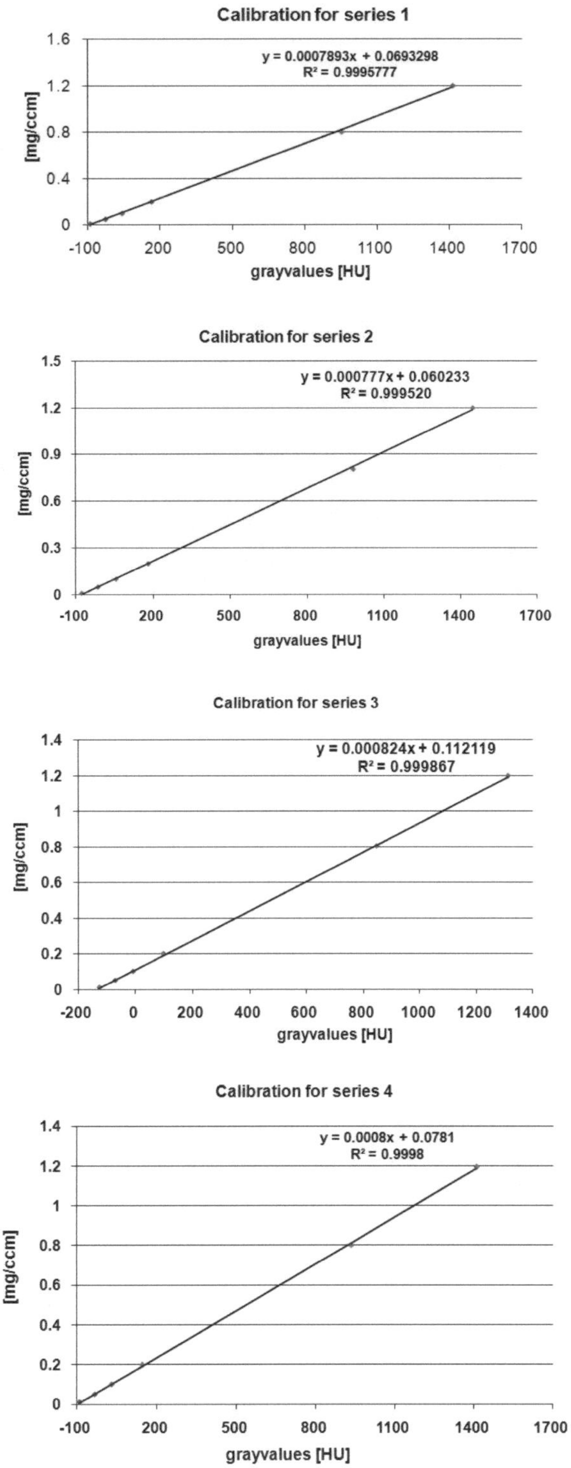

Fig. 5. The calibration curves for different series

2.2 Data from QCT

After radiological examination the images of researched structure are obtained. In the next step these data are conversed to receive information about analyzed bones.
The general course of transforming data is as following:

1. Performing of tomography examinations. As a result the images (sections in different places) of analyzed object are received.
2. Analyzing the X-ray photographs by use specialist software (the dependence between quantity of the absorbed radiation and the radiological density in bone tissue is used). The exemplary tomograms of pelvic bone were presented in Fig. 6.

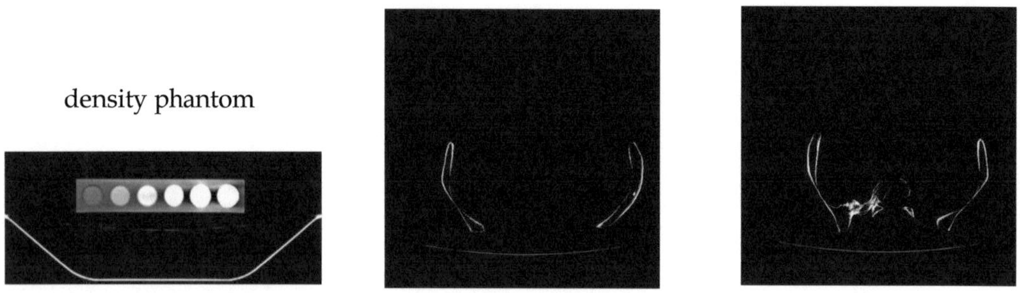

Fig. 6. Exemplary images of human pelvic bone from QCT

3. Standardizing obtained density to Hounsfield scale - HU:

$$1HU = K\frac{\mu_p - \mu_u}{\mu_u} \tag{1}$$

K - amplification factor of images,
μ_p - absorption factor,
μ_u - absorption factor of reference object,

4. On the base of HU density determining the density of bone tissue [7]

$$\rho = 1.122 \cdot HU + 47 \tag{2}$$

5. Delimitation of the material properties of bone tissue, especially elastic modulus (on the basis of experimental research the dependences between bone density and material properties were developed) [2], [14]. It is important step because in numerical simulations we need material properties from the beginning.

$$E = 1.92\rho - 170 \tag{3}$$

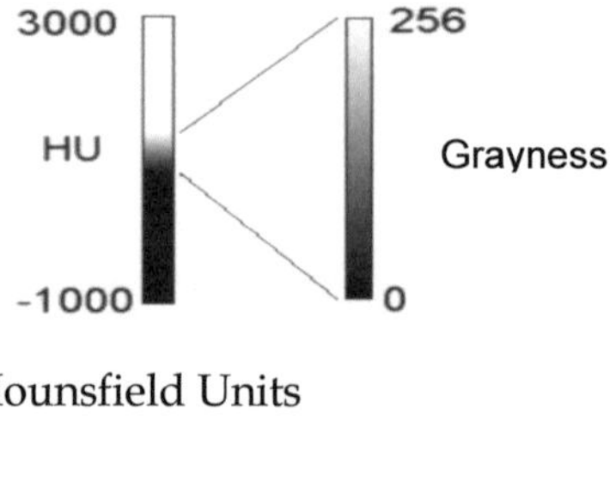

Fig. 7. The gray scale and the Hounsfield Units

2.3 Conversion of data from QCT to create numerical model

During modeling of biological structures occur difficulties connected with representation of geometry and subordinating of material properties to numerical model.
Bones have complicated and non-regular structure. Additional difficulty is mapping of internal structure of bone (there are problems with delimitating of thickness of each layers). Traditional building of geometry in some cases is very hard, time-consuming and created models are over-simplificated. For these reasons during creations of biomechanical structure one use radiological images - on the base data from radiology (e.g. computed tomography) the information about structure of bone are received. If we have section preparations we will obtain geometry from measurement coordination machine, but for living patients it is impossible. As far as problems with representation of geometry were in large part solve in as much determination of material properties to cause bigger difficulties. Biomechanical structures usually belong to non-homogenous and anisotropy material. Reference point is material parameters determinate in experimental researches but in organism conditions they may have different values. Another problem is to estimate material properties during pathological changes. Recognition of these changes and local non-homogenous is a large challenge for medical doctors, biomechanics and manufacturers of diagnosis devices.
For the purpose of assignation material parameters obtained from QCT to numerical model the in-house procedure was used. On the base of QCT images (with resolution 512x512) the matrixes were get.
For every CT image the matrix of values of elastic modulus is determined. When we combine all matrixes for one set of CT images in one big matrix we will prescribed values of elastic modulus in one file. The next step is subordinating values of Young modulus from this matrix to numerical model. Demonstrative show process of converting images from tomography is presented in Fig. 8.

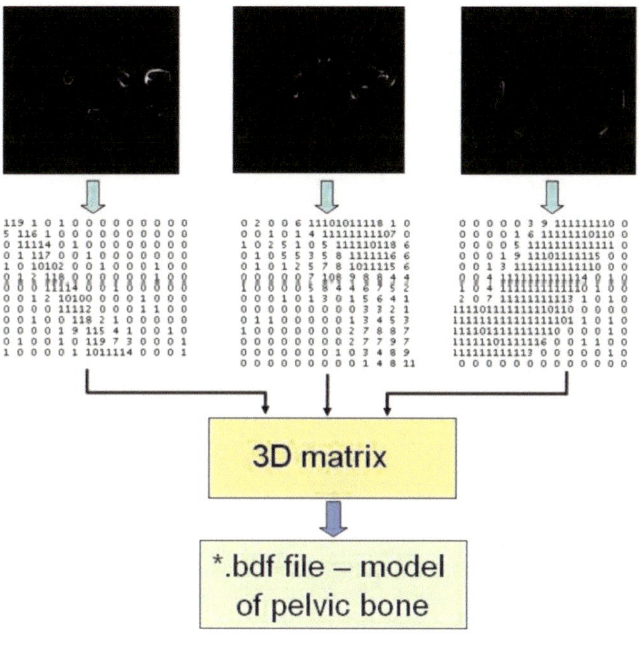

Fig. 8. Procedure to converting images from QCT to create numerical model

Additionally the text files with coordinates of nodes of researched model are created: x.txt, y.txt, z.txt.

Algorithm of the program consists of following steps:

1. Creation of 3D table: [u, v, w] on the base of file combined.txt: coordinate **u** represents coordinate **x**, **v** represents **z** and **w** represents **y** in numerical model.
2. Modification of input file to MSC.Nastran: insertion value of elastic modulus on the base of tomography to numerical model. In this way come into being FEM model in which in every finite element the individual material parameters were subordinated.

The exemplary image from QCT and equivalent cross-section in numerical model are presented in Fig. 9.

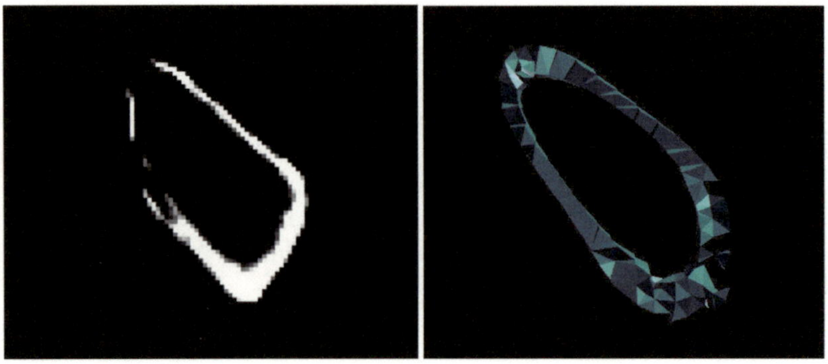

Fig. 9. Tomography image and cross-section in numerical model

Exemplary part of matrix with values of Young modulus is shown in Fig. 10.

```
119 1 0 1 0 0 0 0 0 0 0 0 0 0 0 1 0 0 0 1 1 0 0 1 0 2 0 0 6 11101011118 1 0 0 1 0
5 116 1 0 0 0 0 0 0 0 0 0 0 0 0 0 1 1 0 0 0 0 0 0 0 1 0 1 4 11111111107 0 0 0 0
0 11114 0 1 0 0 0 0 0 0 0 0 0 0 1 0 0 0 0 0 1 0 0 1 0 2 5 1 0 5 111110118 6 0 1 0
0 1 117 0 0 1 0 0 0 0 0 0 0 0 0 0 0 0 0 0 0 0 0 0 0 1 0 5 5 3 5 8 1111116 6 6 0 0
1 0 10102 0 0 1 0 0 0 1 0 0 0 0 0 0 0 0 0 0 0 0 0 0 1 0 1 2 5 7 8 1011115 6 7 1 0
0 1 2 118 0 0 0 0 0 0 1 0 0 0 1 0 0 0 0 0 0 0 0 0 0 0 0 0 7 108 9 8 8 4 4 6 8 0
0 0 0 11114 0 0 1 0 0 0 0 0 0 0 0 0 0 0 0 0 0 0 1 0 0 0 0 5 8 4 4 6 7 5 2 2 111
0 0 1 2 10100 0 0 0 1 0 0 0 0 0 0 0 0 0 0 0 0 0 0 0 0 1 0 1 3 0 1 5 6 4 1 1 104
0 0 0 0 11112 0 0 0 1 1 0 0 0 0 0 0 0 0 0 0 0 0 0 0 0 0 0 0 0 0 3 3 2 1 1 108
0 0 1 0 0 118 2 1 0 0 0 0 0 0 0 0 0 0 0 0 0 0 0 0 1 1 0 0 0 0 0 1 3 4 5 3 2 119
0 0 0 0 1 9 115 4 1 0 0 1 0 0 0 0 0 0 0 0 0 0 0 0 1 0 0 0 0 0 0 0 2 7 8 8 7 5 119
0 1 0 0 1 0 119 7 3 0 0 0 1 0 0 0 0 0 0 0 0 0 0 0 0 0 0 0 0 0 0 0 2 7 7 9 7 10116
1 0 0 0 0 1 1011114 0 0 0 1 0 0 0 0 0 0 0 0 0 0 0 0 0 0 0 0 0 0 1 0 3 4 8 9 11113
0 0 0 1 0 0 3 11115 0 0 1 0 0 0 0 0 0 0 0 0 0 0 0 0 0 0 0 0 0 0 0 1 4 8 1111111
0 0 0 0 1 0 0 1111102 1 0 1 0 1 0 0 0 0 0 0 0 0 0 0 0 0 0 0 0 0 0 1 2 6 119 11110
0 1 0 0 1 0 0 8 11119 5 4 1 1 0 0 0 0 0 0 0 0 0 0 0 0 0 0 0 0 0 4 4 7 119 11110
0 0 1 0 0 0 0 1 111110118 1 1 0 0 0 0 0 0 0 0 0 0 0 0 0 0 0 0 1 3 6 7 111111110
0 0 0 0 0 0 1 0 9 111111101 0 0 0 0 0 0 0 0 0 0 0 0 0 0 0 0 0 0 0 1 6 8 111111110
0 0 0 0 1 0 0 0 0 111111115 0 0 0 0 0 0 0 0 0 0 0 0 0 0 0 0 0 0 0 1 5 11111111110
0 0 0 0 0 0 0 0 0 101111119 1 0 0 0 0 0 0 0 0 1 0 0 0 0 0 0 0 0 0 3 101111118 0
0 0 0 0 0 0 0 0 0 0 1111117 2 1 0 1 1 0 0 1 0 0 0 0 0 0 0 0 0 0 1 0 2 111111115 0
0 0 0 0 0 0 0 0 0 0 111011107 1 0 0 0 0 0 1 0 0 0 0 0 0 0 0 0 0 0 1 3 111111101 0
0 0 0 0 0 0 0 0 0 0 6 111111116 0 0 1 1 0 0 0 0 0 0 0 0 0 0 0 0 0 3 9 111111110 0
0 0 0 0 0 0 0 0 1 0 0 11111011113 1 0 0 0 1 1 0 0 0 0 0 0 0 0 0 1 6 11111110110 0
0 0 0 0 0 0 0 0 0 1 0 6 111111114 0 0 1 1 0 0 0 0 0 0 0 0 0 0 0 5 1111111111111 0
0 0 0 0 0 0 0 0 0 1 0 1 11111011114 0 0 0 1 0 0 0 0 0 0 0 0 0 1 9 11101111115 0 0
0 0 0 0 0 0 0 0 0 0 0 8 11111111119 5 0 0 0 0 0 0 0 0 0 1 3 111111111110 0 0
0 0 0 0 0 0 0 0 0 0 0 0 1111111111111113 0 1 0 2 1 2 1 0 0 4 111111111114 0 1 0
0 0 0 0 0 0 0 0 0 1 0 0 0 4 111111111111106 4 7 9 5 5 3 1 0 4 111111111110 1 0 0
0 0 0 0 0 0 0 0 0 0 0 1 0 1 7 1111111111111111111119 3 3 2 0 7 11111111113 1 0 1 0
0 0 0 0 0 0 0 0 0 1 0 0 1 0 0 111111111111111111111011111011111111110110 0 0 0 0
0 0 0 0 0 0 0 0 0 0 1 0 0 1 1 0 101111111111111111111111111111111111111101 1 0 1 0
0 0 0 0 0 0 0 0 1 0 0 0 0 0 0 0 3 1111111111101111111111111101111111110 0 0 0 1 0
0 0 0 0 0 0 0 0 0 0 0 1 0 1 0 1 0 4 7 11111111111101111111110111116 0 0 1 1 0 0
0 0 0 0 0 0 0 0 0 1 0 0 1 0 0 0 0 0 0 2 6 9 11111111111111111111113 0 0 0 0 0 1 0
0 0 0 0 0 0 0 0 0 0 0 0 0 0 0 0 0 0 0 0 0 0 0 0 0 0 0 0 0 0 0 0 0 0 0 0 0 0 0 0 0
```

Fig. 10. Fragment of table with values of elastic modulus obtained from tomography [GPa]

2.4 Quality of images from QCT

Very important problem is quality of images from radiology examinations. On the base of obtained information, it is deducted about patient's state, disease's progress and it is possible to plan the treatment and check correctness of therapy. In case of QCT, when dates are often converting, quality of tomograms has special meaning. There are a few important features of images, which decide about useful in medical diagnostic: contrast, sharpness, resolution, noise-to-signal ratio, artifacts and distortion of signals.

Occurrence hums and disturbances is one of the characteristic features of signals. In dependence on method there is different kind of hums. Increase of hums level lead to lowering of visibility and the decrease of contrast. In a consequence photographs gives little information and are less useful. Hums are observed on the every stage of transformation data and it would be the best if minimization of disturbances started from the very beginning of creation of images and lasted during whole registration process of the data. Hums and disturbances can influence on incorrect interpretation of photographs. Influence of hums can be limited by using the low-pass filters and locally enlarging the contrast. Unfortunately during reducing of disturbances it can lose the part of information which will influence on level of medical content.

The artifacts are others problems during conversion of photographs from radiology. These are unwanted feature of images appearing in medical modalities. The artifacts do not reflect the properties of researches structures but they are the result of accidental factors. In Fig. 11 the comparison between normal image and image with artifact is shown [4].

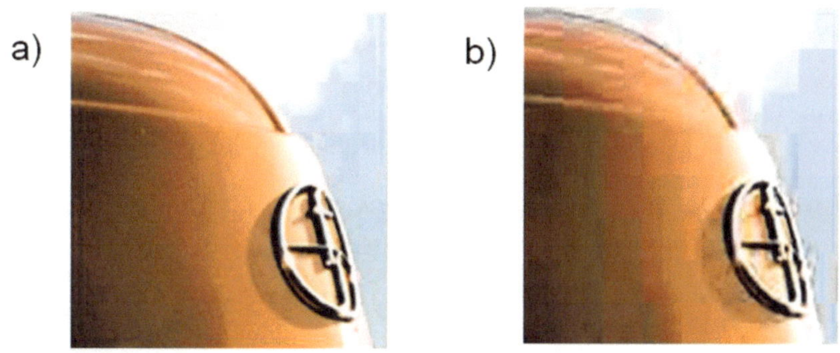

Fig. 11. The differences between: a) correct images and b) images with artifacts [4]

Sometimes it does not influence significantly on perception of diagnostic information, however in some cases it can limit accuracy of interpretation or even mislead (the artifacts pretend features of living structures). Many different factors can cause formation of artifacts e.g.: methods of data processing, algorithms of creation of images, movements of patients or shift of X-ray lamp. During QCT examinations frequent artifacts are appearing defects on boundaries of areas with different density - in images are local decrease of sharpness and contrast, the rise of shadows or the exaggerations. In a consequence it can cause to incorrect estimation of material properties (Fig. 12) [19].

3. Numerical model of human pelvic bone

After performing tomography examination next step is to convert obtained images to get effort state of bone. Data from QCT was used to create the numerical model of human pelvic bone. First, the geometry of the model should be prepared. The geometry from tomography or from measuring coordinate machine can be applied.

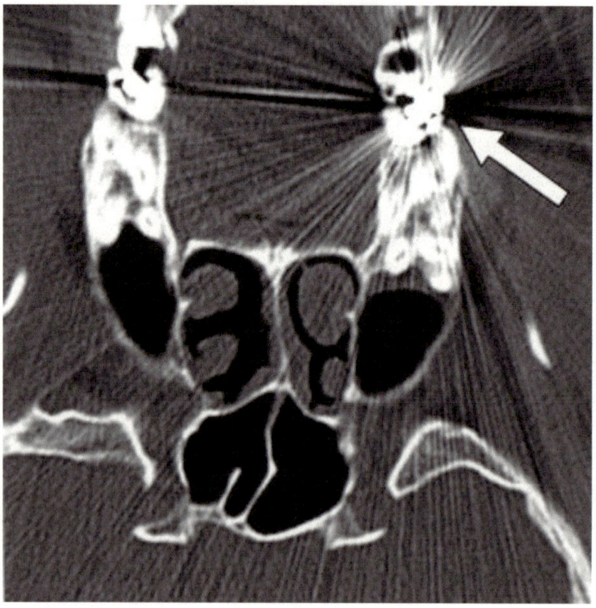

Fig. 12. The artifact caused by metal filling [19]

The model consists of three main parts:
- pelvic bone (compact and trabecular tissue),
- endoprosthesis of hip joint (cement layer and artificial acetabulum),
- femur head (metal or ceramic).

The components and whole model of human pelvic bone are presented in Fig. 13.

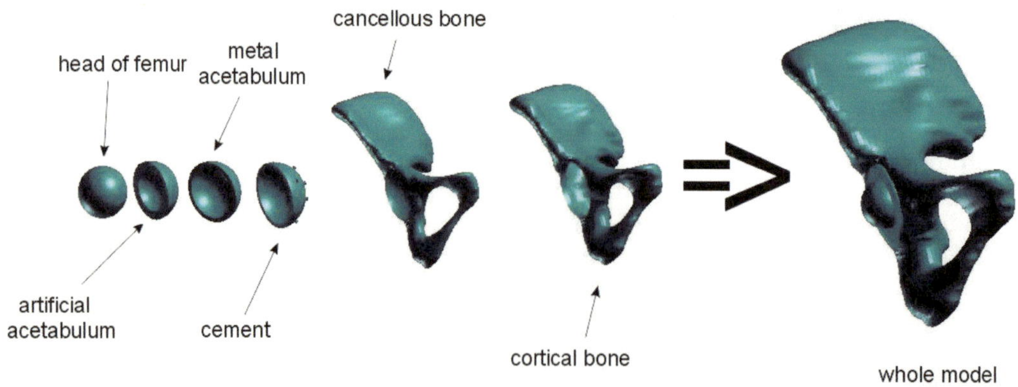

Fig. 13. Component of model of pelvic bone

Characteristic feature of the model is subordinating individual material parameters to each finite element - this represents non-homogenous structure of bone and changes in pelvic bone during osteoporosis (model is closer to real conditions).

After completing prepared model on boundary conditions (it is presented in Fig. 14), the calculations on the base of FEM are performed.
Important problem is to determine the changeability of material properties in numerical model. It was achieved in two approach - they became describe later.

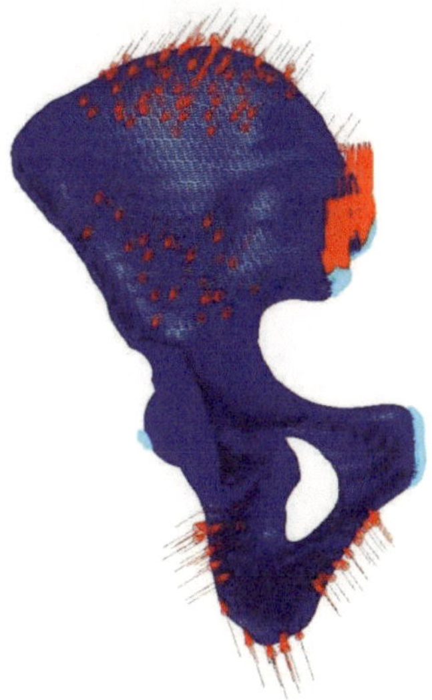

Fig. 14. Meshing and boundary conditions of the model

4. Data collection

4.1 Using of clinical data

Calculations are performed on the base of linear static according to Huber-Von Mises criterion, using data prescribed in chapter 2.3. Important fact is assuming material parameters on the basis of images from tomography.
In Fig. 15, 16 and 17 the distributions of reduced stresses, strains and displacements are presented. The maximum reduced stresses (Fig. 15.) and strains (Fig. 16.) appear in the head of femur and in the joint between sacral and pelvic bone.

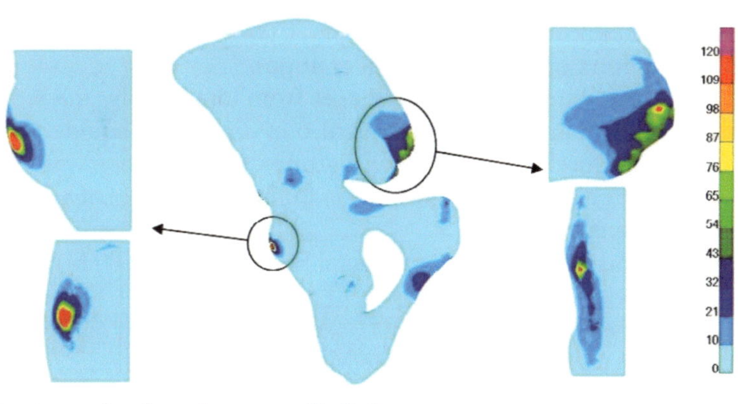

Fig. 15. Distributions of reduced stresses [MPa]

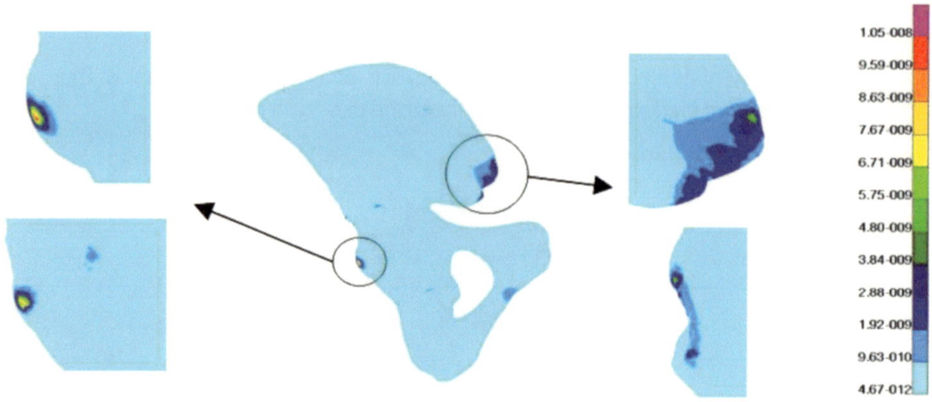

Fig. 16. Distributions of reduced strains

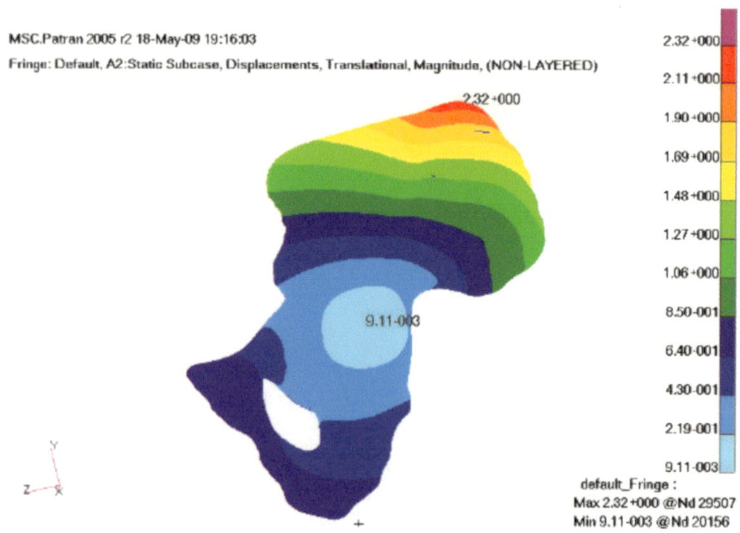

Fig. 17. Distributions of displacements [mm]

4.2 Numerical simulations of osteoporotical changes

In view of difficulties and limited access to images from tomography the numerical models containing osteoporotical changes were created also in different methods. Second approach consist of division whole model to subregions - groups. Cortical bone was divided into five subregions, in each subregions elastic modulus is in the some range of value. In Fig. 18 the subregions of cortical bone are shown:

- Pubic symphysis and joint of pelvic and sacral bone: 15000 –15600 MPa (violet),
- surroundings of acetabulum: 13000–13500 MPa (red),
- upper part of ilium ala: 12000–12600 MPa (brown),
- central part of ilium ala: bone: 13500–14000MPa (yellow),
- ischium and pubis: 14000-14500 MPa (blue).

Cancellous bone was also divided into a couple of part (Fig. 19):

- External layer of bone (2000-2600 MPa):
  - Surroundings of acetabulum (green),
  - Upper and lower part of bone (brown),
- Internal layer of bone:
  - Surroundings of acetabulum: 250–300 MPa (blue),
  - Upper and lower part of bone: 200–250 MPa (yellow).

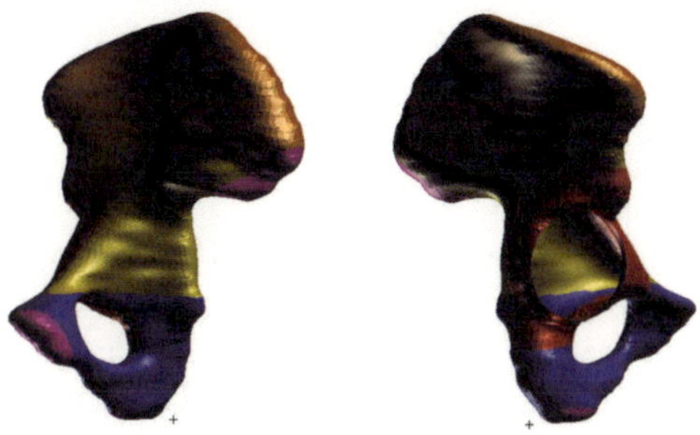

Fig. 18. The subregions of cortical bone

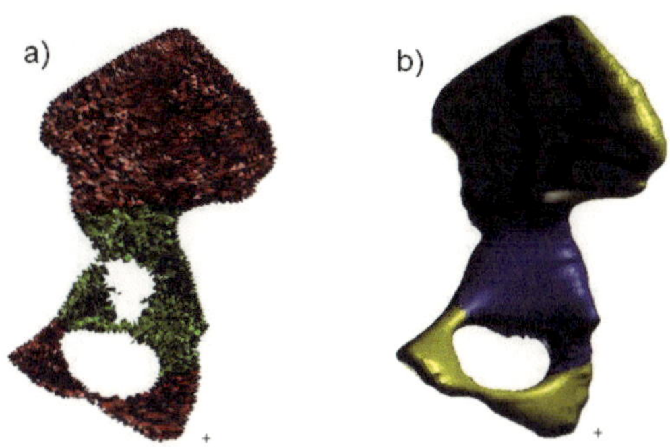

Fig. 19. The groups of cancellous bone: a) external layer, b) internal layer

In each of these groups values of elastic modulus in individual finite element was determined on the base of decreasing of bone mass and the range of changeability of Young modulus (Fig. 20).

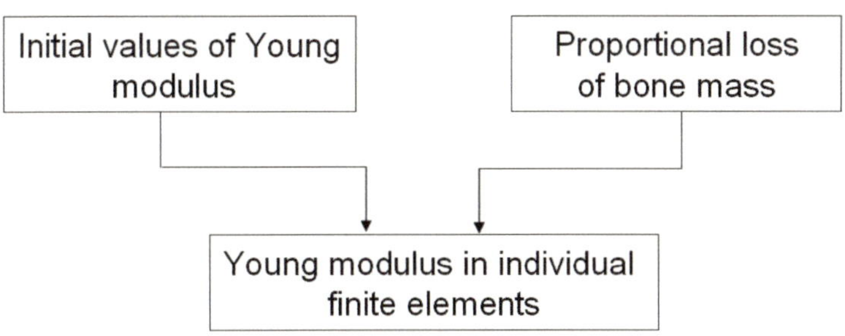

Fig. 20. Determining of elastic modulus in individual finite element

During calculations the following relationship were used:
- for cortical bone - conception of Weinans [12]:

$$E = 4.249 \cdot \rho^3 \tag{4}$$

- for cancellous bone - conception of Mow and Hayes [12]:

$$E = 2.195 \cdot \rho^3 \tag{5}$$

where:
E - elastic modulus,
ρ - radiological density of bone tissue.
It is possible to change these formulas to another and computation distribution of material properties according to different relationships.
The exemplary distributions of stresses, strains and displacements were presented in Fig. 21, 22 and 23. The maximum reduced stresses (Fig. 21.) and strains (Fig. 22.) appear in the head of femur and in the joint between sacral and pelvic bone.

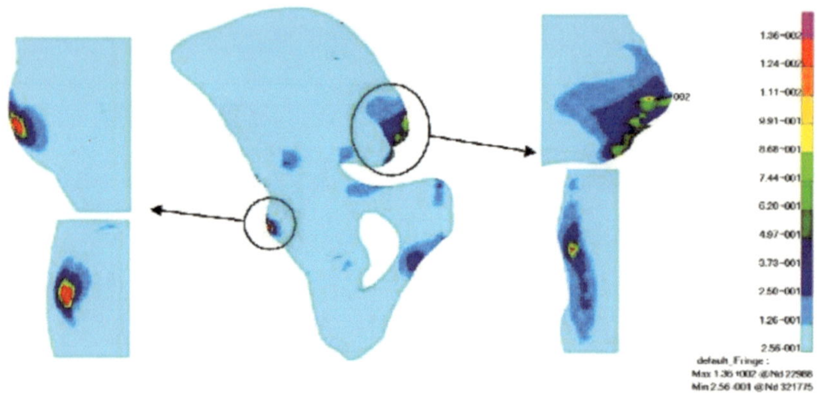

Fig. 21. Distributions of reduced stresses [MPa]

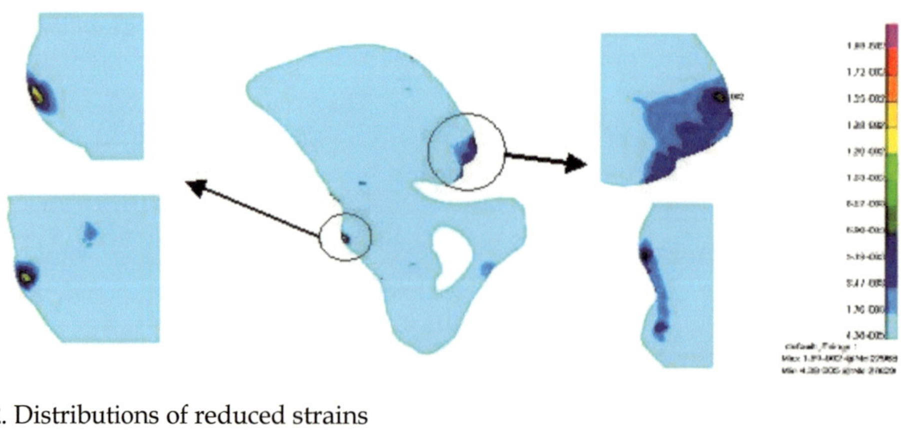

Fig. 22. Distributions of reduced strains

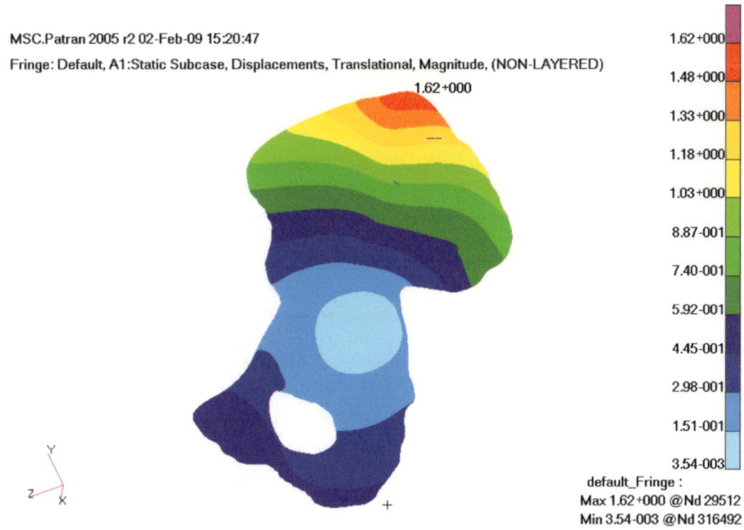

Fig. 23. Distributions of displacements [mm]

Some results of numerical simulations are put into Table 1 and Table 2. The maximum value of displacement and reduced stress in dependence on loss of bone mass (in percent, in upper part of ilium ala) are shown. Next, in Table 2 the same dependence is shown when the loss of bone mass appear in pubic symphysis and sacral joint. Additionally, the value of maximum strain is prescribed.

loss of bone mass [%]	u_{max} [mm]	σ_{max} [MPa]
0	1,38	157
10	1,51	149
20	1,68	140
30	1,89	144
40	2,16	154
50	2,49	164

Table 1. Displacements and stresses for loss of bone mass in upper part of ilium ala

loss of bone mass [%]	u_{max} [mm]	σ_{max} [MPa]	ε_{max}
0	1,38	157	$8{,}00 \cdot 10^{-3}$
10	1,49	148	$1{,}14 \cdot 10^{-2}$
20	1,62	137	$1{,}50 \cdot 10^{-2}$
30	1,79	130	$2{,}00 \cdot 10^{-2}$
40	1,98	144	$2{,}70 \cdot 10^{-2}$
50	2,22	162	$3{,}67 \cdot 10^{-2}$

Table 2. Quantities for loss of mass in pubic symphysis and joint of pelvic and sacral bone

In Fig. 24. the exemplary graph showing relationship between decreasing of bone mass and stresses and displacements. To infer about dangerous state in bone system one should take into attention all of quantities characterizing effort state, e. g. for point A, B and C information about stresses only is not unambiguous (it is not enough information about loss of bone mass) however when we also consider displacements we can determinate how loss of bone mass is in each points.

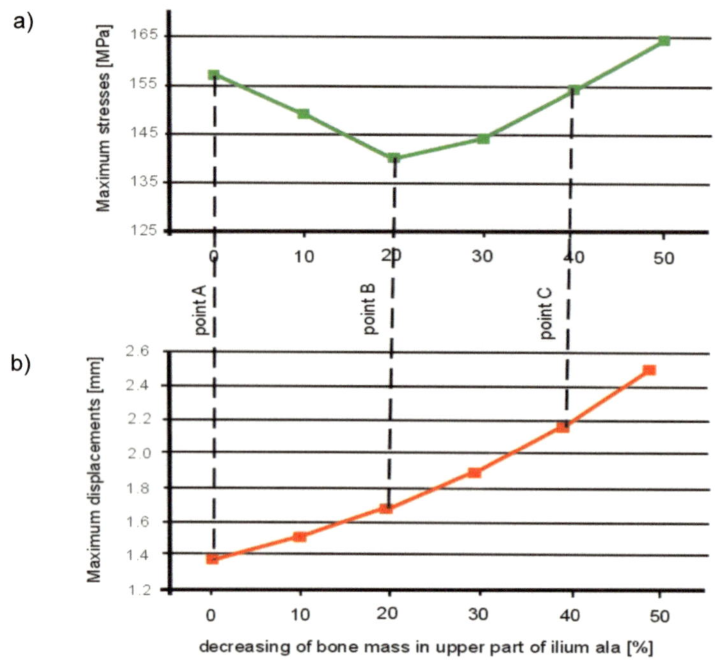

Fig. 24. Relationship between loss of bone mass and: a) stresses, b) displacements

5. Aid of diagnosis osteoporosis in pelvic bone

5.1 Data base

After QCT examinations the tomograms of researches structure are obtained. At the first, it is necessary to determinate the radiological density. To transformation of that quantity one should rescale it to HU. The next step it is delimitation the density of bone tissue (on the base of density in HU). By using relationship between density of bone tissue and material properties it is possible to calculate material parameters of bone tissue in each voxel. From the other hand, on the base of QCT data it is possible to create the geometry of numerical model. When the model is prepared the material properties are inserted and the strength calculation (according to FEM) is performed. On the ground of obtained results (distributions of stresses, strains and displacements) one can get to know about effort in researched bone.

When the large amount of QCT examinations will be realized (the set of data will be converted and strength calculations will be performed) it will be possible to create the base of data. This base will be aid detection of osteoporotical changes in human pelvic bone. This data base one can compare to table - matrix which consists of CT photos: column symbolize images for individual patients, row vector places where images were done. The base one have to divide into two main parts: QCT images and numerical simulations. General structure of data base is shown in Fig. 25.

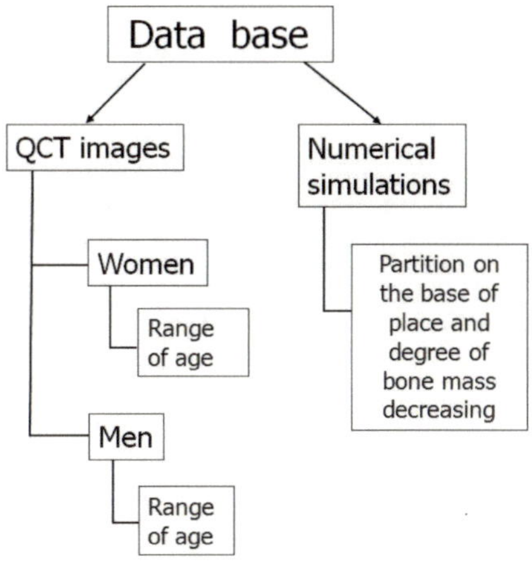

Fig. 25. Schematic structure of data base

The data base makes up folders with suitable data and group with the correct order. The fragment of the base is presented in Fig. 26.

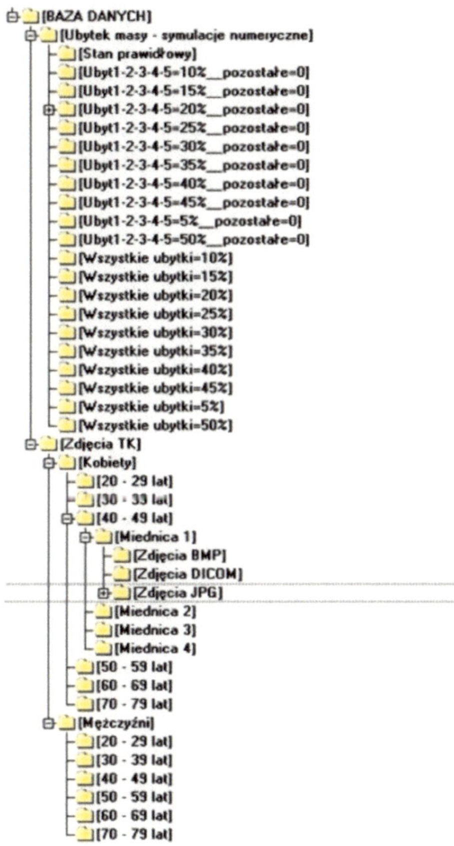

Fig. 26. The part of data base

5.2 Procedure to aid of diagnosis osteoporosis

After building the numerical model the next step of work is to develop procedure to aid of recognizing osteoporotical changes in pelvic bone.

The general principle is as follow: after radiology examination it takes place searching to find the most similar images (searching CT photo from data base). When these images are found the whole model with strength parameters is assigned. Next the results (from strength calculations) are analyzed. As a consequence, particular images from QCT are subordinated to effort of bone. In case of need it is possible to return to searching of base and analyzing the larger number of data. The simplified block diagram of the program is presented in Fig. 27.

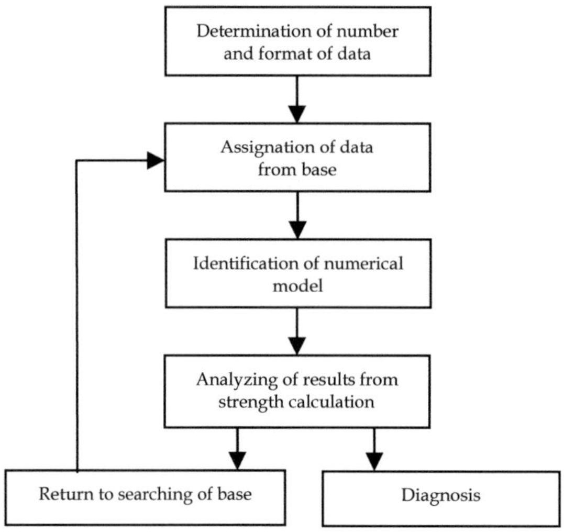

Fig. 27. The block schema of the program

In the program there are available two searching procedures: on the base of tomography images and decreasing of bone mass.

In procedure of searching on the basis of QCT, one can first read image - which will be analyzed, next to read images from data base. When sorting is ready, one should to insert number of image, which is the most similar, to the textbox of the program - the information about dangerous state will appear in the window of the program. This selected views of procedure box are presented in Fig. 28.

In procedure of searching on the basis of loss of bone mass one should indicate the proportional decreasing of bone mass (from the combo box) in each subregions of cortical bone in numerical model of pelvic bone. When all list are ready in the window of the program will appear information about dangerous state and potential dangerous of osteoporosis. This procedure was presented in Fig. 29.

6. Conclusions

- Applied procedure facilitates interpretation of data from QCT and it helps diagnosis what enable earlier detection of osteoporosis and enlarges chance of the treatment.
- Presented procedure delivers additional information about effort state in analyzed bone.
- Information from QCT can be helpful for researching progress of osteoporosis in individual clinical cases (because easier one can find the differences between earlier and later images).

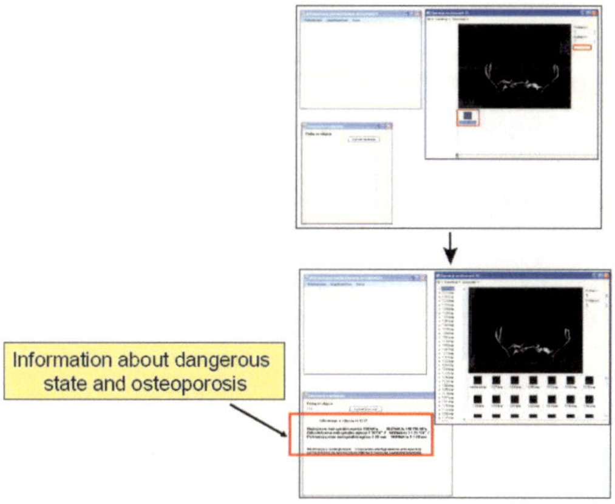

Fig. 28. The algorithm of the searching on the base QCT images

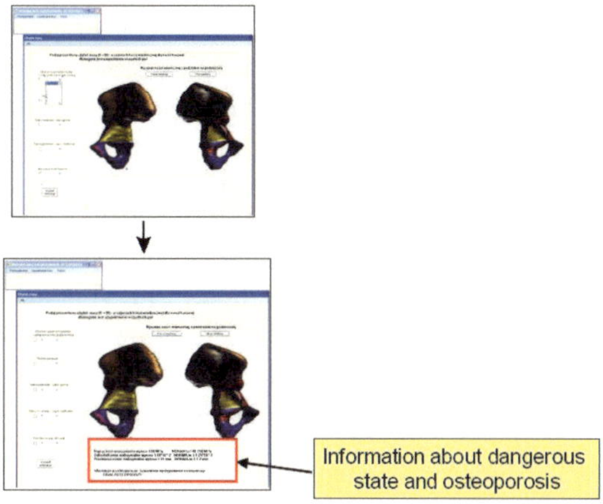

Fig. 29. The algorithm of the searching on the base loss of bone mass

- Subordinating individual images from QCT of effort state provides information about bone system.
- Creation of numerical model on the base of radiological data (especially material properties) increasing it conformance to real conditions.
- Quality of obtained results depends on amount information gathered in the data base.
- Presented procedure enables noticing changes in bones more precisely than standard methods (this is important when the difficulties with clear diagnosis appear).
- Structure of data base enables easy and quick extension.

7. Future plans

- Extension of data base. The structure of data base enables its easy extension. The more data collected in the base it means the bigger possibilities in aid of diagnosis.
- Widening this procedure to another element of bone system. Here, the example of pelvic bone was presented, but one can also applied this procedure to another bone and joint e.g. for the spine or metatarsus bone. To perform this one can dispose data necessary to prepare the numerical models and create proper data base.

8. References

Abrahams P.: The atlas of the human body. Świat Książki, Warszawa 2004 (in Polish)

Adams J. E.: Quantitative Computed Tomography. *European Journal of Radiology* vol. 71, pp. 415–424, 2009

Cierniak R.: Computed tomography. Construction of CT scanners. Reconstrucions algorithms. EXIT, Warszawa 2005 (in Polish)

Engelke K. et al.: Clinical Use of Quantitative Computed Tomography and Peripheral Quantitative Computed Tomography in the Management of Osteoporosis in Adults: The 2007 ISCD Official Positions. *Journal of Clinical Densitometry: Assessment of Skeletal Health*, vol. 11, no. 1, pp. 123-162, 2008

Gregory J. S. & Aspden R. M. Femoral geometry as a risk factor for osteoporotic hip fracture in men and women. *Medical Engineering & Physics*, vol. 30, pp. 1275-1286, 2008

John A., Orantek P., Wysota P. The numerical modeling of osteoporotic changes in selected biomechanical structures, Proceedings of 36th Solid Mechanics Conference SolMech, pp. 36-41, Gdańsk 2008

John A., Wysota P.: Data base to aid of diagnosis of osteoporotical changes in human pelvic bone. Journal of Vibroengineering, Vol. 11, Issue 3, pp. 517-523

John A., Wysota P.: *Procedure to aid of diagnostic of osteoporotical changes in human pelvic bone.* Proceedings of 15th International Conference Mechanika, pp. 199 - 203, Kaunas, 2010

John A., Wysota P.: *Development of computer system to aid of diagnosis osteoporosis in human hip joint region.* Proceedings of International Conference of the Polish Society of Biomechanics 2010, pp. 97-98, Warszawa 2010

Kanis J. A. et al.: European guidance for the diagnosis and management of osteoporosis in postmenopausal women. Osteoporosis International, vol. 19, pp. 399-428, 2008.

Kaneko T. S. et al.: Mechanical properties, density and quantitative CT scan data of trabecular bone with and without metastases. Journal of Biomechanics, vol. 37, pp. 523–530, 2004.

Link T. M., Adams J. E.: The radiologist's important roles and responsibilities in osteoporosis. European Journal of Radiology,vol. 71, pp. 385-387, 2009

McNamara L.M.; Prendergast P.J. & Schaffler M.B.: Bone tissue material properties are altered during osteoporosis. *Musculoskeletal Neuronal Interact*, vol. 5, pp.342-343, 2005

Nayak S., Roberts M.S. & Greenspan S.L. Factors associated with diagnosis and treatment of osteoporosis in older adults. *Osteoporosis International,* vol. 20, pp. 1963-1967, 2009

Rho J.Y., M.C. Hobatho M.C., Ashman R.B., Relations of mechanical properties to density and CT number in human bone bone, Medical Engineering & Physics, vol. 17, pp. 347-355, 1995

Sawada K. et al.: Peripheral quantitative computed tomography (pQCT) is useful for monitoring bone mineral density of the patients who receive hormone replacement therapy. Maturitas, vol. 56, pp. 343–349, 2007

Sawada K. et al.: Peripheral quantitative computed tomography is useful to monitor response to alendronate therapy in postmenopausal women. Journal of Bone Mineral Metabolism, vol. 27, pp. 175–181, 2009

Singer A.: Osteoporosis diagnosis and screening. Clinical Cornerstone: management of osteoporosis, vol. 8, no. 1, pp. 9-18, 2006

Webb W.R., Brant W.E., Major N.M.: Fundamentals of Body CT. *Elsevier Urban & Partner,* Wrocław 2007 (in Polish)

10

Preoperative Virtual Navigation with 3D-CT Volume Rendering for Single Minimum Incision Endoscopic Nephron-Sparing Surgery on Renal Tumors

Takao Kamai et al.*
Department of Urology, Tochigi
Japan

1. Introduction

Thanks to various technical and imaging innovations, pure laparoscopic or hand-assisted laparoscopic surgery is now performed worldwide and is considered to be safe and effective, while also improving the quality of life for patients [1,2]. However, laparoscopy requires three to four incisions, each of which is about 1-2 cm long. Every incision is associated with the potential risk of bleeding, hernia, and/or damage to internal organs, and also incrementally worsens the cosmetic outcome [3,4]. Furthermore, several problems remain to be solved with regard to laparoscopy, including the use of CO_2 pneumoperitoneum, the size of the incision required to retrieve the resected specimen, the need for trocar ports, and the high cost of equipment. Alternatives to conventional laparoscopy include single-site surgery, which is known as laparo-endoscopic single-site surgery (*LESS*), as well as natural orifice transluminal endoscopic surgery (NOTES). In 1998, Kihara *et al.* from Japan reported on minimum incision endoscopic surgery (MIES) performed via a single small incision, which was an attempt to solve the above-mentioned problems with conventional laparoscopic surgery and reduce technical difficulties (Figure 1) [5-9]. MIES is performed via a single small incision that is just large enough to allow extraction of the resected specimen, and is done without gas or trocar ports, making it a safe, reproducible, cost-effective, and minimally invasive treatment option [5-8].

Detection of small renal tumors has continued to increase as a result of improved imaging methods. In patients with a single, small (<4 cm), and localized renal cell carcinoma, nephron-sparing surgery (NSS) has become more common due to advances in renal imaging, improved surgical techniques, and the increasing number of incidentally discovered low-stage carcinomas. As a result, good tumor control and potentially better overall survival have been reported in patients undergoing NSS [10]. Therefore, radical nephrectomy is no longer the standard surgical procedure for such tumors and it has been

* Hideyuki Abe[1], Nobutaka Furuya[1], Tsunehito Kambara[1], Tomoya Mizuno[1], Daisuke Nishihara[1], Yasukazu Shioyama[2], Yoshitatsu Fukabori[1], Tomonori Yamanishi[1] and Yasushi Kaji[2]
[1]*Department of Urology, Tochigi,* [2]*Department of Radiology Dokkyo Medical University, Tochigi, Japan*

recognized that it could even be detrimental [10]. Although its safety is still controversial, use of laparoscopic NSS has been increasing [11]. Single MIES is based on both traditional open surgery and modified hand-assisted laparoscopic surgery [5], so the instruments employed are the same as those used for open or laparoscopic surgery and it only requires a short time to learn the technique [5-7]. Because MIES is performed via a small incision, however, the surgical field is very tight. Accordingly, extensive information about the renal tumor, renal vessels, and adjacent structures needs to be obtained preoperatively so that the surgeon can select the appropriate procedure. Moreover, the renal arteries and veins show anatomical variations that must be clarified before attempting surgical treatment, in order to reduce the risk of unexpected bleeding. It has been reported that CT scanning with three-dimensional (3D) reconstruction of images (3D-CT) and/or 3D-CT angiography (CTA) are useful modalities for viewing the renal arteries with less invasiveness than conventional angiography [12-14], and that these methods can be utilized for navigation when retroperitoneal laparoscopic nephrectomy is performed in patients with renal tumors [15]. We have employed preoperative 3D-CT for evaluation of the renal arteries and veins, as well as the relations between the renal hilar vessels and adjacent structures, in order to improve the outcome of single MIES nephrectomy [16], and have found that single MIES radical nephrectomy can be done more safely by utilizing 3D-CT images to perform virtual surgery, resulting in a shorter operating time and less blood loss.

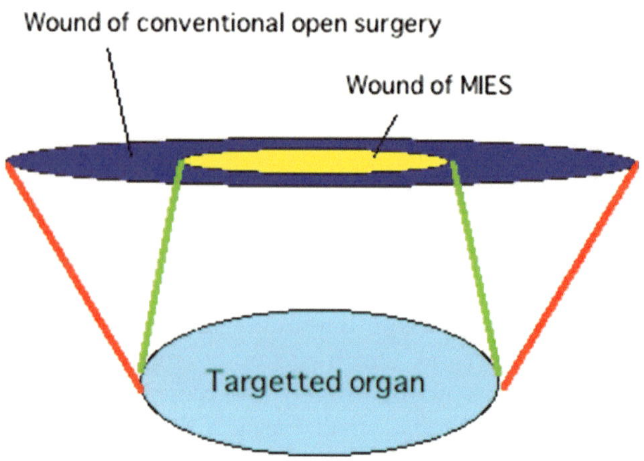

Fig. 1. Schema of single MIES. The length of the wound in MIES is 1/2 - 1/3 in open surgery.

In general, NSS is more difficult than radical nephrectomy and requires more preoperative anatomical data. In particular, detailed preoperative information on the relationship between the tumor and the renal vessels (arteries and veins) is important. It has been reported that 3D-CT provides superior images of the renal vessels and collecting system, and thus is useful for planning NSS [12,13,17]. The technique employed for single MIES nephrectomy of performing preoperative virtual surgery based on 3D-CT images reconstructed by the volume rendering method can also be used when NSS is done by single MIES [16].
In the present study, we reviewed the results of single MIES NSS for renal tumors in 50 consecutive patients treated by one chief operator (T.K*). We also assessed the usefulness of employing 3D-CT images for virtual surgery to decide the approach to the renal tumor during MIES NSS.

2. Methods

2.1 Patients

Fifty Japanese patients aged from 37 to 84 years (mean age: 58.1 years) with cT1aN0M0 renal tumors diagnosed between April 2003 and March 2011 underwent translumbar NSS by single MIES before receiving any other therapy. Patients with tumors located dorsally and very close to the renal hilar vessels were excluded, because such tumors are unsuitable for translumbar MIES. All patients underwent imaging (CT and/or MRI) prior to surgery in order to obtain information for staging. The tumor grade and clinical stage were assigned according to the Fuhrman grading system and the TNM classification, respectively [18,19]. Table 1 summarizes the demographic data, tumor location and size (on CT), operating time, and blood loss. The first 10 NSS procedures were performed without 3D-CT data and the subsequent 40 procedures were done after preoperative virtual surgery employing 3D-CT data. The operating time and blood loss in each group were analyzed in relation to tumor size, side, and location, as well as the length of the skin incision and the body mass index (BMI) [20]. This study was conducted in accordance with the Helsinki Declaration. Institutional Review Board approval was obtained and each patient signed a consent form approved by the Committee on Human Rights in Research of our institution.

	pre-operative axial CT (n = initial 10)	pre-operative 3D-CT (n = subsequent 40)	Surgical procedures (n = 50)
Patient demographics			
No. of patients	10	40	50
Age			58.3 (36 - 81)
Sex (male / female)			32 / 18
Tumor			
Tumor side (right / left)			26 / 24
Tumor size on CT (cm)	2.9 (1.5 - 8)		
MIES Operation			
Operative time (min)			116 (65 - 210)
Blood loss (ml)			212 (25 - 1000)

Table 1. Data collection from 3D-CT and surgical procedures

3. 3D-CT and preoperative virtual surgery

We usually perform NSS via the translumbar approach in patients with relatively small renal tumors. We did not obtain 3D-CT images for the initial 10 patients. However, 3D-CT was done in the subsequent 40 patients (who all had normal renal function and no allergy to contrast medium) in order to plan an appropriate and safe approach to the renal arteries and veins [9]. All of the axial scans (obtained by multidetector row CT) were carefully evaluated before 3D reconstruction was performed, and then 3D images were created by software built into the CT scanner (Leonardo InSpace, Siemens Healthcare, Forchheim, Germany). The arterial phase was used to depict both the renal arteries and veins, since it is the most sensitive phase for the detection of multiple vessels as well as other abnormalities [21]. Data from the CT scans were employed to construct 3D images, after which virtual surgery was performed on a computer. Using the 3D images, the location of the kidney in relation to the lower ribs, iliac crest, and spine was determined to help the surgeon select the best site for making the incision. Possible involvement of adjacent structures by the tumor was also investigated. Images were created that gave an oblique view from the skin incision to the targeted renal artery and vein, in order to allow the surgeon to better understand the anatomical relations between the renal hilar vessels and the surrounding structures. The software (Leonardo InSpace or public domain software OsiriX) allowed the kidney to be freely rotated into different positions and facilitated the creation of any desired cut plane, so that relations between the tumor and the renal vessels or adjacent structures could be demonstrated clearly. Virtual surgery was started by making an oblique intercostal incision between the 11 and 12th ribs. After dissecting between the psoas muscle and Gerota's posterior fascia, we approached the kidney anterior to the psoas muscle. On the right side, we found the posterior surface of the inferior vena cava (IVC) behind the psoas muscle at the level of the lower pole of the kidney. Then we advanced along the IVC toward the liver and identified the right renal artery (RRA). At this level, we also found the right renal vein (RRV) branching from the right side of the IVC. When operating on the left kidney, we initially identified the left renal artery (LRA) running vertical to the psoas muscle at the midpoint of the kidney, after which we identified the left renal vein (LRV) lying behind (ventral to) the LRA. We usually performed simulated surgery from the dorsal to ventral direction as in actual surgery, but we also assessed oblique images in the opposite (ventral to dorsal) direction to better understand relations between the renal vessels and the tumor or adjacent structures.

Because we do not clamp the renal artery for NSS if possible, we need to pay close attention to information about the renal vessels near the tumor in order to preserve renal function. Thus, the renal arteries and veins were followed toward the tumor in order to detect the arterial branches feeding the lesions and the veins draining it (Figure 2 to 5).

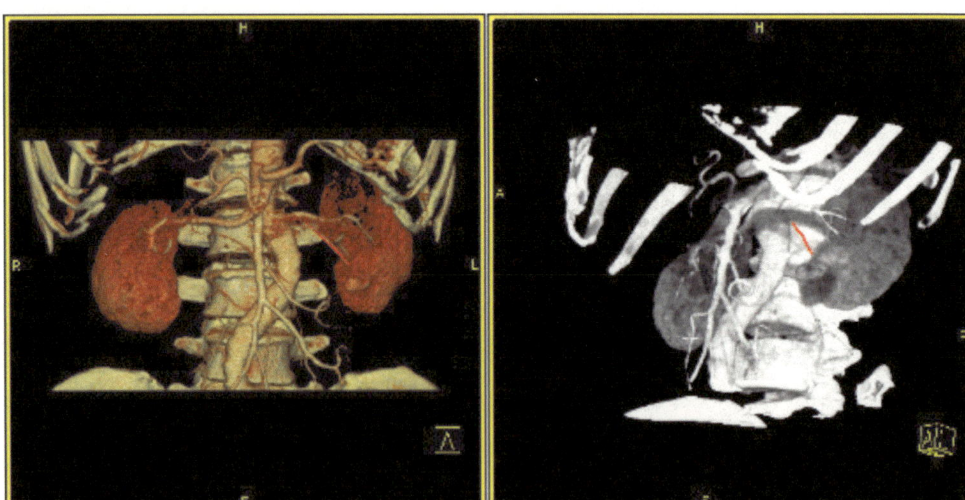

Fig. 2. A left renal tumor. Anterior view (left) and oblique view (right) in the arterial phase. The tumor is located in the ventral lower pole of the kidney. An artery (red) branches off from a proximal vessel and runs toward the tumor. This is the feeding artery.

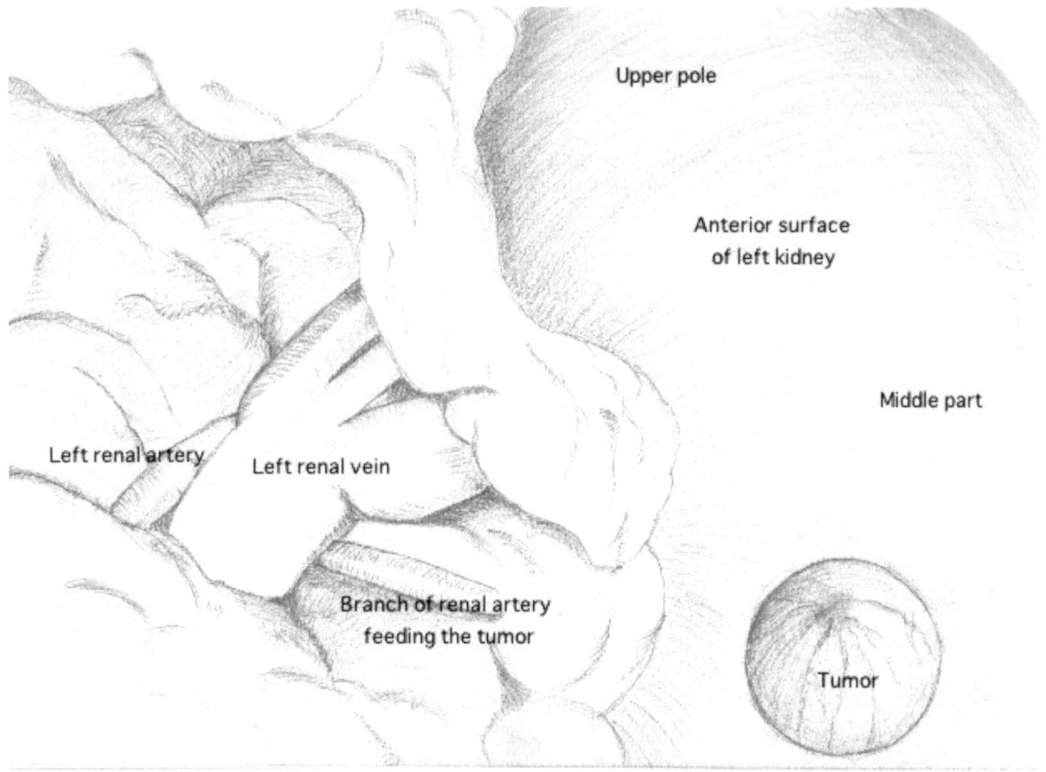

Fig. 3. Sketches of the surgical field viewed through the narrow incision in the Figure 2 for MIES NSS. The tumor is located in the ventral lower pole of the kidney. After dissection between the peritoneum and Gerota's anterior fascia, Gerota's fascia was bluntly dissected to access the renal hilum and the tumor.

4. Surgical technique

We performed NSS by single MIES via the translumbar approach with the patient in the flank position over the break of the operating table according to the reported method [16]. The surgical team consisted of the chief operator and two or three assistants. A flexible high-definition laparoscope (Olympus, Tokyo, Japan) was manipulated by one of the assistants and was moved to the best position for viewing the operating field. The chief operator and first assistant employed a combination of video images and direct vision, while only video images were available for the other assistants.

Based on 3D treatment planning, an oblique intercostal skin incision was made between the 11 and 12th ribs with an average length of about 5 cm (4-6), and a wound retractor (2.5-6 cm in diameter, Applied Medical, CA) was attached. After the external and internal oblique muscles were split, the transversalis fascia was incised, and dissection was performed between the psoas fascia and Gerota's posterior fascia to approach the kidney anterior to the psoas muscle. Gerota's posterior fascia was bluntly dissected and pushed medial to the psoas muscle, achieving immediate access to the renal arteries and veins. We identified the renal artery and vein by manipulation as described previously [16].

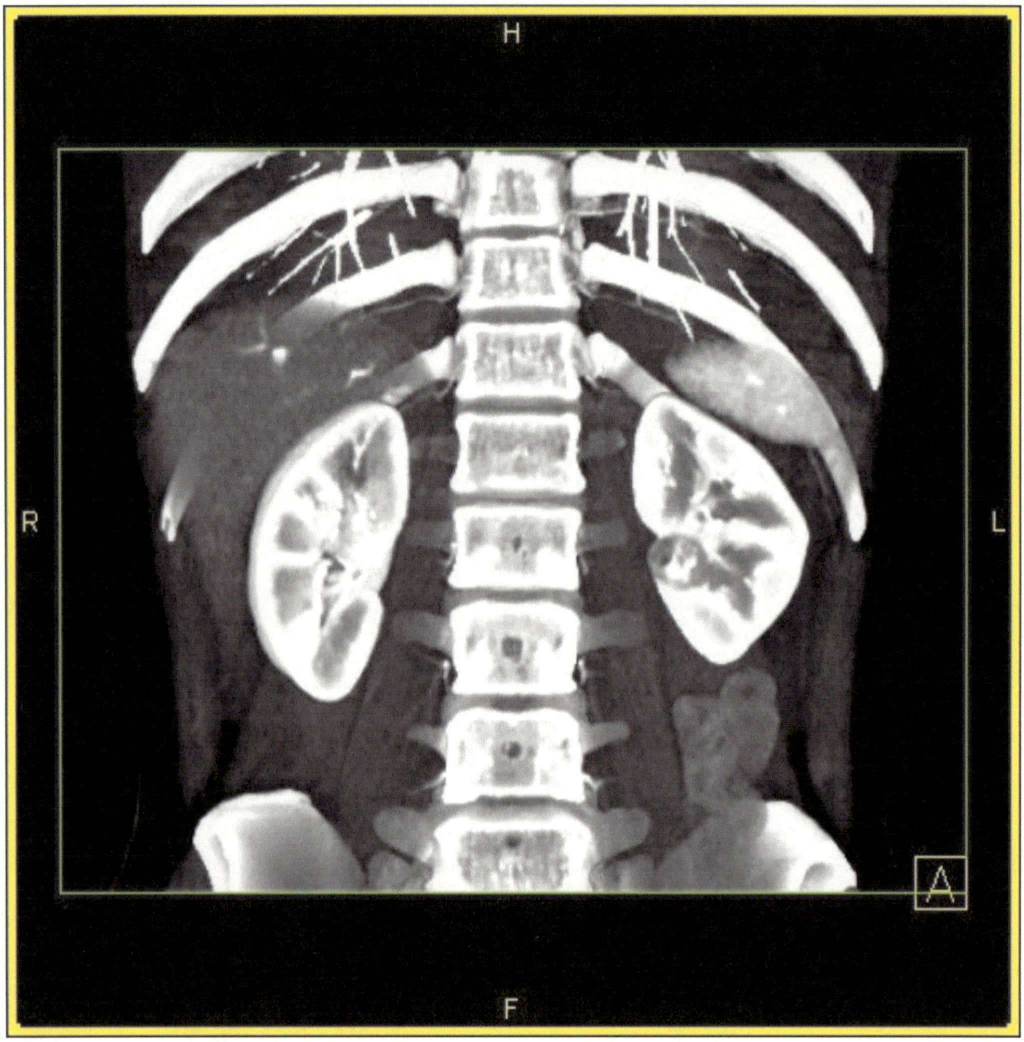

Fig. 4. A left renal tumor adjacent to the renal artery and vein.

After dissecting between the psoas fascia and Gerota's posterior fascia to approach the posterior (dorsal) surface of the kidney, dissection was performed between the peritoneum and Gerota's anterior fascia to approach the anterior (ventral) surface of the kidney. Dissecting both sides of the kidney was useful for mobilization and for approaching the tumor. Gerota's posterior fascia was bluntly dissected and pushed medial to the psoas muscle, achieving access to the renal vessels. Then Gerota's fascia covering the tumor was exposed. We used ultrasonography to find smaller tumors, if necessary. Next, Gerota's fascia was cut close to the tumor and the perinephric fat was dissected to approach the normal renal parenchyma near the lesion. If the tumor was on the posterior (dorsal) side, Gerota's posterior fascia was bluntly pushed medially off the psoas muscle, and the renal pedicle was exposed via the posterior approach. When the tumor was on the anterior (ventral) side, Gerota's anterior fascia was bluntly pushed laterally off the peritoneum and the renal pedicle was exposed via the anterior approach. Microwave tissue coagulation was

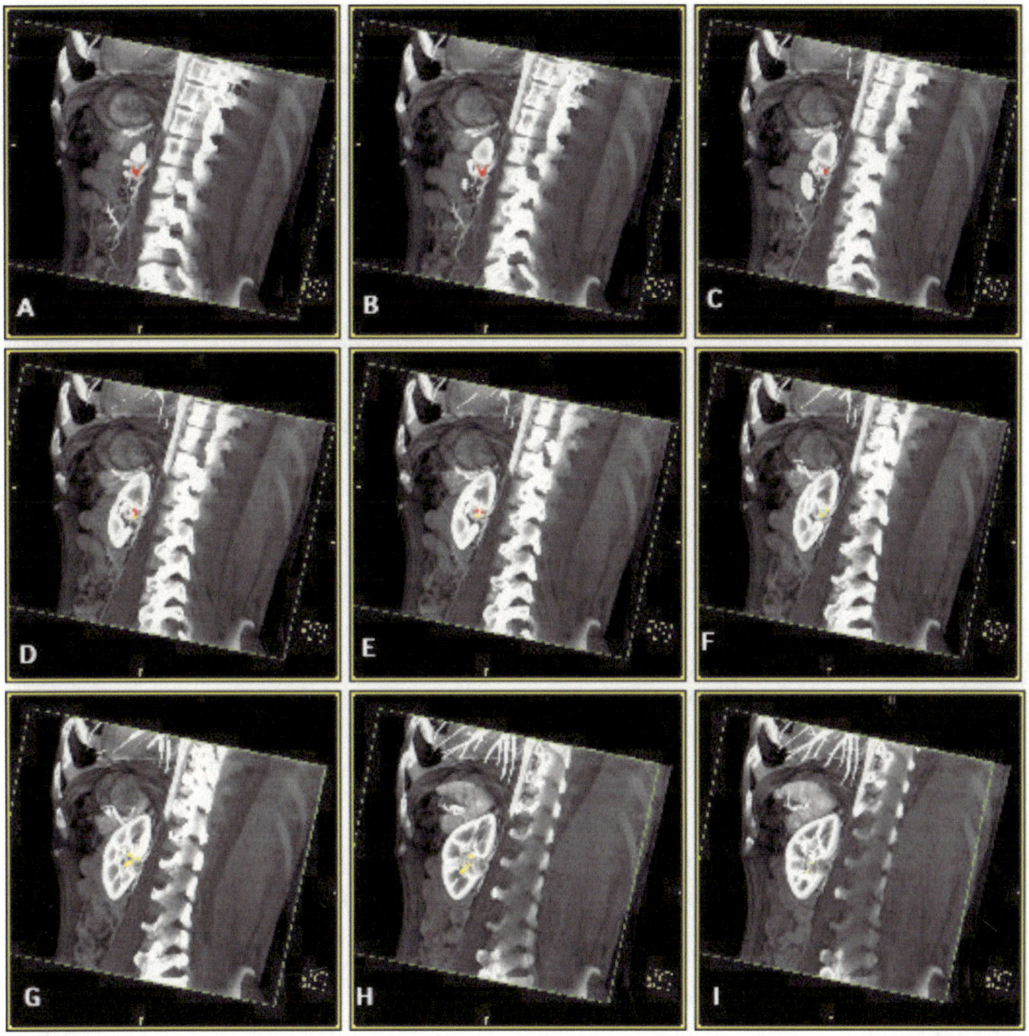

Fig. 5. A left renal tumor very close to the renal hilum (Figure 3). Oblique view from the dorsal to ventral direction in the arterial phase. The CT scans are arranged from central (A) to lateral (I). A, B, C: An artery (red) branches off from a proximal vessel and run toward the periphery. D, E: The artery (red) divides into three small arteries (red, red, and yellow). F: The yellow artery divides into four arterioles (two yellow and two blue). G, H, I: The tumor can be seen in the midportion of the kidney. Two yellow arteries run close to the tumor (T) with a branching artery (green). During NSS, we should pay careful attention to this yellow artery that may feed the tumor.

performed with a Microtaze OT-110 M microwave generator and a needle-type monopolar electrode that was 1.0 to 1.5 cm long and 1 mm in diameter. Coagulation with the electrode was done at 0.5 to 1 cm from the tumor margin. The electrode was inserted into the renal parenchyma at 5 to 10 mm intervals for coagulation at 50 W for 45 seconds, followed by 15 seconds of rest. If the tumor was located close to the renal pedicle, coagulation of the parenchyma was limited to avoid injury to the renal artery or vein and the tumor was excised with scissors or a harmonic scalpel by cutting along the middle of the coagulated zone. The renal artery was clamped, if necessary. After transected vessels were ligated and the collecting system was sutured, indigocarmine was injected intravenously to confirm that there was no significant leakage of urine. An argon beam coagulator was applied to achieve complete hemostasis of the cut surface, if required. All renal defects were filled with perinephric fat and the resected tumor was retrieved thorough the incision. After placing a drain tube within Gerota's fascia, the skin was closed.

5. Statistical analysis

Since the data did not show a normal distribution, the results were analyzed by employing the non-parametric Mann-Whitney *U* test for comparison between two groups and the non-parametric Kruskal-Wallis test to compare three groups. Because Boneferroni's correction is generally employed for multiple comparisons, the Mann-Whitney *U* test was corrected by this method. A probability (P) value of less than 0.05 was considered significant. Analyses were done with commercially available software.

6. Results

NSS was performed successfully by single MIES in all 50 patients. The baseline demographic, clinicopathological, intraoperative, and postoperative data of the subjects are summarized in Table 2. Although there were no operative complications, the incision was extended by 1 to 2 cm in three patients to control hemorrhage. Bleeding was successfully arrested in all three patients and none of them required blood transfusion.

Preoperative 3D reconstruction of volume-rendered images was done in 40 patients, but the first 10 procedures were performed without 3D-CT data. The 50 patients were divided into three groups. There were no differences of tumor size among the groups (data not shown). The operating time (mean ± S.D.) for the initial 10 NSS performed without virtual surgery was 141.9±40.7 min, and there was a significant decrease in the second (117.9±25.7 min, P=0.0440) and third (102.36±19.4 min, P=0.0024) groups that received NSS after preoperative virtual surgery (Figure 6A). Furthermore, the operating time in third group was shorter than in second group (P=0.0353). In contrast, there was tendency toward smaller blood loss in the second group (192.4±110.2 ml) and the third group (191.5±103.2 ml) than in the first group (303.1±291.5 ml), but there was no statistical difference (Figure 6B). There were no differences between tumors on the right and left sides with regard to the operating time (data not shown) or blood loss (data not shown).

We also analyzed the influence of tumor size and location on the operating time and blood loss. Tumors that were located at the upper pole (132.4±34.2 min) and middle part (115.3±33.8 min) required a longer operation time than those at the lower pole (132.4±34.2 min, P=0.0323, Figure 6C). Similarly, tumors that were located at the lower pole (154.0±57.2 ml, P=0.0037) had a smaller blood loss than those at the upper pole (311.2±216.0 ml) and middle part (193.5±145.9 ml, Figure 6D).

There was no difference of the operating time between the ventral side (118.9±34.0 min) and the dorsal side (110.6±15.7 min, P=0.3602, Figure 6E), and but the blood loss of the ventral side (193.9±174.4 ml) was smaller than those of the dorsal side (243.9±115.1 ml, P=0.0347, Figure 6F).

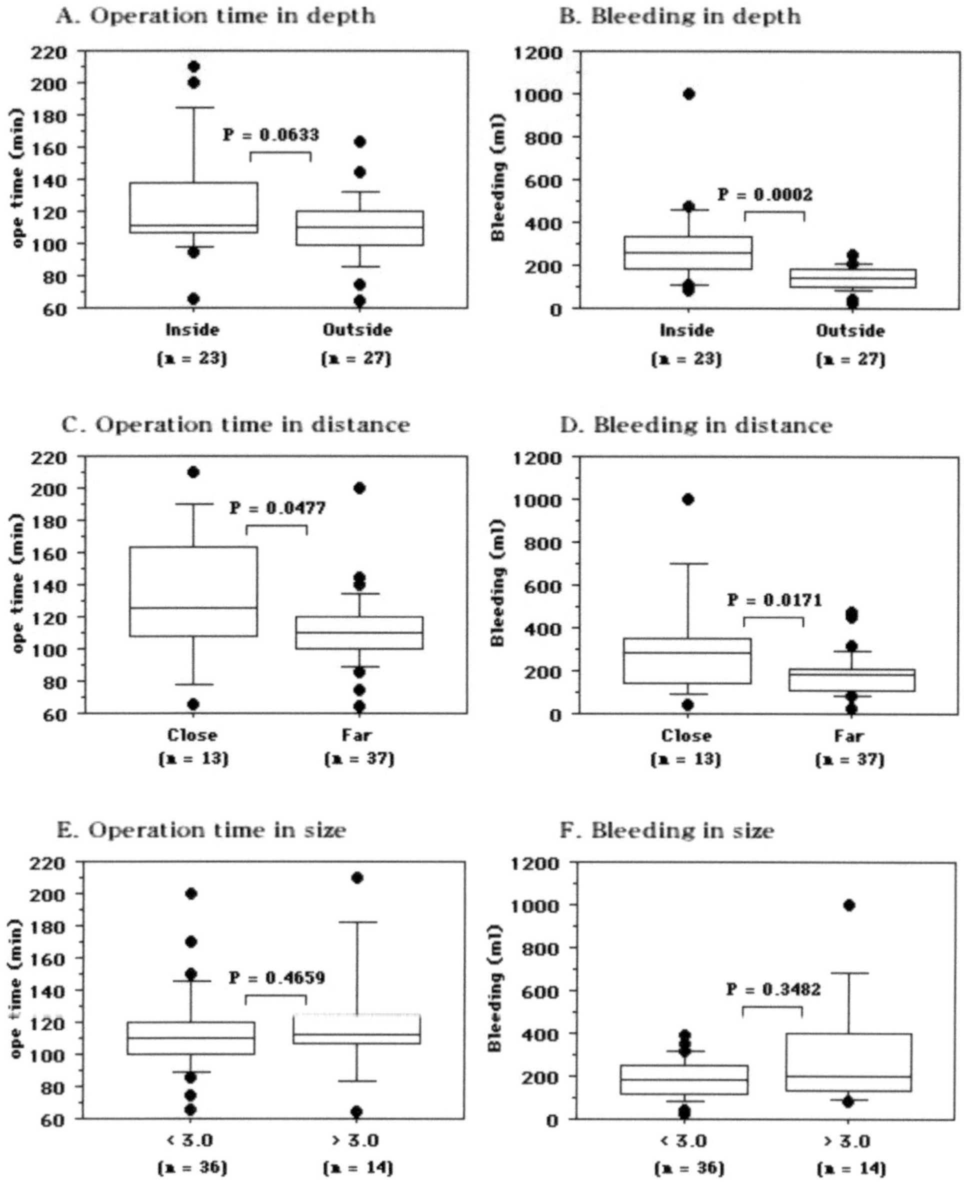

Fig. 6. Comparison of the first to third NSS groups with regard to operating time (A), blood loss (B). Comparison of tumor location between patients with lower pole, middle part, upper pole, dorsal (Dor), and ventral (Ven). Median values are shown in the box plots. Bold circled P values were obtained by comparing the three groups with the Kruskal-Wallis test.

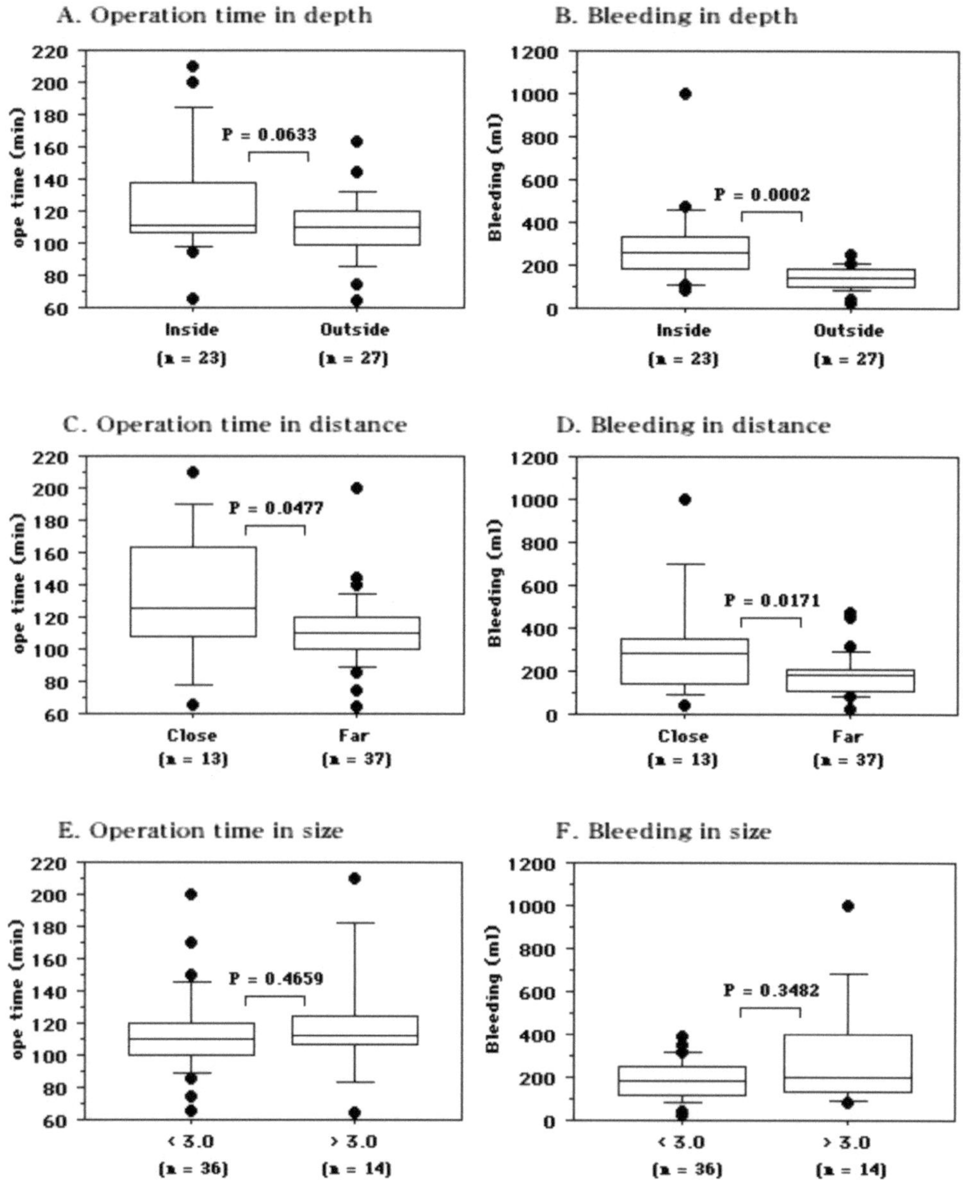

Fig. 7. Operating time and bleeding in relation to tumor location and size. A,B: Tumor depth. Equator of tumor was below (Inside) and above (Outside) the kidney surface. C,D: Tumor is close to (Close) or far from the renal hilum (Far). E,F: Tumor smaller or larger than 3 cm in diameter.

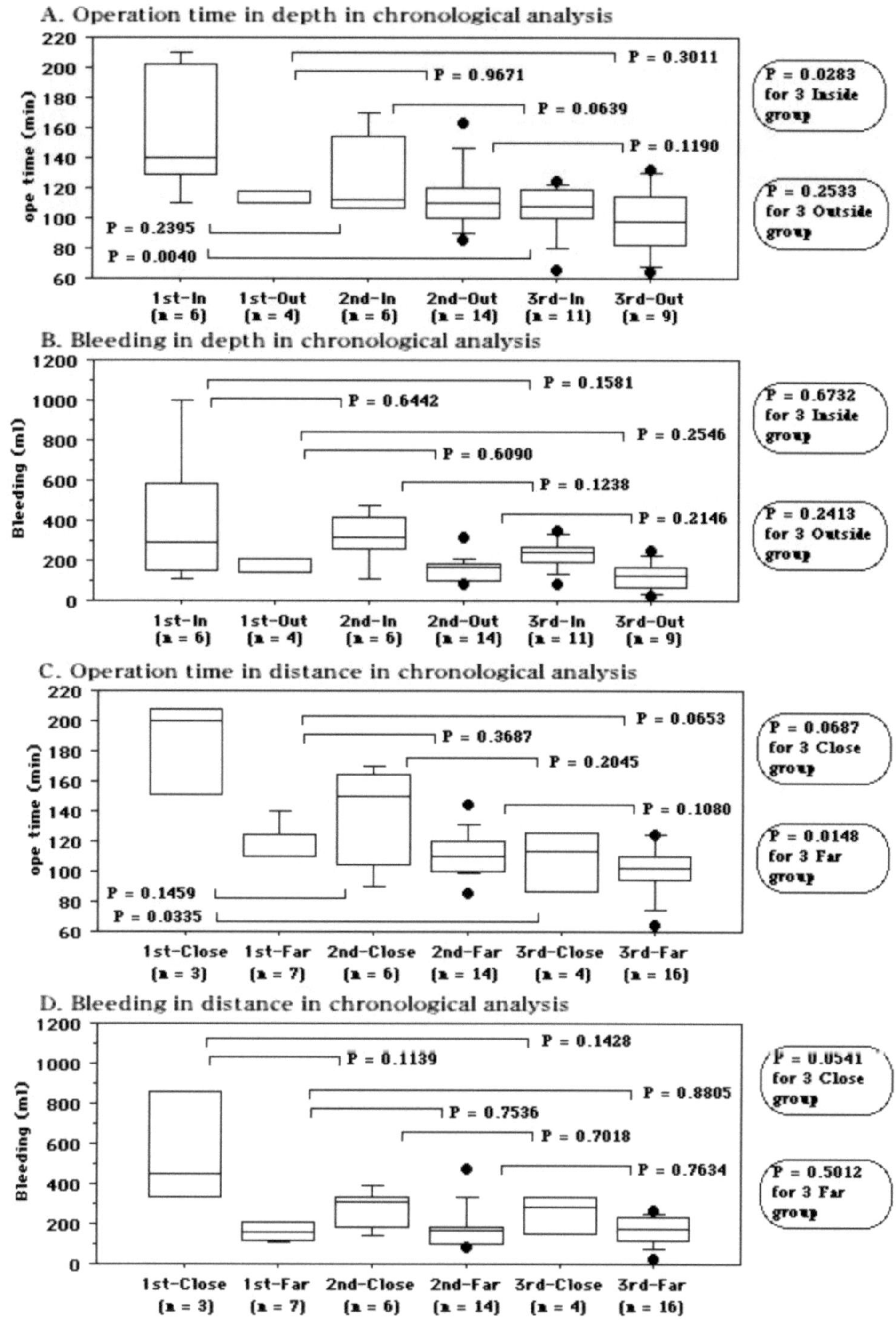

Fig. 8. Comparison of operating time and bleeding in relation to tumor depth (Inside or Outside) and distance (Close or Far) between the first to third NSS groups. Bold circled P values were obtained by comparing the three groups with the Kruskal-Wallis test.

The tumors that were relatively deeply (inside) located required longer operation time and larger blood loss (124.9±34.9 min, 296.8±197.8 ml) than those relatively superficially (outside) located (108.8±21.1 min, P=0.0633; 143.6±54.7 ml, P=0.0002, Figure 7A,B)
Tumors that were located close to renal hilum required a longer operation time (131.8±42.4 min) and a greater blood loss (314.1±264.8 ml) than those far from hilum (111.4±22.6 min, P=0.0477; 182.5±95.5 ml, P=0.0171, Figure 7C,D).
There were no difference of the operating time and blood loss between tumor size (Figure 7E,F).
In the chronological analysis, the operating time in the tumor that was inside (Figure 8A) and far from the hilum (Figure 8C) was dramatically shorter when the procedure was done after preoperative virtual surgery than when it was done without simulation. There was also shorter operating time and less blood loss in the tumor close to the hilum when NSS was done after virtual surgery (Figure 8C,D).

7. Discussion

Since we were familiar with the anatomical frame, landmarks, and operating technique for radical nephrectomy of cT1-3aN0M0 renal tumors via the translumbar approach, we also employed this approach for NSS by single MIES. The present results demonstrate that NSS can be performed safely by single MIES. The extraperitoneal subcostal translumbar approach avoids the risk of peritoneal contamination and also results in earlier resumption of normal bowel function after surgery. We used 3D-CT images to display the location of the kidney in relation to the lower rib cage, iliac crest, and spine, thereby helping the surgeon to accurately plan the initial incision. The position of the kidney and the location and size of the tumor determined the length of the incision.
Preoperative 3D imaging of the renal arteries and veins has been reported to provide useful information for laparoscopic nephrectomy [15,16]. Single MIES is performed via a single small incision, so detailed anatomical information is required in order to approach the renal artery and vein safely as the operation progresses step-by-step with manipulation of the endoscope and instruments in the narrow surgical field. We performed preoperative CT and used the volume rendering method for reconstruction of 3D images because it retains all data by summing the contributions from each voxel along a line set at any viewing angle through a stack of axial images. After 3D images are created, two-dimensional images can also be obtained. Thus, the 3D-CT images can be employed to view the kidney in different positions and 2-dimensional images can be created in any desired plane for clear demonstration of the relations between the tumor and the renal vessels or adjacent structures. In addition, performing virtual surgery is likely to provide the surgeon with more information than that gained from careful study of standard axial CT scans.
We think that the most important point for NSS is to avoid damage to the renal arteries and veins, particularly when the tumor is close to the hilar vessels (Figure 7). It is also difficult to manipulate the tumors whose equator was below (Inside) the kidney surface (Figure 7). Resection of upper pole tumors took longer and was associated with more blood loss (Figure 6).
Comparison between our first 10 NSS procedures and the subsequent 40 with preoperative virtual surgery revealed that latter group had a shorter operating time and smaller blood loss in the tumors whose equator was below (Inside) the kidney surface or close to the renal hilum (Figure 8). Based on data from preoperative 3D simulation, intraoperative experience,

and re-evaluation of our surgical technique by reviewing operative videos for the subsequent 40 patients, we have developed a successful method for approaching the tumor and handling the feeding artery and the hilar vessels. As described in Methods, our approach to the feeding artery and hilar vessels was improved by review of 3D-CT information. These results may reflect both the feedback effect and the learning curve related to accumulation of experience with virtual surgery and actual NSS, indicating that virtual surgery based on 3D-CT data is useful for identifying the feeding artery and renal hilar vessels and for assessing their relations to the tumor, allowing NSS to be performed more safely by single MIES. However, a randomized trial comparing the outcome of patients with or without preoperative virtual surgery should be performed in order to confirm that simulation based on 3D-CT images is useful.

Single MIES is based on standard open surgery, but we use a flexible high-definition laparoscope for easy identification of tissue planes and to allow more precise dissection with minimal trauma. Many of the longer instruments used in open surgery can be inserted into the narrow incision for MIES, so it has a lower cost than conventional laparoscopic surgery (30-40% less). Moreover, the assistants at our hospital are now performing single MIES as chief operators. Because of their experience with this technique, including direct vision and viewing video images as assistants during many single MIES procedures, they had a relatively short learning period. Another advantage of single MIES is that the incision can be extended quickly if required.

Since we have no experience of *LESS* or NOTES, we could not determine whether or not those procedures are superior to single MIES for NSS. However, any of these new single-site laparo-endoscopic procedures and robotic-assisted methods may be a potential alternative to conventional open or laparoscopic surgery.

8. Acknowledgement

The authors are grateful to Junka for her excellent sketches of the surgical field, and Kazumoto Kimura, PhD, for his constructive suggestions regarding statistical analysis.

9. Conclusion

NSS can be performed more safely by single MIES after utilizing 3D-CT images to carry out preoperative virtual surgery, resulting in a shorter operating time and less blood loss.

10. References

Dunn MD, Portis AJ, Shalhav AL, Elbahnasy AM, Heidorn C, McDougall EM, Clayman RV : Laparoscopic versus open radical nephrectomy: a 9-year experience. *J Urol* 2000, 164 : 1153-1159.

Rassweiler J, Frede T, Henkel TO, Stock C, Alken P : Nephrectomy: a comparative study between the transperitoneal and retroperitoneal laparoscopic versus the open approach. *Eur Urol* 1998, 33 : 489-496.

Raman JD, Cadeddu JA, Rao P, Rane A : Single-incision laparoscopic surgery: initial urological experience and comparison with natural-orifice transluminal endoscopic surgery. *BJU Int* 2008, 101 : 1493-1496.

Kommu S, Kaouk JH, Rane A. Laparo-endoscopic single-site surgery; preliminary advances in renal surgery. *BJU Int* 2008, 103 : 1034-1037.

Kihara K, Kawakami S, Fujii Y, Masuda H, Koga F : Gasless single port access endoscopic surgery in urology: Minimum incision endoscopic surgery, MIES. *Int J Urol* 2009, 16 : 791-800.

Kihara K, Kageyama Y, Yano M, Kobayashi T, Kawakami S, Fujii Y, Masuda H, Hyochi N : Portless endoscopic radical nephrectomy via a single minimum incision in 80 patients. *Int J Urol* 2004, 11 : 714-720.

Kageyama Y, Kihara K, Ishizaka K, Okuno T, Hayashi T, Kawakami S, Masuda H, Suzuki M, Hyochi N, Arai G : Endoscopic minilaparotomy radical nephrectomy for chronic dialysis patients. *Int J Urol*, 2002, 9 : 73-76.

Kageyama Y, Kihara K, Kobayashi T, Kawakami S, Fujii Y, Masuda H, Yano M, Hyochi N Portless endoscopic adrenalectomy via a single minimum incision using a retroperitoneal approach: Experience with initial 30 cases. *Int J Urol* 2004, 11 : 693-699.

Kamai T, Yoshida K : Portless endoscopic radical nephrectomy. *Urology View*, Tokyo, 2006, 4 : 66-72.

Novick AC : Open surgery of the kidney. In Wein AJ, Kavoussi LR, Novick AC, Partin AW, Peters CA., editors. Campbell-Walsh Urology. 9th Edition. Philadelphia: Saunders Elsevier; 2007. P.1686-1758.

Gill IS, Kamoi K, Aron M, Desai MM. 800 laparoscopic partial nephrectomies: a single surgeon series. *J Urol* 2010, 183 : 34-41.

Chernoff DM, Silverman SG, Kikinis R, Adams DF, Seltzer SE, Richie JP, Loughlin KR : Three dimensional omaging and display of renal tumors using spiral CT; a potential aid to partial nephrectomy. *Urololgy* 1994, 43 : 125-129.

Coll DM, Uzzo RG, Herts BR, Davros WJ, Wirth SL, NOVICK AC : 3-Dimensional volume rendered computerized tomography for preoperative evaluation and intraoperative treatment of patients undergoing nephron sparing surgery. *J Urol* 1999, 161 : 1097-1102.

Coll DM, Herts BR, Davros WJ, Uzzo RG, Novick AC : Preoperative use of 3D volume rendering to demonstrate renal tumors and renal anatomy. *Radiographics* 2000, 20 : 431-438.

Marukawa K, Horiguchi J, Shigeta M, Nakamoto T, Usui T, Ito K : Three-dimensional navigator for retroperitoneal laparoscopic nephrectomy using multidetector row computerized tomography. *J Urol* 2002, 168 : 1933-1936.

Kamai T, furuya N, Kambara T, Abe H, Honda M, Shioyama Y, Kaji Y, Yoshida K : Single minimum incision endoscopic radical nephrectomy for renal tumors with preoperative virtual navigation using 3D-CT volume-rendering. *BMC Urology*, 2010, 10: 1471-2490-10-7.

Ueda T, Tobe T, Yamanoto S, Motoori K, Murakami Y, Igarashi T, Ito H : Selective intra-arterial 3-dimensional computed tomography angiography for preoperative evaluation of nephron-sparing surgery. *J Comput Assist Tomogr* 2004, 28 : 496-504.

Fuhrman SA, Lasky LC, Lmas C : Prognostic significance of morphologic parameters in renal cell carcinoma. *Am J Surg Pathol* 1982, 6 : 655-663.

Sobin LH, Wittekind CH editors. : International union against cancer. UICC, *In* TNM classification of malignant tumors, 6rd ed. New York, Wiley-Liss, 2002.

WHO. Obesity: preventing and managing the global epidemic. Report of a WHO Consultation. WHO Technical Report Series 894. Geneva: World Health Organization. 2000.

Herts BR, Coll DM, Lieber ML Streem SB, Novick AC : Triphasic helical CT of the kidneys: contribution of vascular phase scanning in patients before urologic surgery. *Am J Roentgenol* 1999, 173 : 1273-1277.

11

Spatial Anatomical Variation of Segmental Hepatic Vasculature and Bile Duct Assessed by Integrated 3D CT Images for Right Lateral Sector Graft Liver Transplantation

Koji Okuda and Atsushi Yoshida
Department of Surgery, Kurume University School of Medicine, Kurume
Japan

1. Introduction

In adult living donor liver transplantation (LDLT), a right lateral sector graft is newly introduced to overcome graft-size disparity of the right lobe graft or left lobe graft[1-3). However, it is obvious that the procurement of right lateral sector has technical difficulties. High number of either unrecognized or extemporaneously handled biliary and vascular variants poses high risk both to the donor and the recipient[4)]. Thus, understanding of the anatomical variations of sectoral and segmental bile duct, hepatic artery and portal vein of the donor and recipient are a prerequisite.
Diagnostic imaging with multidetector computed tomography (MD-CT) allows accurate and noninvasive preoperative evaluation of the hepatobiliary anatomy[5,6)]. And, three-dimensional (3D) representation of anatomic structures is thought to improve understanding of complex spatial interactions[7,8)].
We investigate anatomical variations of the segmental portal vein, artery and bile duct for the right lateral sector, including not only variant of each structures but also 3D relationship, based on the integrated 3D images, for guideline of safe right lateral sector graft transplantation.

2. Patients

Seventy-three patients underwent contrast enhanced dynamic MD-CT and MD-CT cholangiography. Among these, 66 patients who met the following inclusion criteria were selected: age over 20 years, no tumor in the liver/hepatic hilum, no tumor located in peripheral sites in the liver which is more than 30mm in diameter, no previous hepatic or biliary surgery. 3D images of the portal vein, hepatic artery and bile duct were reconstructed in all. 14 patients were excluded from the study because of the poor quality of 3D images. Consequently, 52 patients were enrolled in this study. There were 40 men and 12 women with age ranged from 42- 78 (mean 65) years. There were 24 patients with hepatocellular carcinoma, 4 with cholangiocellular carcinoma, 7 with extrahepatic bile duct cancer, 3 pancreatic cancer, 1 papilla vater carcinoma, 5 with gall bladder cancer, 1 adenomyomatosis, 5 stone, , 1 chronic hepatitis, 1 liver hemangioma.

3. Imaging technique

All dynamic CT studies were performed with MD-CT (Asteon multi ver. 1.5 Toshiba, Tokyo or LightSpeed Plus, GE Yokogawa, Tokyo). Patients received 100 ml of iopamidol with an iodine concentration of 370 mg/ml (Iopamiron 370; Nihon Schering, Osaka, Japan) as intravenous contrast for vascular imaging. The contrast medium was injected at a rate of 4 ml/sec. with an automatic power injector. Three or four phase scanning was performed with a single breath-hold helical technique at 3 mm collimation, 3.5 helical pitch and 0.75 second gantry rotation speed. Data from the artery dominant phase and the portal vein dominant phase were used to reconstruct the 3 D images.

For biliary imaging, in 38 cases, CT scan was acquired 30 minutes after intravenous infusion of 100ml of biliary contrast agent (Meglumine isotraxate, Biliscopin; Shering, Berlin, germany) at a rate of 0.1ml/sec (DIC-CT). In all 38 cases, DIC-CT and dynamic CT scan were performed on different days because of the possible accelerated adverse effects of the vascular and the biliary cotarst media. Each scan was performed with the same focus of view. In 14 cases having percutaneous transhepatic biliary drainage (PTBD) tube, biliary enhanced CT was performed after administering 3- 15 ml of 6 % biliary contrast agent (Biliscopin) through the PTBD tube (PTBD-CT). The adequate volume of contrast agent was determined by the previously performed PTBD cholangiography. MDCT cholangiography was performed by intravenous injection of a biliary contrast agent in 38 cases, and by injection from percutaneous biliary drainage tube in 14.

4. Image interpretation

Analysis of the image data was performed based on source images and 3D postprocessing images on commercially available workstations (Intage rvse, KGT, Tokyo and VertualPlace, AZE, Osaka). 3D reconstruction of the hepatic vasculature was made using a volume rendering algorithm. The volume rendered images were obtained in projections selected to depict the course of hepatic vasculature best. The resulting 3D images of the hepatic artery, portal vein and the bile duct rendered for each step of the artery dominant phase, portal vein dominant phase and the DIC-CT/PTBD-CT respectively were carefully reviewed and compared with the axial source images to ensure that no important structure was inadvertently deleted from the 3D images. 3D images of the hepatic artery, portal vein and the bile duct (Fig 1-A, Fig 1-B, Fig 1-C) which were adjusted to position each other focusing at the hepatic hilum on 2D axillary, sagital and coronary imaging sequences, were further integrated into a single image (Fig 1-D).

5. Diagnostic examination

In 52 of the 66 evaluated patients, the MD-CT studies were considered as diagnostic. The study was not diagnostic in the remaining 14 patients because of the poor timing of the contrast and image acquisition. 5 patients had poor arterial phase images, 13 had poor biliary images and 4 had both. Portal imaging was satisfactory in all patients.

The advantages of MD-CT are mainly faster capability, improved temporal resolusion, improved spatial resolusion and increased effectiveness of the intravascular contrast agent. Reliability of the 3D MD-CT on the anatomical evaluation has been reported in several articles[5,6,9,10)]. However, a problem is that 3D reconstruction imaging does not protect

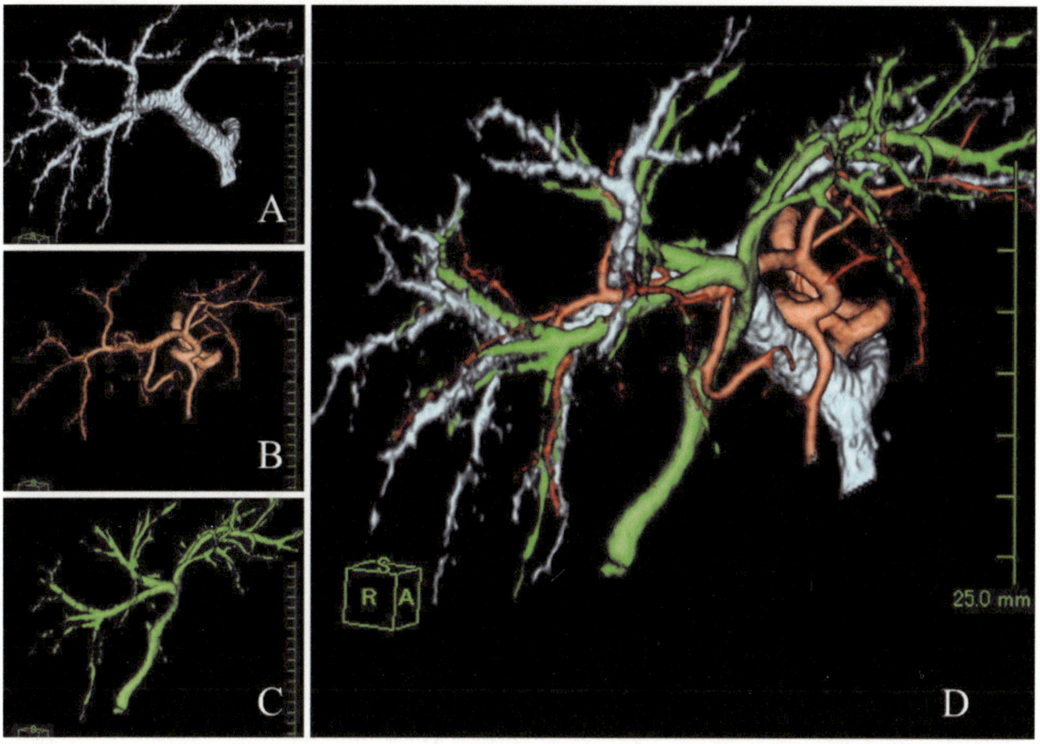

A:portogram reconstructed from portal dominant phase data, B:angiogram reconstructed from artery dominant phase data, C:cholangiogram reconstructed from DIC-CT data, D:integrated image of the 3Dportogram, angiogram and cholangiogram

Fig. 1. Integrated 3D image of vasculature and biliary system

against potential misinterpretation during post-processing. To increase the reliability of vascular imaging, authors, who are an expert in the anatomy of hepatic structures, checked and pick up the missing branches on sequential 2D images after automatic reconstruction of 3D vascular images.

6. Anatomical variant of portal veins

Ramification pattern of the right portal vein was defined into 5 types according to Nakamura's classification[11] (Figure 2). It is reported that ramification of the portal vein has a few anomalies compared with the bile duct and the artery [6]. Nevertheless, as to the right lateral portal vein (RLP), the single portal vein cases were only 30 cases, 57.7% and others had dual RLPs with (10 cases, 19.2%) or without (12, 23.1%) a common ostia at origin (Fig. 3).

7. Anatomical variant of biliary system

The pattern of branching of the biliary system in the right lobe is classified into 7, based on tributary from the right lateral sector (Figure 4). 49 cases have single right lateral duct (RLD), and 3 have dual RLDs. Pattern I is normal anatomy in which RLD and the right

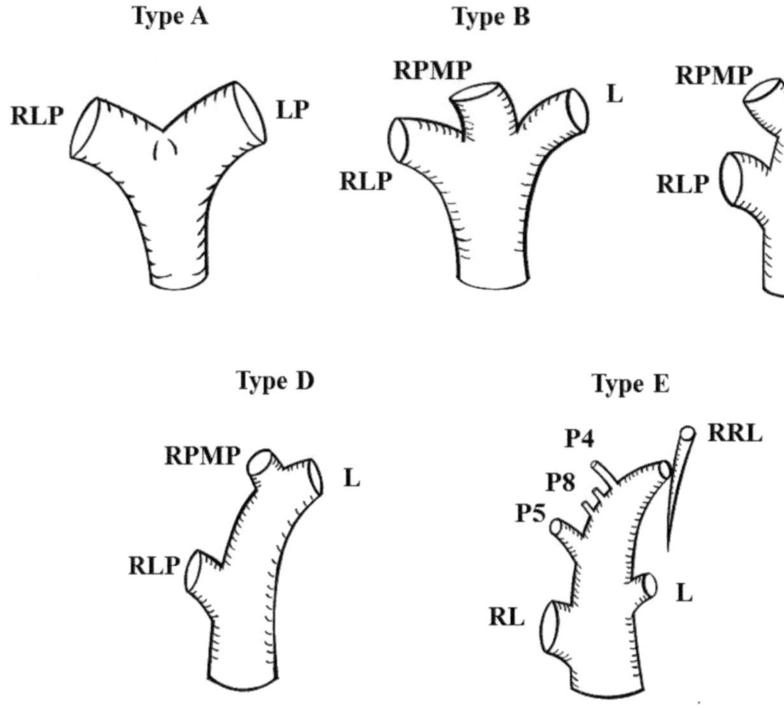

Type A: 42cases, 80.8%, type B: 3 cases, 5.8%, Type C: 6 cases, 11.5%, Type D: 1 cases, 1.9%, Type E: 0 cases
*RPMP: right paramedian portal vein, RLP: right lateral portal vein, RP: right portal vein, LP: left portal vein, P5:portal vein for the segment 5, P8: portal vein for the segment 8, P4: portal vein for the segment 4, RRL: right sided round ligament

Fig. 2. Ramification pattern of portal vein for the right lobe

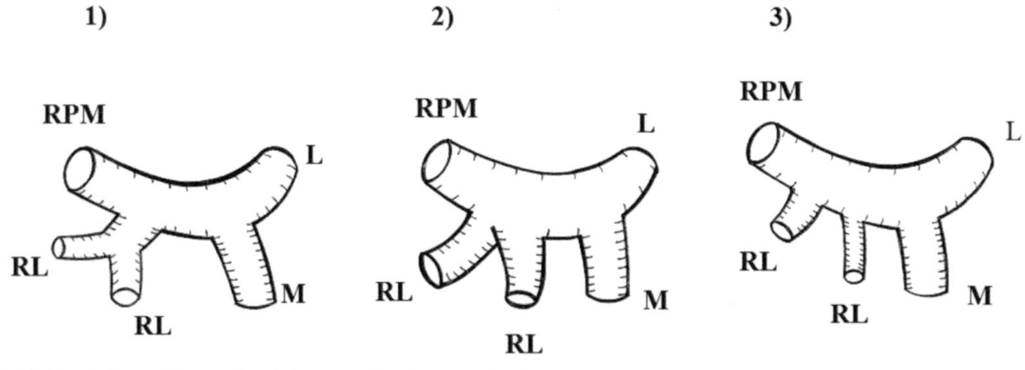

1) RLP originated from the right portal vein as a single trunk: 30 cases, 57.7%, 2) dual RLPs originate from the right portal vein by a common ostia: 10 cases, 19.2%, 3) dual RLPs originate from the right portal vein independently through separate ostia: 12 cases, 23.1%
*RPMP: right paramedian portal vein, RLP: right lateral portal vein, MP: main portal vein, LP: left portal vein

Fig. 3. Anatomical variants of right lateral portal vein

paramedian duct (RPMD) join to form the right hepatic duct which further joins the left hepatic duct to form the common hepatic duct. Pattern II is trifurcation of RL, RPMD and the left hepatic duct. In Pattern III, RLD joins the left hepatic duct. Pattern IV is the joining of RLD to the common hepatic duct. Pattern V, VI and VII are dual RLDs. Pattern V is dual RLD insertion into RPMD independently. In Pattern VI, there are two right hepatic ducts each formed by the joining of separate RPMD and RLD. Pattern VII is multiple RLDs and RPMDs. Incidence of each type in our series were Pattern I: 33 patients, 63.5%, Pattern II: 8, 15.4%, Pattern III: 5, 9.6%, Pattern IV: 3, 5.8%, Pattern V: 1, 1.9%, Pattern VI: 1, 1.9% and Pattern VII: 1, 1.9%.

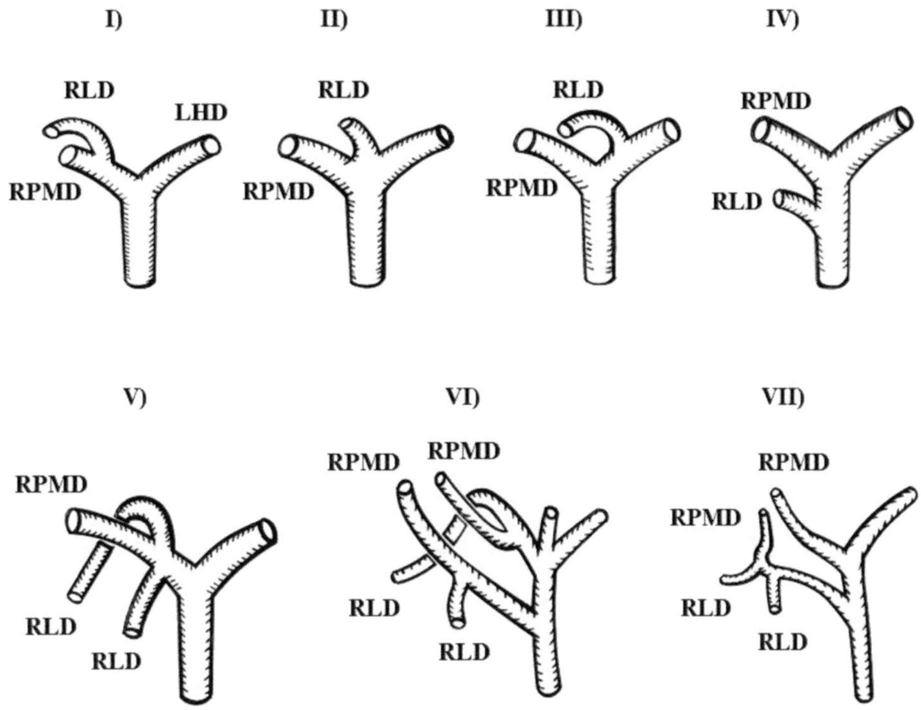

I) normal anatomy: 33 cases, 63.5%, II) trifurcation: 8 cases, 15.4%, III) RLD joins the left hepatic duct: 5 cases, 9.6%, IV) RLD joins the common hepatic duct: 3 cases, 5.8%, V) dual RLDs insert to RPMD independently: 1 case, 1.9%, VI) two right hepatic ducts each is formed by the joining of separate RPMD and RLD: 1 case, 1.9%, VII) multiple RLDs and RPMDs: 1 case, 1.9%
*RPMD: right paramedian duct, RLD: right lateral duct, LHD: left hepatic duct

Fig. 4. Anatomical variants of right lateral bile duct

8. Anatomical variant of arteries

The branching pattern of the right lateral artery (RLA) is demonstrated in Figure 5. The single RLA was observed in 38 patients (73.1%) and dual RLAs in 14 (26.9%). A single RLA arising from the right hepatic artery was seen in 33 patients. RLA was originating from a replaced right hepatic artery from the superior mesenteric artery in 3 patients and from the gastroduodenal artery in one patient. RLA arising from the middle hepatic artery as an accessory artery was seen in another patient (Fig.5-d). Among patients with dual RLAs, in 9, arteries were originating independently from the right hepatic artery (Fig.5-e). In 4 patients, dual arteries were taking off independently from the replaced right hepatic artery from the superior mesenteric artery (Fig.5-f). Combined supply from a right lateral branch of the right hepatic artery and a branch of the gastroduodenal artery was also seen in another patient (Fig5-g).

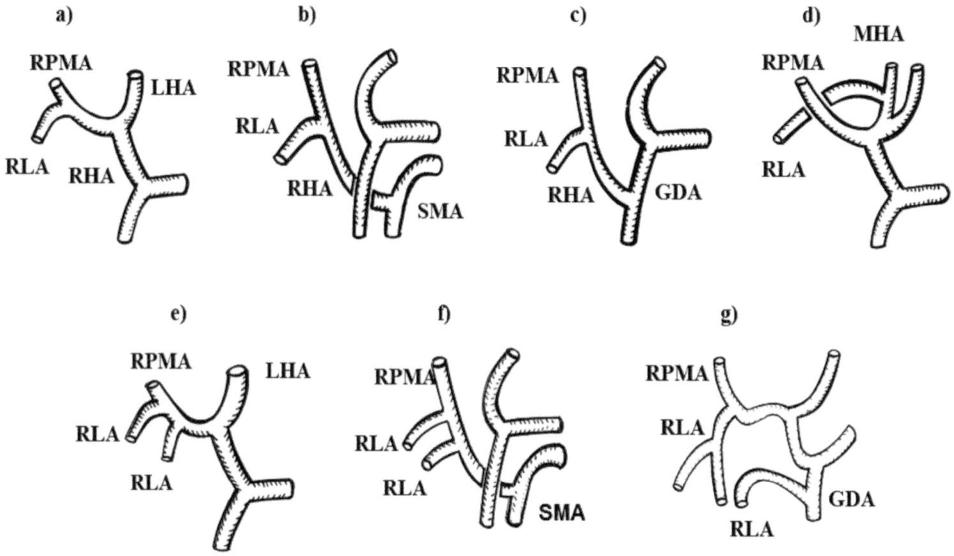

a) normal anatomy:33 cases, 63.5%, b) RLA from replaced RHA from SMA: 3 cases, 5.8%, c) RLA from replaced RHA from GDA: 1 cases, 1.9%, d) RLA from MHA: 1 case, 1.9%, e) dual RLAs from RHA: 9 cases, 17.3%, f) dual RLAs from replaced SMA: 4 cases, 7.7%, g) dual RHAs from RHA and from GDA: 1 case, 1.9%

*RLA: right lateral artery, RPMA: right paramedian artery, RHA: right hepatic artery, SMA: superior or mesenteric artery, MHA: middle hepatic artery, GDA: gastroduodenal artery

Fig. 5. Anatomical variants of right lateral artery

9. 3D relationship of the artery, bile duct and portal vein for right lateral sector

3 D relationship of the artery and bile duct to the right lateral sector with reference to the portal vein branches were studied. We defined the right lateral bile duct/artery which run dorsally and superiorly to RMPV as a 'north-turning' duct/artery and the bile duct/artery which run ventrally and inferiorly to the right portal vein and RMPV was defined as a 'south-turning' duct/artery[12] (Fig 6). In 49 patients with single RLD, 44 had the 'north-turning' duct and 5 had the 'south-turning' duct. In 3 patients with multiple RLDs, one had both of 'south-turning' variety and the other two showed a combination of 'north-turning' and 'south-turning' ducts. Among 38 cases of single RLA, 8 had 'north-turning' artery and 30 had 'south-turning' artery. Out of 14 dual RLAs cases, in 6, a combination of 'north-turning' and 'south-turning' arteries were observed. In the remaining 8 cases, all demonstrated 'south turning' arteries.

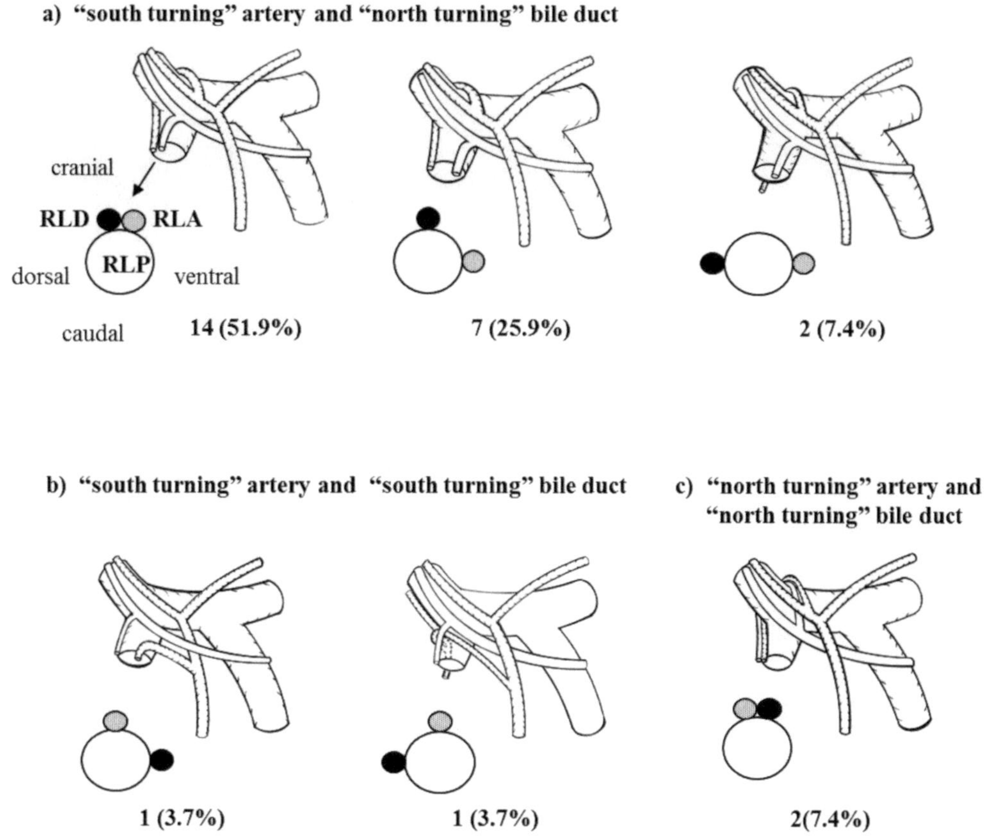

*RPD: right paramedian duct, RLD: right lateral duct, RPMP: right paramedian portal vein, RLP: right lateral portal vein

Fig. 6. Running pattern of the light lateral duct/artery

In 27 patients of the single artery-bile duct- portal vein for the right lateral sector, the combination of "south-turning" artery and "north turning" bile duct was the most frequent pattern (22 cases) (Fig. 7). In all of them, the artery was running cranial or ventral to the bile duct and the portal vein at the sectional plane of origin of RLPV. The bile duct was sited cranial to the portal vein in 20 cases and dorsal in 2. The "south turning" artery – "south turning" bile duct combination was observed in 3 cases and the "north-turning" artery - "south-turning" bile duct combination in two. Among these patients with these two patterns, 4 had the artery sited dorsally or cranially to the bile duct.

10. Application for right lateral sector transplantation

Although reconstruction of multiple portal veins and bile ducts has been challenging in LDLT, it is recently reported that multiple branches can be reconstructed safely using technical modifications in the right lobe or left lobe graft transplantation. Kyoto team reported that dual portal branches can be reconstructed safely with or without interposed venous graft[11]. They also described that all the biliary variants were successfully reconstructed with an acceptable complication rate, those are 9.3% bile leaks and 8.5% of

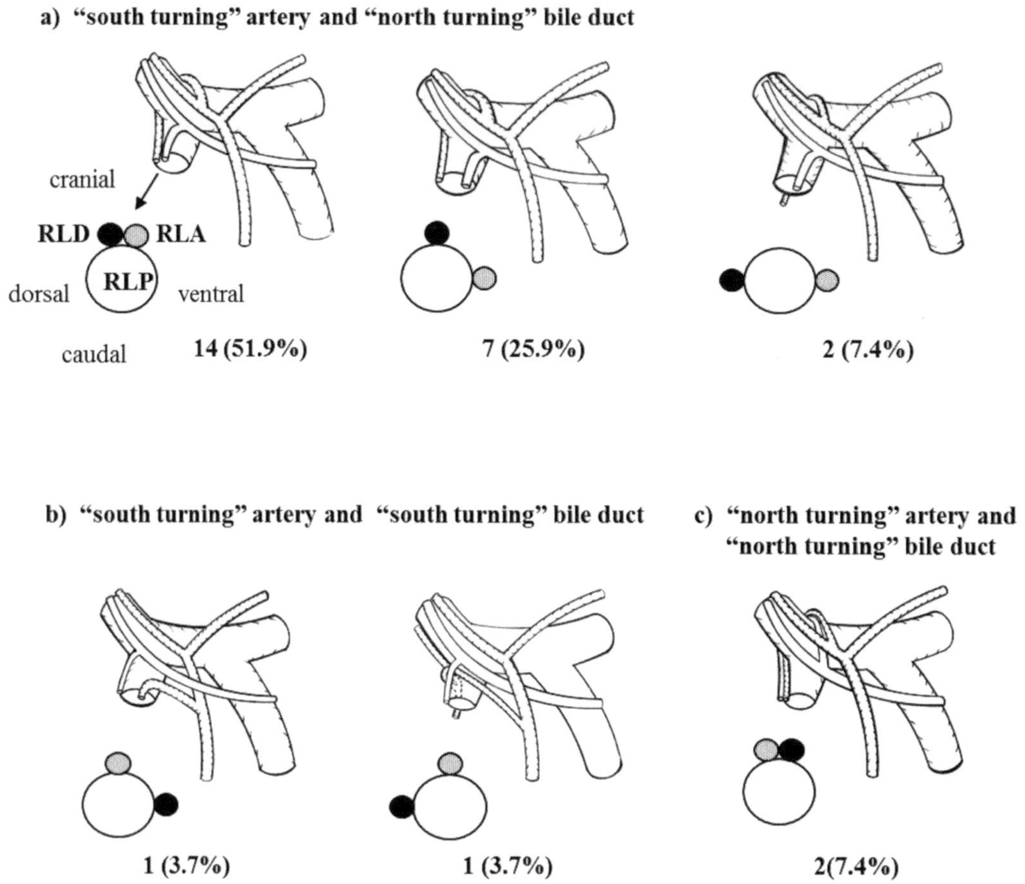

a) "south-turning" artery and "north-turning" bile duct; both artery and bile duct run through the cranial side of RLP: 13 cases, 48.1%, artery runs through the ventral side with bile duct running through cranial side: 7 cases, 25.9%, and with bile duct running through the dorsal side: 2 cases, 7.4%
b) "south-turning" artery runs through the cranial side with "south-turning" bile duct running through the ventral side: 2 cases (7.4%), and with bile duct running through the dorsal side: 1 case, 3.7%
c) "north-turning" artery runs through the cranial with "north-turning" bile duct running through the cranial side: 2 cases, 7.4%
*RLA: right lateral artery, RLD: right lateral duct, RLP: right lateral portal vein

Fig. 7. 3D relationship of artery, bile duct and portal vein for right lateral sector, Scheme of the sectional plane of the orifice of RLP are presented at the right inferior corner of each figure.

stenosis, in grafts with multiple biliary orifices. However, the branches of portal vein and bile duct for right lateral sector are smaller and its variants are more complicated. In dual duct cases especially when one duct runs dorsally to RLPV and other ventrally, reconstruction of dual ducts partitioned by the portal vein should be unacceptably difficult. We observed 2 cases with this anomaly. Even in the cases of single RLD, 3 cases had RLD run dorsal side of the RLPV. This anomaly is also difficult to be reconstructed because duct reconstruction should be interfered by the ventrally located RLPV.

This study revealed 14 cases, 26.9%, had dual RLA. The branch or branches for the right lateral sector are thinner and shorter than those of the right lobe graft or left lobe graft. Reconstruction of all dual arteries may be difficult in right lateral sector transplant. How to reconstruct multiple graft arteries remains controversial. Some institution recommended that livers with aberrant arteries should not to be used because these graft require multiple arterial reconstructions with high incidence of postoperative arterial thrombosis[13-15]. On the other hand, Ikegami et al.[16] recommended to reconstruct only thickest artery if intraoperative doppler shows pulsatile arterial flow and arterial signal in the corresponding segment of the non-anastomosed arteries. Even though, preoperative precise identification of the arterial variants by imaging and the accurate assessment of the feasibility are essential components of a successful right lateral graft LDLT.

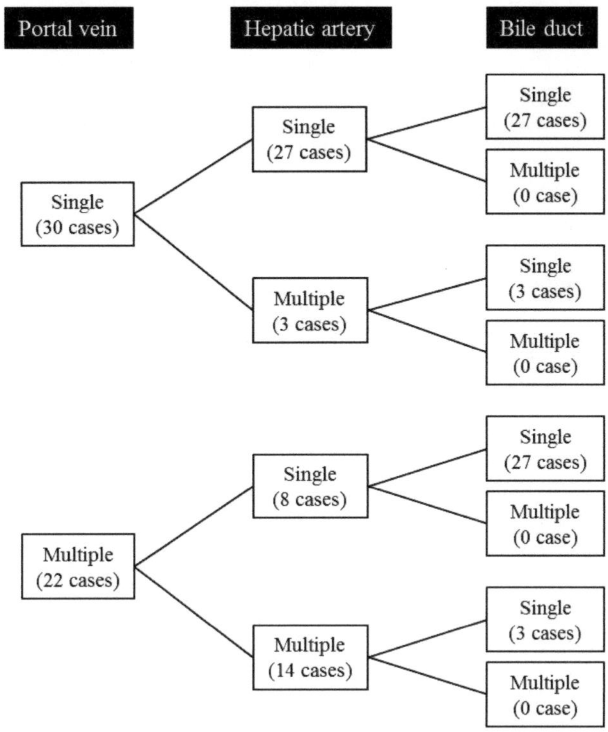

Fig. 8. Combination of anatomical variants of right lateral portal vein, bile duct and artery

11. Conclusion

In 9-18% of potential donors, the right lateral sector has volumetric advantage compared to the left lobe[2,3]. However, anomalies of the hepatic vasculature cause further limitation for the feasibility of transplantation. In our study, cases having single portal vein, single artery and single bile duct are only 27 among 52 (Fig.8). Therefore, to increase safe right lateral sector LDLT and to overcome donor shortage, accurate preoperative anatomical evaluation and excellent surgical technique coping with the particular anatomical variants are required. Anatomical understanding based on the 2D images is not sufficient[8]. The understanding of the 3D vascular and biliary anatomy will contribute to a better definition of the anatomical contraindications for transplantation, and to achieve successful right lateral sector LDLT.

12. References

[1] Sugawara Y, Makuuchi M, Takayama T, Mizuta K, Kawarasaki H, Imamura H, Hashizume K. Liver transplantation using a right lateral sector graft from a living donor to her granddaughter. Hepatogastroenterology. 2001;48:261-263

[2] Hwang S, Lee SG, Lee YJ, et al. Donor selection for procurement of right posterior segment graft in living donor liver transplantation. Liver Transpl. 2004;10:1150-1155.

[3] Leelaudomlipi S, Sugawara Y, Kaneko J, Matsui Y, Ohkubo T, Makuuchi M. Volumetric analysis of liver Segment in 155 living donors. Liver transpl. 2002;8:612-614

[4] Imamura H, Makuuchi M, Sakamoto Y, Sugawara Y, Kawasaki S, Takayama T. Anatomical keys and pitfalls in living donor liver transplantation. J Hepatobiliary Pancreat Surg 2000;7:380-394

[5] Sakai H, Okuda K, Yasunaga M, Kinoshita H, Aoyagi S. Reliability of hepatic artery configuration in 3D CT angiography compared with conventional angiography--special reference to living-related liver transplant donors. Transpl Int. 2005;18:499-505

[6] Schroeder T, Radtke A, Kuehl H, Debatin JF, Malago M, Ruehm SG. Evaluation of living liver donors with an all-inclusive 3D multi-detector row CT protocol. Radiology. 2006;238:900-910

[7] Uchida M, Ishibashi M, Sakoda J, Azuma S, Nagata S, Hayabuchi N. CT image fusion for 3D depiction of anatomic abnormalities of the hepatic hilum. AJR 2007;189:W184-W191

[8] Beermann J, Tetzlaff R, Bruckner T, et al. Three-dimensional visualization improves understanding of surgical liver anatomy. Medical Education 2010; 44: 936-940

[9] Chen YF, Lee TY, Chen CL, Huang TL, Chen YS, Lui CC. Three-dimensional helical computed tomographic cholangiography: application to living related hepatic transplantation. Clin Transplant. 1997 11:209-213

[10] Yeh BM, Breiman RS, Taouli B, Qayyum A, Roberts JP, Coakley FV. Biliary tract depiction in living potential liver donors: comparison of conventional MR, mangafodipir trisodium-enhanced excretory MR, and multi-detector row CT cholangiography--initial experience. Radiology. 2004;230:645-651.

[11] Nakamura T, Tanaka K, Kiuchi T, et al. Anatomical variations and surgical strategies in right lobe living donor liver transplantation: lessons from 120 cases. Transplantation 2002;73:1896-1903.

[12] Kawarada Y, Das BC, Taoka H. Anatomy of the hepatic hilar area: the plate system. J Hepatobiliary Pancreat Surg 2000;7:580-586

[13] Soin AS, Friend PJ, Rasmussen A, et al. Donor arterial variations in liver transplantation: management and outcome of 527 consecutive grafts. Br J Surg 1996;83:637-41

[14] Kosteric JK, Piper JB, Leef JA, et al. Angiographic selection criteria for living related liver transplantation. Am J Roenterol 1996;166:1103-1108

[15] Broelsch CE, Whitington PF, Emond JC, et al. Liver transplantation in children from living related donors. Surgical techniques and results. Ann Surg 1991 214:428-437

[16] Ikegami T, Hashikura Y, Nakazawa Y, et al. Risk factors contributing to hepatic artery thrombosis following living-donor liver transplantation. J Hepatoboliary Pancret Surg 2006;13:105-109

12

Fully Automatic Technique for Liver Segmentation from Abdominal CT Scan with Knowledge-Based Constraints

Nader H. Abdel-massieh
Menoufia University
Egypt

1. Introduction

The proposed fully automatic technique and method to segment liver structure is divided into two sections: first section is *Pre processing steps and rough (initial) segmentation;* the second section is *refined segmentation (snake step),* see Figure 1. The proposed automatic technique to detect tumor in liver parenchyma is also divided into two sections: first section

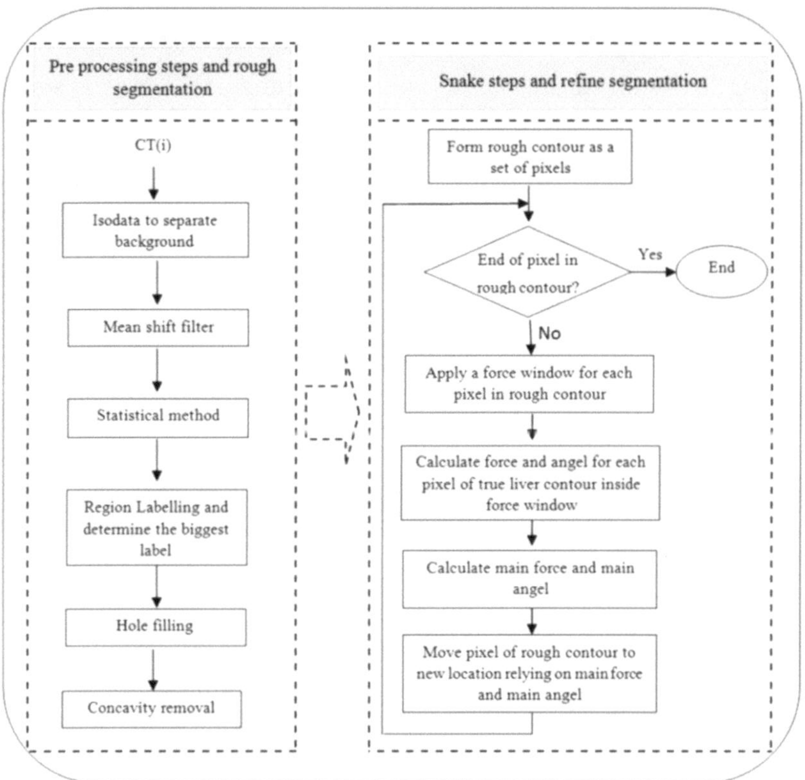

Fig. 1. Block diagram for the proposed fully automatic liver segmentation technique

liver tumor segmentation to detect any lesions; the second sections is *tumor classification* to differentiate between possible tumor and any other defect in CT slices, see Figure 2.

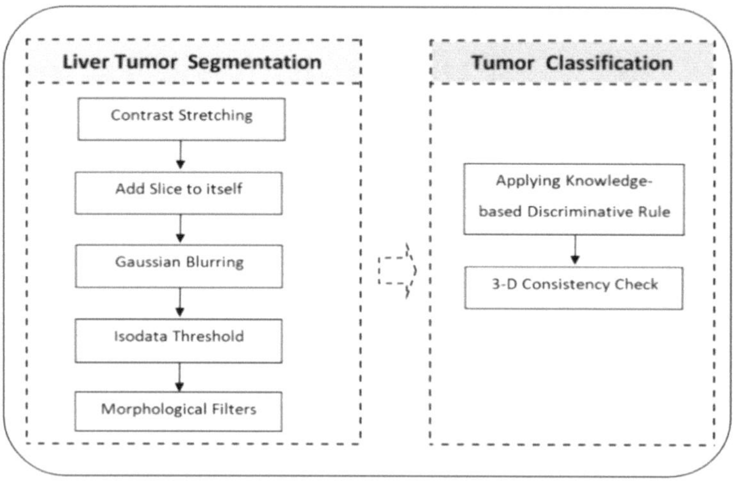

Fig. 2. Block diagram of the proposed automatic liver tumor detection technique

2. Liver segmentation

2.1 Preprocessing and rough segmentation

2.1.1 Isodata

Before beginning the rough segmentation, the background of CT slice is separated using Isodata algorithm which it is one of the thresholding segmentation techniques. Isodata stands for Iterative Self-Organizing Data Analysis Techniques. The threshold is chosen from the brightness histogram of CT slice. The histogram is initially segmented into two parts using a starting threshold value such as θ_0 (where θ is threshold value), half the maximum dynamic range. The sample mean $(m_f, 0)$ of the gray values associated with the foreground pixels and the sample mean $(m_b, 0)$ of the gray values associated with the background pixels are computed, see Figure 3. A new threshold value θ_1 is now computed as the average of these two sample means. The process is repeated, based upon the new threshold, until the threshold value does not change any more. In formula:

$$\theta_k = \frac{m_{f,k-1} + m_{b,k-1}}{2} \quad until\ \theta_k = \theta_{k-1} \tag{1}$$

After applying Isodata algorithm the outer area around patient's body will be eliminated, as seen in Figure 4. , and this help in the reduction in computation time needed for following steps.

2.1.2 Mean shift filter

In order to remove noise caused by patient breathing and the defects of CT scanner, Figure 5. Mean shift filter is used for edge-preserving smoothing. Convolution and rank filters (such as median filter, mean filter, etc.) could reduced the image noise, but they do not preserve the details and will blur the edges as well.

Mean Shift is a powerful and versatile non parametric iterative algorithm that can be used for lot of purposes like finding modes, clustering, edges etc. Mean Shift was introduced in Fukunaga and Hostetler and has been extended to be applicable in other fields of

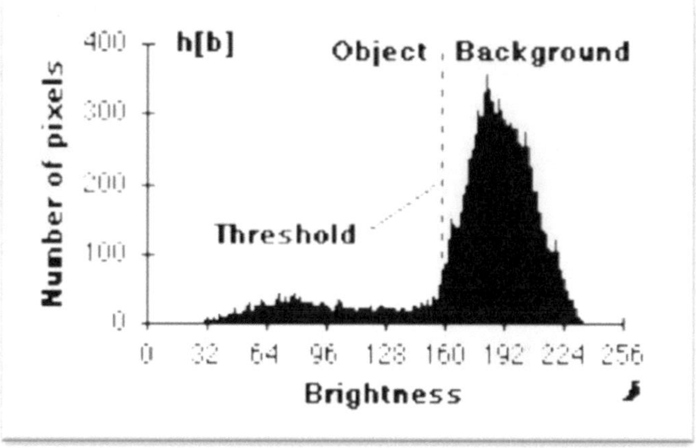

Fig. 3. An example of brightness histogram

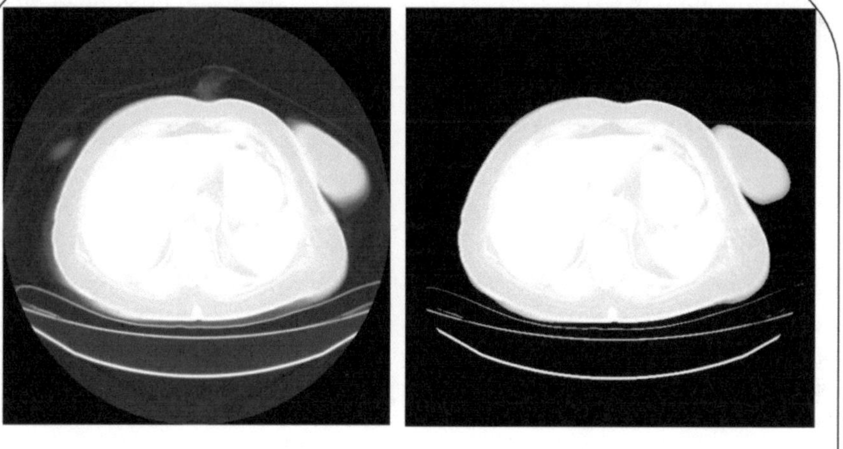

(a) Original CT image before background separation

(b) CT image after applying Isodata

Fig. 4. Block diagram of the proposed automatic liver tumor detection technique

Computer Vision. Mean shift filtering is a data clustering algorithm commonly used in computer vision and image processing. For each pixel of an image (having a spatial location and a particular color), the set of neighboring pixels (within a spatial radius and a defined color distance) is determined. For this set of neighbor pixels, the new spatial center (spatial mean) and the new color mean value are calculated. These calculated mean values will serve as the new center for the next iteration. The described procedure will be iterated until the mean of both spatial and the color (or grayscale) stops changing. At the end of the iteration, the final mean color will be assigned to the starting position of that iteration.

Given an image map $I(i,j)$ (matrix of which each element represents its corresponding pixel's grey level intensity), a set of data points can be constructed by simply assigning each pixel's location in the map as the first two coordinates, and setting the third coordinate to be the normalized value of the pixel's intensity: for the (i,j) th pixel of the image, the corresponding data point will be:

$$I(i,j) \longrightarrow (i,j,I(i,j) * C) \quad (2)$$

where C is the normalization constant, chosen to be - [average of width and height of image]/[max intensity]:

$$C = \frac{height + width}{2} \times \frac{1}{255} \quad (3)$$

The mean shift iteration can be given explicitly by:

$$y_{k+1} = \frac{1}{n_k} \sum_{X_i \in S_h(y_k)} X_i \quad (4)$$

In the $(k+1)$ th iteration, we shift the current location by the mean position of all data points contained within the sphere of radius h, centered at y_k .

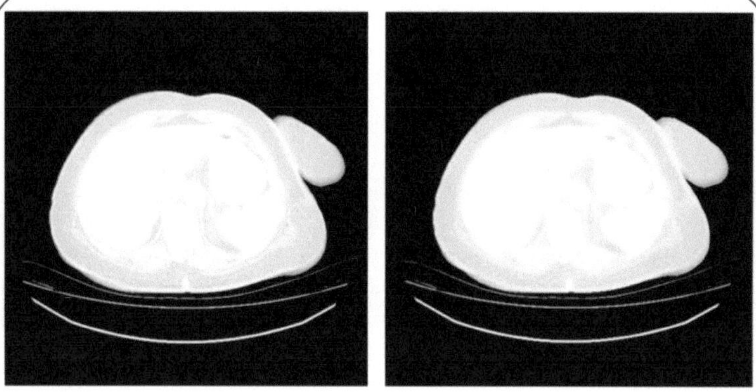

(a)CT image before applying Mean Shift (b)CT image after applying Mean Shift

Fig. 5. CT slice before and after Mean Shift smoothing

2.1.3 Statistical model

A 3D approach based on statistical information of images and associated to an adaptive threshold technique was implemented in order to recognize the voxels belonging to the liver tissue.

Proper identification of a specific region of interest (ROI) and corresponding definition of the reference key statistics are often crucial points for full automation of algorithms. A technique was developed to find fully automatically this ROI for preventing user dependencies. The proposed algorithm identifies the most liver representative region in the volume dataset as described in the following.

First, each slice of the pre-processed volume is divided into 64 squared regions, as shown in Figure 6., on which the mean image intensity and its standard deviation are calculated (the number and size of these regions had been chosen based on the statistical relevance of estimation samples).

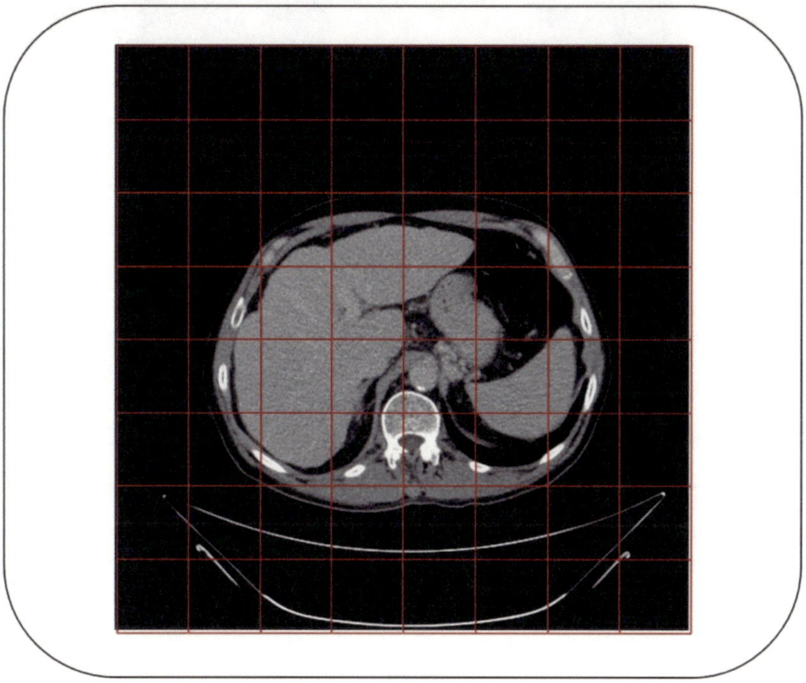

Fig. 6. CT slice is divided into 64 squared regions

Then, the internal abdominal regions having minimal standard deviation (defined as those values lower than 1% of the peak value of corresponding histogram without background) are separated from all volume slices and sorted out in ascending order of mean values. Since the liver is the biggest organ of the abdomen and is homogeneous in terms of image intensity, the great majority of those regions belong to the liver, as shown in Figure 7. Therefore, the μ_{ROI} representing the liver tissue is finally selected in this group by choosing the region with the median value of the above-mentioned homogeneous μ_{ROIs}.
Its statistical information permitted to implement an automatic adaptive histogram-based thresholding technique used to partition images. Therefore, liver voxel recognition depends on patient-specific image datasets since it is calculated automatically through the statistics of the ROI, and not from general learning data analysis. In this work, the threshold was evaluated by using the mean μ_{ROI} and the standard deviation σ_{ROI}. Then, a gate function G is applied to the volume to select the voxels belonging to the liver tissue in function of their image intensity value, defined as follows:

$$G(x,y,z) = \begin{cases} 1 & if\ \mu_{ROI} - 2\sigma_{ROI} \leq I(x,y,z) \leq \mu_{ROI} + 2\sigma_{ROI} \\ 0 & else \end{cases} \tag{5}$$

where $I(x,y,z)$ is the volume intensity value of the voxel (x,y,z) in the mean shift-filtered image.

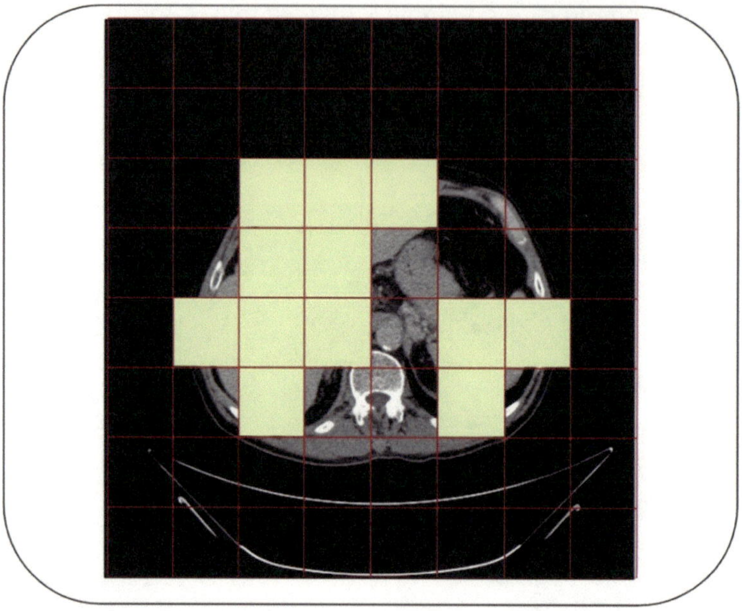

Fig. 7. Determining the squared regions with calculated liver mean (μ_{ROI})

The result of statistical method is a binary image with liver and some parts of organ with similar gray level as black blobs on white background see Figure 8.

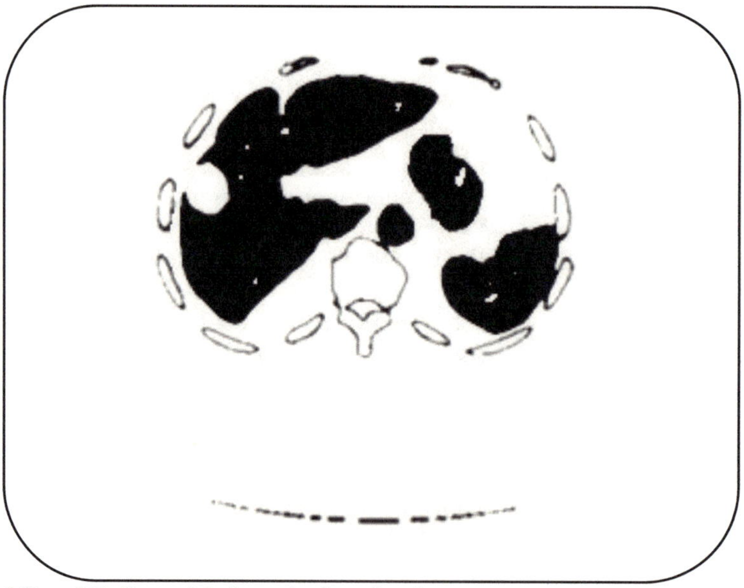

Fig. 8. Thresholding CT slice with the calculated value μ_{ROI}

2.1.4 Region labeling

In this step, liver is needed to be extracted from other blobs which are the other tissues and organs that share same gray level and turned to be binary. A knowledge-based rule that in the main slice, where liver is as big as possible, liver structure is the biggest organ in the slice; and so in order to extract the liver region labeling algorithm is used and the biggest label will be that of liver, as shown in Figure 9.

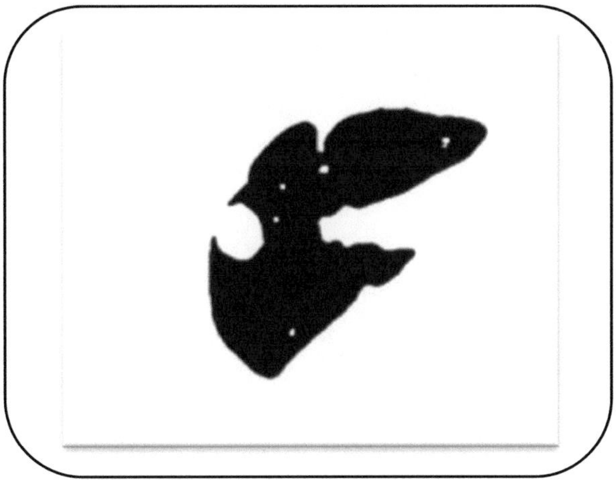

Fig. 9. Labeling the biggest blob

2.1.5 Holes filling

The output of last stage is a black structure with is mostly liver along with some neighboring tissue attached to it because it has close gray level on white background. This black structure contains holes due to existence of vessels, lesion or defects inside liver and when the gate function in statistical model stage is used the irregular pixels of lesion inside liver with will not be considered belonging to liver. The existence of these holes inside liver may hinder the work or snake algorithm that will be used later in following stage to refine final segmentation contour, see Figure 10.

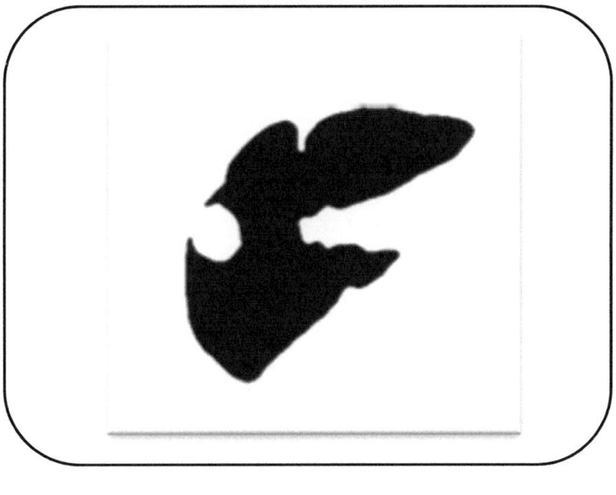

Fig. 10. Hole filling of liver structure

2.1.6 Concavity removal

One of the problems that face segmenting liver structure from CT images is the existence of tumor near the edge of liver. In this case, when applying the statistical method to discriminate liver parenchyma from other tissues, tumor tissue will be excluded and hence this will appear like a concave at the edge of segmented liver; That concave may hinder the grow of snake in a following step. A vacancy completely surrounded by liver tissue can be easily filled using simple region filling. However, cancerous tissue is often located adjacent to the border of the liver, as shown in Figure 11.; in this case the area cannot simply be filled as it is open on one side. The proposed method solves this problem using shape information, as the region near the missed area forms a shape like a bay and convex corners remain near the bay.

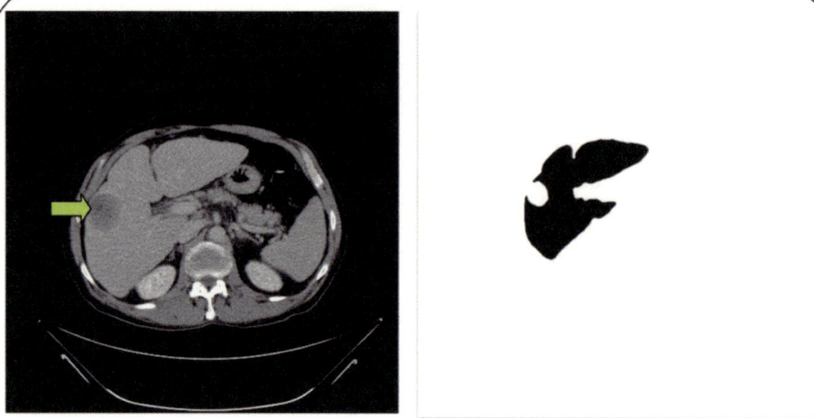

(a) Liver CT slice with tumor near edge (b) Thresholded liver CT slice with

Fig. 11. An example of concave near liver edge due to existence of tumor

Concavity removal consists of three steps; the first step is to identify the outstanding corners around liver structure; the second step is to specify the pair of corners near the missed concave, and the third is filling the missed region to completely recover the liver.

a. *Identifying the outstanding corners*...The result of hole filling step is first smoothed; then we subtract the smoothed image from the original image (before smoothing) to have image of main corners as a result of subtraction, Figure 12.
b. *Specifying the pair of corners near the missed concave*...a line between each two pairs of corners is made, and for each line we check for two conditions :
   i. If the line wholly lies outside live structure.
   ii. If there is a vacant region inside the line. The vacant region is determined relaying on concavity rate which can be calculated using the formula:

$$Concavity\ ratio = \frac{length\ of\ perpendecular\ \text{line}\ between\ corners\ line\ and\ liver\ boundary}{distance\ between\ pair\ of\ corners} \tag{6}$$

If the concavity ratio exceeds 125% (empirically predefined value), that vacant is a concave that need to be filled. If there is a line meets these two conditions; that line is probably a line between two corners around concave, shown in Figure 13.

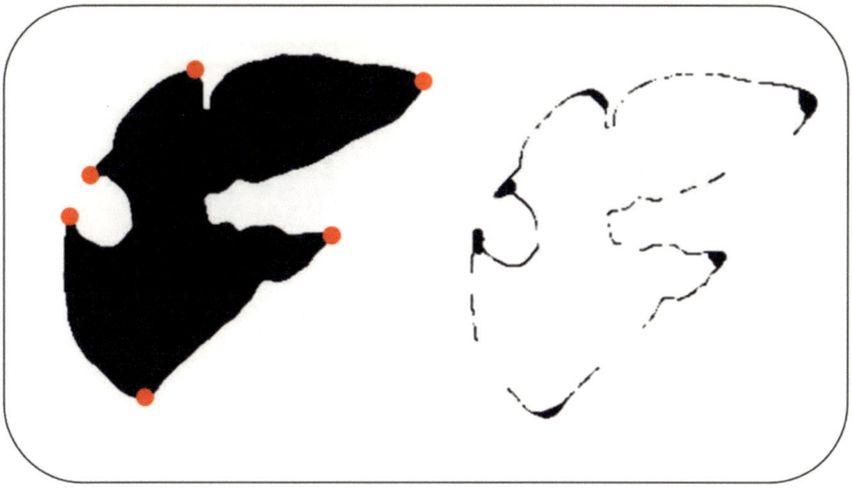

Fig. 12. Identifying the outstanding corners around liver structure

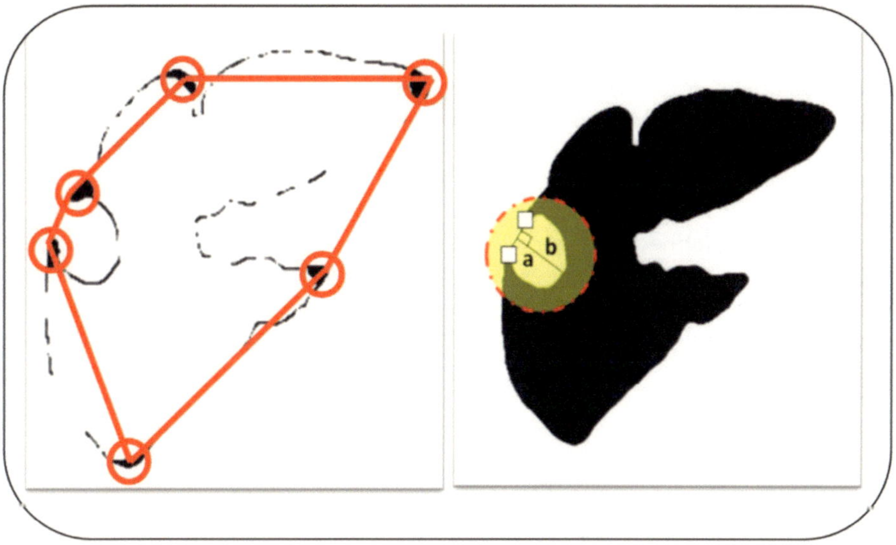

Fig. 13. Specifying the pair of corners near the missed concave

c. *Filling the missed region…* the pair of points will be linked by an arc (or line) and the region inside an arc is filled the diameter of the arc is determined from the diameter of liver border assuming that the left side of the liver border approximately forms an arc. Using these technique most of missed lesion areas can be successfully corrected.

2.2 Refined segmentation

2.2.1 Detection the initial contour

After filling the holes inside liver and the concaves near the outer edge of liver, a simple edge detection algorithm is needed to extract the edge of rough segmentation; then the edge

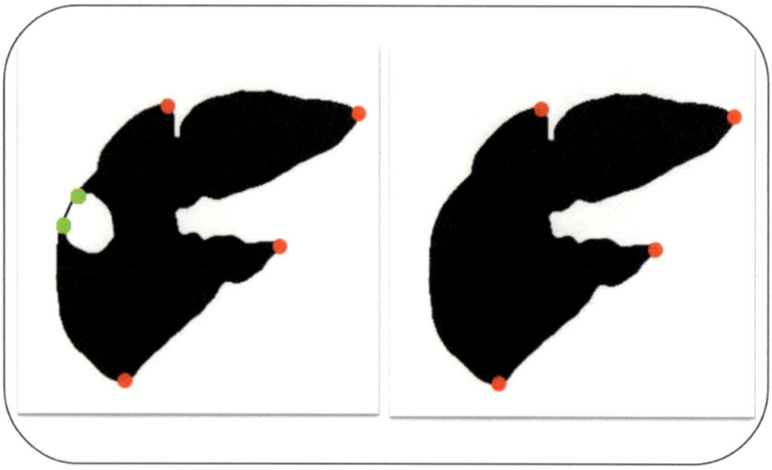

Fig. 14. Filling the concave in liver structure

is treated as a sequence of pixel. The rough segmented contour of liver will be refined in the next stage.

2.2.2 The proposed snake algorithm

The concept of active contours models was first introduced in 1987 and has later been developed by different researchers. An active contour is an energy minimizing spline that detects specified features within an image. It is a flexible curve which can be dynamically adapted to required edges or objects in the image.

It consists of a set of control points connected by straight lines, as it is showed in Figure 15. The active contour is defined by the number of control points as well as sequence of each other. Fitting active contours to shapes in images is an interactive process. The user must suggest an initial contour, which is quite close to the intended shape. The contour will then be attracted to features in the image extracted by internal energy creating an attractor image.

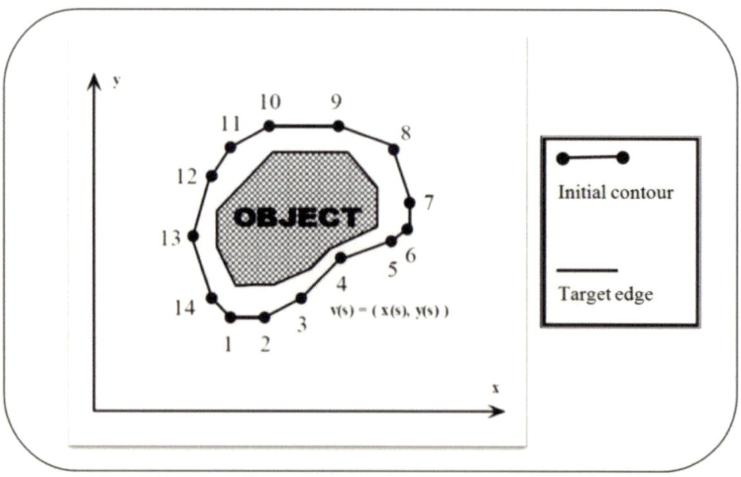

Fig. 15. Snake movement towards final edge

In this study the refinement to the rough segmentation is performed by a new proposed optimized snake technique. The proposed snake algorithm relies mainly on simple computed force not for the entire image, but for specific pixels in a window centered on each pixel of the initial contour; this process in done iteratively and in each iteration the window centered on pixels of initial contour is reduced as the contour approach the final edge of liver.
Snake algorithm begins by forming a window and center on each pixel of the initial contour. For each pixel of the final edge which intersects with the window centered on pixels of initial contour, a force is computed using the equation (7):

$$\text{force} = \frac{\text{constant}}{(\text{distance})^2} \tag{7}$$

$$\sin\theta = \frac{\text{opposite}}{\text{distance}} \tag{8}$$

$$\cos\theta = \frac{\text{beside}}{\text{distance}} \tag{9}$$

Then, for each pixel of the true contour of liver in the window we calculate the angels with the pixel of the rough contour centered in the window using the formulas (8) and (9) and as shown in Figure 16.

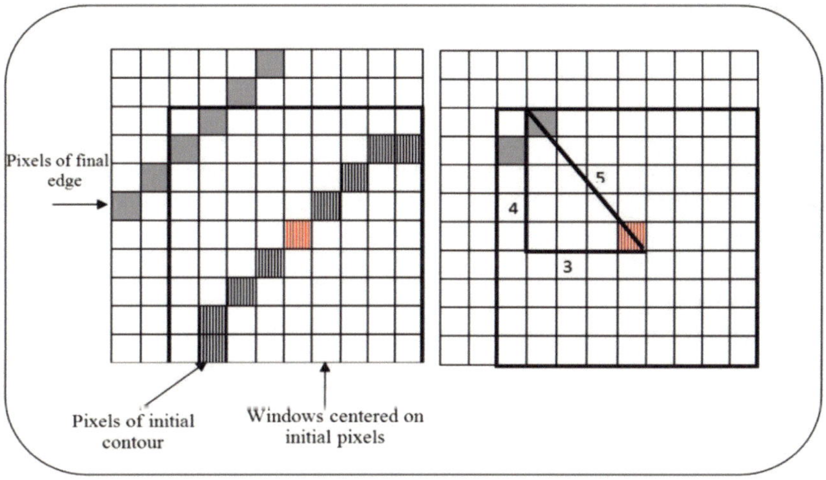

Fig. 16. Calculating force and angel for each pixel of true contour of liver

We use the force and the angel in order to calculate force at X and Y direction (X_f, Y_f) using formulas (10) and (11):

$$X_f = \text{force} \times \cos\theta \tag{10}$$

$$Y_f = \text{force} \times \sin\theta \tag{11}$$

Then we calculate main force and main angel for all pixels in true contour using formulas (12) and (13):

$$\text{main force} = \sqrt{\sum X_f + \sum Y_f} \tag{12}$$

$$\text{main angel} = \arctan(Y_f \,/\, X_f) \tag{13}$$

Using the calculated main force and the main angel, the pixel of initial contour will move to a new location approaching the final edge. The window move to the next pixel and the main force and main angel is calculated again for each pixel of the final edge which intersects with the window centered on the next pixel. After the window finish moving on all the pixels of the initial contour causing the pixels to move a step towards the final edge, the window will iterate over all the pixels of initial contour till it stops moving.

3. Liver tumor segmentation

3.1 Tumor detection

3.1.1 Contrast stretching

Having segmented the liver structure in the CT image, the next step is to enhancing the contrast of the segmented slices as liver parenchyma and tumor tissue have similar gray levels. For selecting the stretching range, there is a trade-off between reducing the noise in the image and avoiding over-enhancement.

Linear contract stretching is used to increase the difference between liver tissue and tumors. Among several methods of contract stretching, such as Selective histogram equalization, direct stretching with the linear relationship, linear stretching according to the fitting curve and nonlinear stretching with the logarithmic transformation, direct stretching with the linear relationship shows good result, which can be performed with formula (14):

$$I' = \frac{I'_{max} - I'_{min}}{I_{max} - I_{min}} (I - I_{min}) + I'_{min} \tag{14}$$

where, Iand I' are the gray levels before and after transformation, respectively. I'_{max} and I'_{min} are the highest and lowest gray level after transformation, I_{max} and $I_{min}$are the maximum and minimum gray level in the liver region before the transformation, respectively.

3.1.2 Add slice to itself

After finishing with contrast enhancement stage, the difference in gray level between liver and tumor is now clear. The gray levels of liver parenchyma are higher than that of tumor tissue as shown in Figure 17. (b). The following step is to add the enhanced image to itself.

$$R(i,j) = I'(i,j) + I'(i,j) \tag{15}$$

After contrast enhancement the pixels of liver parenchyma is brighter, in range between 140 and 160, so that when the value of each pixel is added to itself the value of addition will reach 255 and will appear as white. On the other hand, the pixels which represent tumor tissue is dark with gray level in range between 15 to 40, and so when the value of each tumor pixel is added to itself according to formula (15), the result gray level will be between 30 to 80 appearing as dark spots as shown in Figure 18.

3.1.3 Gaussian blurring

The result of addition is image background as well liver tissue that appears as white background with some pepper noise, and tumors that appear as dark spots with range of

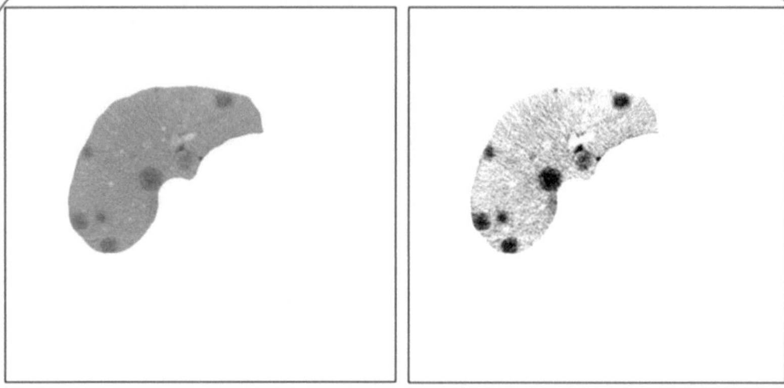

(a) Segmented liver from CT slice (b) Contrast enhanced slice

Fig. 17. CT slice before and after contrast enhancement

Fig. 18. Result of adding contrast enhanced image to itself

gray levels. In order to remove the noise and make the region of tumor more homogeneous as shown in Figure 19. (a), Gaussian smoothing is used as in formula (16), where x is the distance from the origin in the horizontal axis, y is the distance from the origin in the vertical axis, and σ is the standard deviation of the Gaussian distribution.

$$G(x, y) = \frac{1}{\sqrt{2\pi\sigma^2}} e^{-\frac{x^2+y^2}{2\sigma^2}} \tag{16}$$

3.1.4 Isodata threshold

As mentioned before, Isodata is a thresholding method which does not need a given threshold value instead the method automatically determine the optimal threshold value. The image after applying Gaussian blurring is a white background with gray blobs which represent liver tumor. When Isodata thresholding technique is applied, the gray blobs will be transformed to be black on white background as sown in Figure 19. (b).

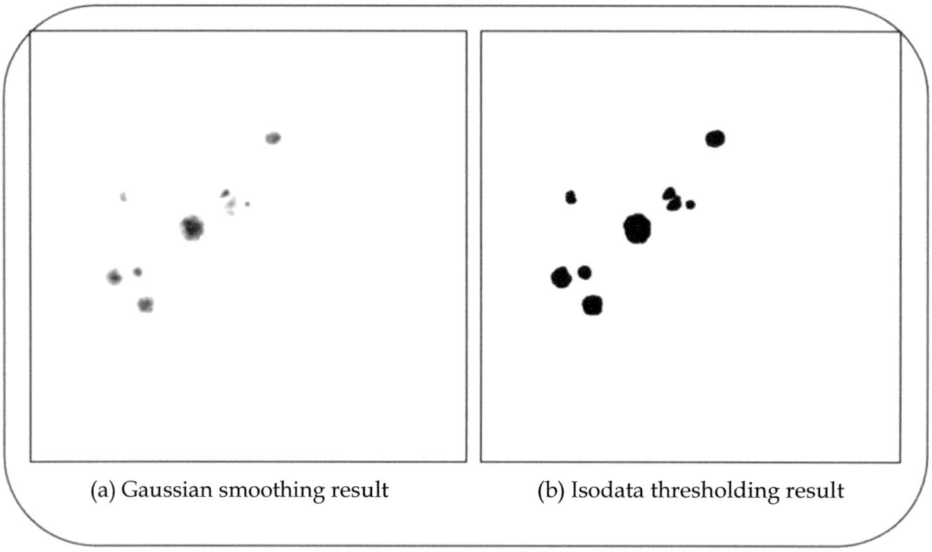

Fig. 19. CT slice before and after Isodata threshold

3.1.5 Morphological filters

When Isodata technique is applied the gray blob representing liver tumor along with some scattered noise gray pixels will be turned to black color. In order to remove the noise like pepper pixel, morphological erosion then dilation are used sequentially.

3.2 Tumor classification

3.2.1 Discriminative rule

The final stage is to eliminate the erroneous segmented tumors. In order to differentiate between a true segmented tumor and CT image defects, a discriminative rule is applied based on medical knowledge that lesion forms a circle-like mass. The circularity of the segmented mass can be defined as in formula number (17):

$$\text{Circularity} = \frac{\text{area of intersection between blob and circle}}{\text{area of formed circle}} \tag{17}$$

The area of the segmented blob is calculated, and then a circle with the same area of the blob is formed. We want to center the circle inside the blob so that all or majority of the circle will be inside the segmented blob. Although there are some algorithms used to detect the center of a blob, yet the irregular shape of blobs may cause misleading result. A simple but effective technique is used; we centered the circle on each pixel of the blob and calculate the intersection between the circle and the blob, we scan with the circle till we get the largest intersection area; hence the center of the blob is obtained. If the circularity is more than 85%, the segmented blob will be considered as circle-like shape and so it is probably a tumor, as shown in Figure 20.

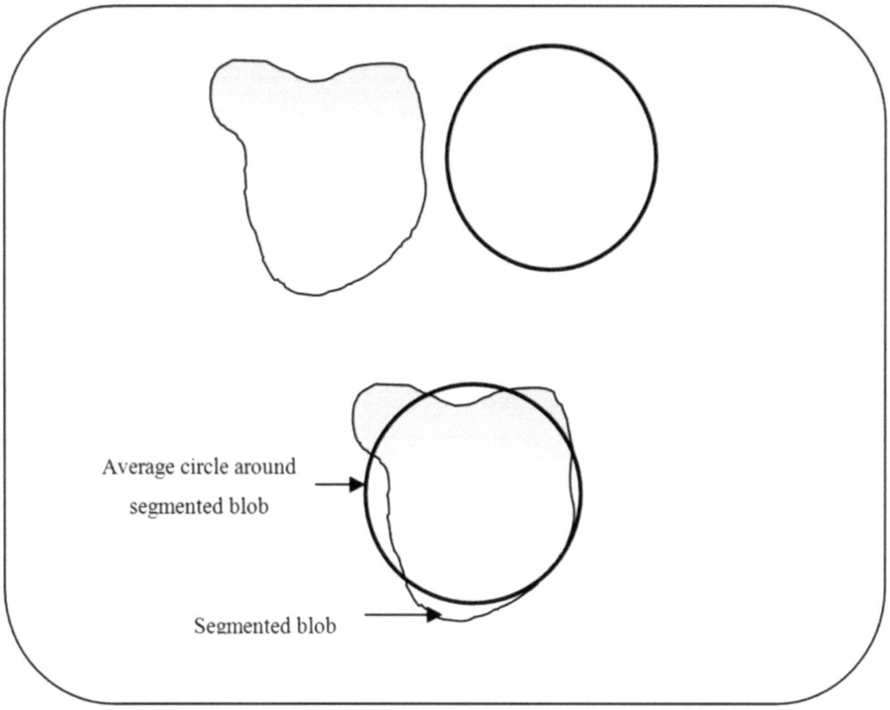

Fig. 20. Knowledge-based circularity rule

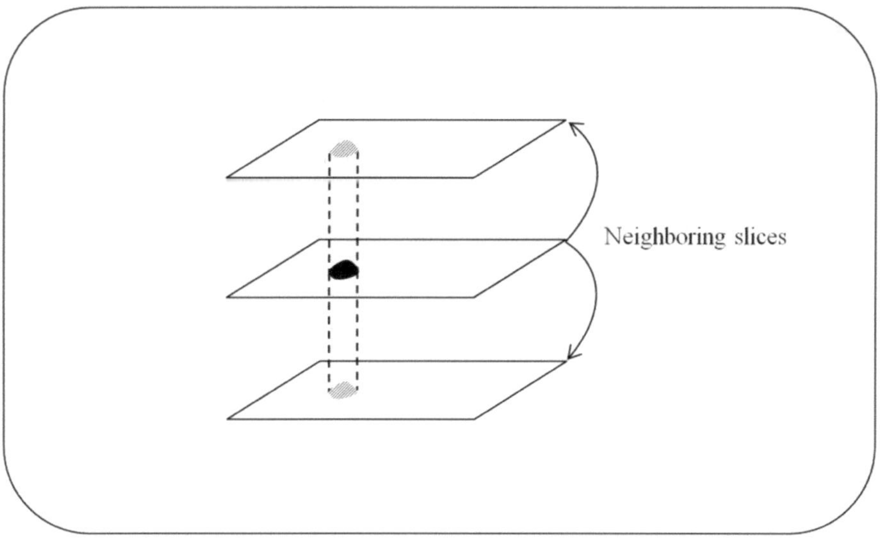

Fig. 21. 3D consistency check with neighboring slices

3.2.2 3-D consistency check

Another discriminative rule relies on 3-D consistency check is performed based on three-dimensional information that a lesion mass cannot appear in a single slice independently. If a slice has a suspicious tumor and this slice has no interaction with other suspicious tumors in the neighboring slices, this slice with a suspicious tumor will be considered erroneous and the selected blob will be disregarded, Figure 21.

4. References

J.-S. Hong, T. Kaneko, R. Sekiguchi, and K. H. Park, "Automatic Liver Tumor Detection from CT," in Automatic Liver Tumor Detection from CT- IEICE- TRANSACTIONS on Information and Systems, 2001, pp. 741-748.

Y. Liang, *et al.*, "Image enhancement for liver CT images," Shanghai, China, 2009, pp. 75130K-8.

L. Massoptier, and S. Casciaro, "Fully automatic liver segmentation through graph-cut technique," *Conf Proc IEEE Eng Med Biol Soc,* vol. 2007, pp. 5243-6, 2007.

L. Massoptier, and S. Casciaro, "A new fully automatic and robust algorithm for fast segmentation of liver tissue and tumors from CT scans," *Eur Radiol,* vol. 18, no. 8, pp. 1658-65, Aug, 2008.

K. Fukunaga, and L. Hostetler," The estimation of the gradient of density function, with applications in pattern recognition". IEEE transactions on Information Theory, 21(1), 1975, 32–40.

F. Liu, B. Zhao, P. K. Kijewski, L. Wang, L. H. Schwartz, "Liver segmentation for CT images using GVF snake," *Med Phys*, vol. 32, no. 12, pp. 3699-706, Dec, 2005.

P. Rodrigues, J. L. Vilaca, and J. Fonseca. "An image processing application for liver tumour segmentation". in Bioengineering (ENBENG), 2011. ENBENG 2011. 1st Portuguese Meeting in. 2011.

X. Jian-Wu, and K. Suzuki. Computer-aided detection of hepatocellular carcinoma in hepatic CT: False positive reduction with feature selection. 2011 IEEE International Symposium on Biomedical Imaging: From Nano to Macro, 2011.

M. Rudzki, "Automatic image contrast enhancement method for liver vasculature detection". 2011 Proceedings of the 18th International Conference in Mixed Design of Integrated Circuits and Systems (MIXDES), 2011.

A. H. Foruzan, R. A. Zoroofi, M. Hori, and Y. Sato, "A knowledge-based technique for liver segmentation in CT data," *Comput Med Imaging Graph.*, Vol. 33, pp. 567-587, Dec. 2009.

Jie L, Lin S, Min D, Yu SCH, Pheng Ann H: "An interactive approach to liver segmentation in CT based on deformable model integrated with attractor force," 2011 International Conference on Machine Learning and Cybernetics (ICMLC), 2011: 1660-1665.

Haiming A, Chunlan Y, Shuicai W, Yi Z, Song B: "Automatic Segmentation and 3D Reconstruction of Human Liver Based on CT Image," 2010 4th International Conference on Bioinformatics and Biomedical Engineering (iCBBE), 2010: 1-4.

13

MicroCT: An Essential Tool in Bone Metastasis Research

Bethany A. Kerr and Tatiana V. Byzova
Lerner Research Institute, The Cleveland Clinic
United States of America

1. Introduction

Microcomputed tomography (microCT) is an essential tool for the study of small animal osseous and soft tissue structures. While several other technologies can be used to image bone, vasculature, and other soft tissues, microCT alone provides high spatial resolution of both hard and soft tissues. Prior to the development of microCT imagers, small animal research was conducted in clinical CT scanners; however, a consequence was poor resolution of the smaller tissues. The development of microCT permitted enhanced small animal imaging resolution and increased use of microCT in preclinical studies. Recent improvements to X-ray detector sensitivity have resulted in the ability of microCT, in combination with contrast agents, to be used in soft tissue studies. In clinical scanning, barium or iodine are typically used for soft tissue assessment; while in small animals, intraperitoneal injections of non-ionic water-soluble contrast medium or intravenous injections of a barium/gelatin mixture can be used for the visualization of soft tissues and vasculature (Paulus et al., 2000). This chapter will focus on the use of microCT to scan osseous tissues. The use of microCT has been well characterized in the study of bone development, fracture repair, biomaterial integration, osteoporosis, and, more recently, cancer bone metastasis.

MicroCT allows for the creation of three-dimensional images of the bone which can be processed both qualitatively and quantitatively. MicroCT analysis quantifies several bone structural indices: bone mineral density (BMD), bone volume to total volume ratio (BV/TV), bone surface area (BSA), trabecular number (Tb.N), trabecular thickness (Tb.Th), and trabecular spacing (Tb.Sp). In addition, since microCT is non-destructive, the same specimens can then be used for mechanical testing, histological analysis, or further experiments. MicroCT scanning is the ideal method for assessing bone structure compared with magnetic resonance imaging (MRI), positron emission tomography (PET), X-rays, or bone histomorphometry (Table 1).

Magnetic resonance imaging (MRI) is non-ionizing and ideal for soft tissue scanning, but not for osseous tissue. Although overall changes in the bone architecture can be seen, MRI cannot provide a structural analysis of bone tissue (Jiang et al., 2000). In addition, small animal MRI devices have micrometer spatial resolution, similar to microCT, but low sensitivity compared with highly sensitive microCT (Mayer-Kuckuk & Boskey, 2006). Overall, MRI has been used extensively for bone research and can provide some information on the bone structure and its level of mineralization, but is not as quantitative as microCT scanning. Finally, microCT scanners for small animals are considerably smaller and less expensive than MRI machines.

Parameter	MicroCT	MRI	PET	X-ray	Histomorphometry
Small animal	Yes	Yes	Yes	Yes	Yes
Sensitivity	High	Low	High	Low	N/A
Spatial Resolution	Micrometer	Micrometer	Millimeter	Millimeter	Micrometer
Structural Quantification	Yes	Minimal	No	Minimal	Yes
Mineralization Levels	Yes	Yes	No	Minimal	Yes
Non-destructive	Yes	Yes	Yes	Yes	No

Table 1. Comparison of imaging technologies for assessing bone structure. MicroCT: microcomputed tomography, MRI: magnetic resonance imaging, PET: positron emission tomography.

Positron emission tomography (PET) is useful for functional imaging and gene expression studies; however, it requires the use of radiolabeling. Single photon emission computed tomography (SPECT) also requires the use of isotopes, but has improved resolution compared with PET. Small animal PET and SPECT have high sensitivity and easy signal quantification, but cannot provide anatomical information and thus are not as effective in assessing the bone structure and mineralization as microCT. In addition, the spatial resolution of PET is at the millimeter level, which is very low for imaging small animals and thus does not provide as detailed a picture of the bone structure in small animals compared with microCT (Mayer-Kuckuk & Boskey, 2006; Paulus et al., 2001). Thus, while PET and SPECT are sensitive imaging methods, their use of isotopes and low spatial resolution prevent these imaging methods from being ideal choices for studying the bone architecture.

x-ray technology provides a two-dimensional image of the bone structure. While bone mineralization is often measured by X-ray, the accuracy of measurements is much greater using microCT. For example, a larger change in BMD must occur to be measured by x-ray, compared with microCT. In fact, microCT scanning can measure a change in cortical thickness of 10-20% which would be undetectable using x-ray imaging. In addition, microCT can distinguish between fractured and non-fractured vertebrae better than x-rays (Genant et al., 2008). Further, while radiography can indicate a loss of mineral, only microCT can differentiate between a thin layer of highly mineralized tissue and a thick layer of less mineralized tissue (Gielkens et al., 2008). Additionally, microCT analysis allows for the cortical and trabecular bone to be analyzed separately, which cannot be done with x-rays (Ravoori et al., 2010). Thus, microCT analysis presents a complete picture of the bone structure, which cannot be accomplished using x-rays.

Quantitative bone morphometry originally was determined from two-dimensional bone biopsies and used to measure structural indices of the bone. MicroCT allows for three-dimensional measurements of a majority of the same structural indices. Bone volume density and bone surface density can be measured equally well by histomorphometry and microCT. However, only microCT can accurately measure Tb.Th, Tb.Sp, and Tb.N, which must be assumed using "ideal" plates and rods in histomorphometry (Muller, 2009). Further, microCT detects bone loss earlier than histomorphometry (Laib et al., 2000). An advantage of histomorphometry is the evaluation on a cellular level (Gielkens et al., 2008); however advances in microCT are improving resolution to the cellular level and negating this advantage.

2. A history of microCT in bone research

The advantages of microCT scanning over other methods have resulted in improved qualitative and quantitative analysis of small animal bone structure leading to the increased prevalence and utilization of microCT to study the bone structure over the past decade. Quantitative microCT measurements are highly reproducible in both rats and mice (Nishiyama et al., 2010). This reproducibility, in combination with the availability of transgenic animals, has led to important studies elucidating the mechanisms of various proteins and genes controlling bone development, bone healing, osseointegration, osteoporosis, and the progression of primary and metastatic bone cancers.

2.1 MicroCT bone research applications

Most orthopaedic research examines the development, maintenance, and repair of skeletal tissues and utilizes microCT scanning for structural analysis during these processes. MicroCT scanning relies on the mineralization of bone to detect the bone architecture and thus cannot be used to study cartilage or other soft materials. However, changes in the bone architecture or bone mineralization can be used to describe alterations in bone development, bone healing, biomaterial integration, or osteoporosis. The measurement of these changes by microCT allows for the development of therapeutics and an understanding of the molecular mechanisms governing these processes.

2.1.1 Bone development

Bone development occurs through one of two processes: intramembranous or endochondral ossification. Endochondral ossification is the development method of the long bones, during which a cartilaginous anlagen is remodelled and replaced by bone, while intramembranous ossification is used predominantly by the skull. The process of bone development and the genes and proteins involved have been extensively studied using knock-out mice. Using these transgenic mice, the importance of genes and proteins in controlling the structure and mineralization of the skeleton produced by intramembranous or endochondral ossification can be studied using microCT analysis. MicroCT analysis permits quantification of developmental delays in the formation of bones throughout the body in response to changes in developmental cues. In addition, the progression and genetic etiology of osteogenesis imperfecta, a genetic disorder of fragile bones, can be studied by microCT scanning. Using various genetically altered mice, the developmental changes resulting in osteogenesis imperfecta have been elucidated. In addition, possible interventions and treatments for the disease can be tested using microCT to measure changes in mineralization. Thus using microCT scanning and genetically altered mice, factors controlling bone mineralization, skull and vertebral development, and developmental bone architecture have been elucidated.

2.1.2 Bone healing and fracture repair

After a bone fracture, a non-union space is often left, which must be healed through a proliferative process, part of which can be visualized by microCT imaging. The distance between the bones and the angle of fracture govern the speed of healing and both of these parameters can be measured shortly after fracture by microCT. During the healing process, the first, reactive phase is marked by increased inflammation and granulation tissue formation. In the second, reparative phase, chondrocytes and osteoblasts migrate into the gap. Chondrocytes begin to lay down a cartilaginous callus, which is then mineralized by osteoblasts producing woven bone through endochondral ossification, which recapitulates bone development. In the final, remodelling phase, osteoblasts and osteoclasts remodel the woven bone into cortical and trabecular bone with a similar shape and mechanical strength to the original bone. MicroCT imaging can be used during the reparative and remodelling phases to assess the healing process. MicroCT analysis provides information on the temporal and topographical changes which occur as the callus is reorganized into bone and during the final remodelling phase (Freeman et al., 2009). Further, microCT scanning can be used to determine the effectiveness of different treatments and interventions in accelerating or improving the bone healing process. In particular, the use of low-intensity pulsed ultrasound to accelerate fracture healing has been studied extensively using microCT analysis (Freeman et al., 2009). Thus, microCT scanning can be used to assess the fracture healing process and to measure the effectiveness of therapeutics aimed at accelerating the process.

2.1.3 Biomaterial research

The osseointegration of bone tissue with implants and scaffolds is integral to bone regeneration and to prevent loosening, rejection, and microdamage to the bone surrounding the implant which could result in fatigue fractures and catastrophic failures. Scaffolds and implants need to encourage bone growth into the porous portions without the formation of fibrous capsules around the implant, which prevent osseointegration. MicroCT analysis has several functions in the design of scaffolds and implants (Rolf et al., 2010). MicroCT scanning can be used to produce 3D images of the scaffold or implant pores to properly measure the porosity which affects permeability, cell migration and bone ingrowth. In addition, the pore interconnect diameter and number of connections per pore can also be measured. An ideal scaffolding material will have porosity and interconnection size and number similar to that of trabecular bone, which can be compared directly using microCT (Jones et al., 2009). After implantation of an implant or scaffold, the levels of mineralized tissues within the pores over time can be measured using microCT; although this measurement can be difficult if the implant material is similar to the ingrowing bone. Nonetheless, changes in pore size can still be measured and any changes would correlate with bone ingrowth (Jones et al., 2009; Reynolds et al., 2009). In a recent study using titanium foam to coat implants, microCT scanning was used to first measure the differences in porosity of dense titanium and foam covered implants and was then used to measure the amount of bone ingrown into the implant after 2 weeks (Wazen et al., 2010). Further, microCT analysis can be used to diagnose osteomyelitis, which is caused by peri-prostethic infection and is a leading cause of implant rejection. The coating of implants with antibiotics to prevent infection is currently being studied. This implant coating prevents the growth of bacteria after implantation and inhibits the associated bone destruction, which can be measured non-invasively by microCT (Adams et al., 2009). Thus, microCT analysis can also be used to study the osseointegration of various biomaterials.

2.1.4 Osteoporosis

MicroCT imaging is especially important for the study of osteoporosis, particularly disease progression and treatment efficacy, as it is one of the few imaging techniques which can provide information on the bone mineral content and density. In addition, scanning is non-invasive and images can be registered to assess changes over time (Ruegsegger et al., 1996). For example, microCT has been used to measure changes in BV/TV, Tb.Th, and Tb.N in the iliac crest of human bone biopsy specimens to determine the extent of osteoporosis and the effects of various drug interventions. Additionally, microCT is used to study osteoporosis in small animals. To study the effects of hormones and preclinical treatments, mice and rats undergo ovariectomies and are monitored for changes in the bone structure including decreased trabecular connectivity and decreased BV/TV which can result from decreased hormones (Genant et al., 2008). In addition, the use of estrogen replacement therapy to rescue ovariectomized mice has been measured using microCT and has shown that BV/TV is restored, but that the connectivity of the trabeculae remains decreased (Jiang et al., 2000). To further study osteoporosis prevention, the role of mechanical stress was assessed by subjecting mice to hindlimb unloading by tail suspension for 2 weeks and bone architecture was monitored using microCT scanning. Using this method, mechanical stress was shown to be integral to maintaining the bone structure and density (Martin-Badosa et al., 2003). Using ovariectomies and hindlimb unloading, several therapies and the importance of mechanical stress, representing exercise, have been validated in mouse models leading to improved treatment and prevention of osteoporosis.

2.1.5 Primary bone cancers

Primary bone cancers can be either benign (osteochondromas) or malignant. Malignant bone tumors include chondrosarcomas, Ewing's sarcoma, and osteosarcomas. Although uncommon, these primary bone cancers have a high incidence of recurrence and can be difficult to diagnose. MicroCT density measurements can be used to differentiate between chondrosarcomas and osteosarcomas in patient samples, as chondrosarcomas were found to have a lower density within the tumors compared with osteosarcomas, although the trabecular densities were similar (Langheinrich et al., 2008). Further, since osteosarcomas occur in the bone osteoid, they are most often studied using microCT. In these tumors, microCT scanning is often performed to monitor tumor growth and lesion characteristics. In addition, the presence of further disease progression and the development of metastases can also be determined using repeated microCT scanning (Yang et al., 2007). Thus, microCT imaging can be used to assist in the diagnosis and monitoring of primary bone cancers.

2.1.6 Bone metastasis

Several cancers metastasize to the bone, specifically: breast, kidney, lung, prostate, thyroid, and multiple myelomas. The process of bone metastasis has been primarily studied in breast, myelomas, and prostate cancers, which display preferences for the bone environment in human metastasis. In small animal models, bone metastasis is often studied via the injection of cancer cells intravenously, intracardiacally, orthotopically or intratibially. These injected cells can then colonize the bone and these metastatic tumors are either osteoblastic, osteolytic, or a combination of both. MicroCT has been used primarily to study changes in the bone microenvironment in response to a metastatic tumor, as discussed in detail in the following section. In some cases, human bone has been implanted subcutaneously in immunodeficient mice and acts as a preferential metastatic site for intracardiacally injected human cancer cells. In these studies, microCT can still be used to analyze changes in the implant structure during bone metastasis progression (Rosol et al., 2003). Thus, microCT scanning can be used to study the interaction between metastatic cancer and bone during the development and progression of metastases.

2.2 MicroCT in metastatic cancer-bone interactions

As cancer progresses, metastasis occurs. Many cancers can metastasize to bone; however, metastatic multiple myelomas, breast carcinomas and prostate carcinomas, show a particular preference for the bone microenvironment. MicroCT has been used extensively to examine the interaction between metastatic tumors and the bone in both patient biopsies and animal models. Patient biopsies from bone bearing metastatic breast carcinomas, prostate carcinomas, or myelomas were analyzed by microCT to determine changes in the bone architecture, which could be used to diagnose malignancy. MicroCT scanning of metastatic biopsies was demonstrated to be quick and accurate in assessing excess bone turnover due to either increased resorption or formation due to malignant growth (Chappard et al., 2010). While the use of microCT to diagnose patient metastases is significant, a majority of published studies focus on the use of microCT to determine the factors responsible for the metastasis of primary cancers to bone using animal models (Table 2).

Model Types	Injection Sites	Bone Phenotypes
Spontaneous Syngeneic Xenograft Chemical Transgenic Reconstitution	Subcutaneous Intracardiac Intratibial Tail vein Orthotopic	Osteoblastic Osteoclastic Combination

Table 2. Animal models used in bone metastasis research. The different models, injection sites, and possible resulting bone phenotypes are listed. These diverse methods to trigger bone metastasis have had various rates of success and resulted in distinct bone phenotypes.

2.2.1 Multiple myelomas

Multiple myelomas are associated with osteolysis of the bone, which can be measured using microCT. In patients, microCT is used to measure changes in trabecular BV, as well as to visualize cortical lesions in three dimensions. In addition, microCT can be used to scan for metastatic myeloma lesions, which cause a derangement in the bone architecture. Mouse models of multiple myelomas have been established and are used to determine the consequences of malignant growth on the bone microenvironment. Using microCT, metastatic tumor lesion locations and the subsequent changes in the bone structure were accurately measured (Fowler et al., 2009; Postnov et al., 2009). Using these models, multiple myeloma lesions in the bone have been characterized as osteolytic, with a high number of lesions in the cortical bone, leading to decreased trabecular BV/TV (Fowler et al., 2009). This model may be used for further studies of multiple myeloma metastases.

2.2.2 Breast cancer

Breast cancer bone metastases occur in 80% of patients with advanced disease and are predominantly osteolytic. MicroCT has been used successfully on patient biopsies to study treatment efficacies and to measure metastatic progression resulting in osteolysis. Correspondingly, microCT has been used to measure osteolysis during metastatic tumor growth in several breast cancer small animal models. When malignant breast carcinoma cells were injected into the femur of rats, decreases in trabecular and cortical bone mineral content were measured by microCT. Further, BV/TV, Tb.N, and Tb.Th were lower in limbs of mice with metastatic breast cancer (Kurth & Muller, 2001). In addition, several chemical agents can induce breast cancer in mice and rats. After rats were injected with N-methyl-N-nitrosourea to induce breast cancer, microCT was used to measure changes in the bone structure in a model of spontaneous cancer formation. Bone health was decreased in animals that developed tumors and both Tb.N and Tb.Th were decreased compared with control rats (Thorpe et al., 2010). These studies demonstrate that microCT imaging can be used to examine alterations in the bone architecture in response to metastatic breast cancer and to test the effectiveness of treatments to prevent tumor-induced osteolysis.

2.2.3 Prostate cancer

Prostate cancer metastasizing to the bone often results in osteoblastic lesions or a combination of osteoclastic and osteoblastic lesions. By comparing normal human bone tissue, osteosclerotic tissue, and osteoblastic metastatic lesions using microCT *ex vivo*, prostate cancer metastasis was shown to increase Tb.N and connectivity compared with benign osteosclerosis, but these lesions were found to have decreased BMD compared with normal and benign tissues (Sone et al., 2004). Prostate cancer metastasis is studied *in vivo* using rat, mouse, and dog models. While some instances of spontaneous prostate cancer exist in these models, a majority of prostate cancers are injected. Murine models of prostate cancer can be syngeneic in immunocompetent mice or xenograft models in immunocompromised mice, as well as a few spontaneous tumor models. Metastatic tumors in mice are largely osteolytic or a combination of osteoblastic and osteolytic (Singh & Figg, 2005). Using microCT, intratibial injections of prostate cancer cells was shown to result in extensive osteolysis of the trabeculae, followed by periosteal bone deposition (McCabe et al., 2008). By scanning the same region of bone over time, the rate of osteolysis can be measured and used to approximate the kinetics of tumor growth. The use of transgenic mice has also led to the identification of various proteins and genes involved in metastatic progression and initiation. Using transgenic mice, several bone proteins, including SPARC, were demonstrated to play important roles in the progression of metastatic prostate cancer lesions. A loss of SPARC protein resulted in enhanced osteolysis upon tumor challenge, as demonstrated by decreased BV/TV, Tb.Th, Tb.N, and BSA measured using microCT (McCabe et al., 2011). Also using microCT, this osteolysis was shown to be specific for prostate cancer, as intratibial injection of melanoma cells did not produce the same effect (McCabe et al., 2011). These studies underscore the importance of microCT scanning as a tool to measure bone structural indices during bone metastasis.

3. Primary tumor growth stimulates bone turnover

While prostate cancer metastases are osteoblastic, patients without visible metastases experience abnormal bone formation and resorption (Kingsley et al., 2007). Interestingly, prostate cancer cells are more likely to colonize bone during the remodelling period (Gomes et al., 2009); thus, it would benefit the tumor to stimulate bone turnover prior to metastasis. Although alterations in bone remodelling in patients with distant, primary cancers have been described, the mechanisms behind this pre-metastatic bone turnover have not been elucidated. Having previously established that intratibial injection of prostate cancer cells stimulates osteolysis (McCabe et al., 2008; McCabe et al., 2011), we wanted to determine the effects of primary tumor growth on the bone microenvironment. We used subcutaneous injections of prostate cancer cells to simulate a primary tumor and performed microCT scanning to assess changes in the bone structure.

3.1 Basic methods and considerations

The design of microCT experiments to study bone metastasis in small animals requires the consideration of various factors. The species, the age, the anesthetization of animals, the number of cells injected, and the time of tumor growth must be optimized prior to beginning experimentation. Further, several parameters of the microCT scanning procedure must be considered when planning experiments. Once these parameters have been optimized, as described below, microCT scanning of animals bearing tumors can be performed with both consistency and precision. Guidelines for microCT image acquisition and reporting of results were recently published (Bouxsein et al., 2010) and should be considered when designing experiments.

3.1.1 Animals

When planning microCT experiments, the choice of small animal must first be made. Most commonly, mice or rats are used in microCT experiments. The availability of a variety of transgenic mice results in their being highly used as experimental subjects. In mice, significant age-related trabecular bone loss begins by 24 weeks of age, and this must be accounted for when choosing animals. In addition, some variations in bone structure occur seasonally (Delahunty et al., 2009). Performing microCT scanning prior to tumor implantation or other intervention diminishes the seasonal and age-related alterations in bone architecture.

In our study, the mice used were six- to twelve-week-old and sex- and age-matched immunocompetent C57BL/6 (WT) or immunodeficient NOD/SCID mice (Jackson Laboratories, Bar Harbor, ME). All animal procedures were performed in accordance with an approved institutional protocol according to the guidelines of the Institutional Animal Care and Use Committee of the Cleveland Clinic.

3.1.2 Tumor injections

When preparing for tumor injections, the number of cells to be implanted and the time of growth vary by tumor type. The aggressiveness of the tumor cells or the cancer type can affect the rates of cell growth. In a previous study, we demonstrated the efficacy of different injections and injected cell numbers on the development of bone metastases (McCabe et al., 2008). In addition, we have found that murine melanoma cells must be injected in higher numbers than murine prostate cancers to grow equally (Feng et al., 2011). Further, the use of xenograft models in immunodeficient animals results in diminished cell growth and longer incubation times necessary to obtain similarly sized tumors as those from syngeneic models. We have found that while human prostate cancers and murine prostate cancers can be injected at the same cell density, human prostate cancers require at least an extra week of growth to form palpable tumors (Feng et al., 2011). The main factor regulating cancer cell growth in mice is the health of the cells prior to implantation. Healthy cells below confluence will grow more readily than highly confluent cells. Thus, optimization must be performed to determine the best conditions for tumor cell growth and implantation.

In this study, cells are implanted subcutaneously with microCT scanning performed a day before injection. WT mice were injected subcutaneously (s.c.) with $4x10^5$ RM1 murine prostate cancer cells and sacrificed 12 days post implantation (5 mice/group). Separately, NOD/SCID mice were injected s.c. with $4x10^5$ LNCaP-C4-2 (C4-2) human prostate cancer cells and sacrificed 20 days post implantation (5 mice/group).

3.1.3 MicroCT scanning

The microCT scanning process requires several parameters to be optimized before scanning: the amount and type of anesthesia and restraint, the effects of ionizing radiation dosing, and the variables affecting repeated image acquisition. To obtain clear scans, mice must be restrained and/or anesthetized. Insufficient anesthesia can result in the subject moving during scanning, while excessive anesthesia can result in death (Paulus et al., 2001). When planning repeated scans, the effect of ionizing radiation dosing should be considered. Ionizing radiation doses can affect bone growth and may also affect tumors. A single scan produces radiation doses approximately 5% of the LD_{50} for mature mice (Paulus et al., 2001). However, repeated scans could result in changes in the tumor growth or bone resorption kinetics. To minimize the dosing effects, microCT scanning should be done at a specific interval. When performing repeated microCT scanning, several factors must be optimized to minimize differences between scans. Repeated image acquisition requires special considerations including positioning, scanning medium (for *ex vivo*), image resolution, and uniform regions of interest (Stock, 2009). During processing, samples are filtered, segmented, registered, and uniform regions of interest are applied to create masks for differentiating between cortical and trabecular bone. Phantom calibration must be performed regularly to calibrate the scanner values for the measurement of morphometric parameters. Phantom values are calculated for materials whose dimensions and geometries are known (Stoico et al., 2010). For bone research, values are measured using phantoms for air, water, and bone. The registering of bones results in increased reproducibility between scans and is necessary to measure changes in the bone structure across different time points (Nishiyama et al., 2010). By optimizing all of these scanning parameters, changes in the bone structure can be measured and registered over time.

In our study, mice are anesthetized by i.p. injection of 100 mg/kg ketamine and 10 mg/kg xylazine prior to cell implantation and microCT scanning. MicroCT analysis of the proximal tibiae was performed one day prior to cell implantation, 3 days later, and then every 7 days until experimental termination to minimize the effects of multiple radiation doses. Scans were conducted in the Cleveland Clinic Biomedical Imaging and Analysis Core Center on a GE eXplore Locus microCT (GE Healthcare, Piscataway, NJ) and 360 X-ray projections were collected in 1° increments (80 kVp; 500 mA; 26 min total scan time). Projection images were preprocessed and reconstructed into 3-dimensional volumes (1024^3 voxels, 20 μm resolution) on a 4PC reconstruction cluster using a modified tent-FDK cone-beam algorithm (GE reconstruction software). Three-dimensional data was processed and rendered (isosurface/maximum intensity projections) using MicroView (GE Healthcare). For each volume, a plane perpendicular to the z-axis/tibial shaft was generated and placed at the base of the growth plate. A second, parallel plane was defined 1.0 mm below and the entire volume was cropped to this volume of interest for quantitative analysis. Image stacks from each volume of interest were exported for quantitative analysis. Cancellous bone masks were generated in MicroView and 3D trabecular structural indices were extracted using custom MatLab (The MathWorks, Inc, Natick, MA) algorithms. Tb.Th and Tb.Sp were determined by previously reported methods (Hildebrand et al., 1999). Tb.N was calculated by taking the inverse of the average distance between the medial axes of trabecular bone segments. BV/TV (total bone voxels divided by total cancellous bone mask voxels) and BSA (sum of pixels along edges of trabecular bone) were also calculated for each VOI. Phantom calibrations are perfomed regularly using air, water, and bone phantoms.

3.2 Representative results and discussion

Using subcutaneous tumor implantation and microCT scanning, we assessed the consequences of primary tumor growth on bone metabolism. We found that injection of murine prostate cancer cells (RM1) in immunocompetent mice results in enhanced bone formation compared with sham injected mice after 12 days of tumor growth. Reconstructions of the microCT scanned bones demonstrate increased trabecular bone in RM1 injected mice (Figure 1). When changes in the bone structural indices were quantified,

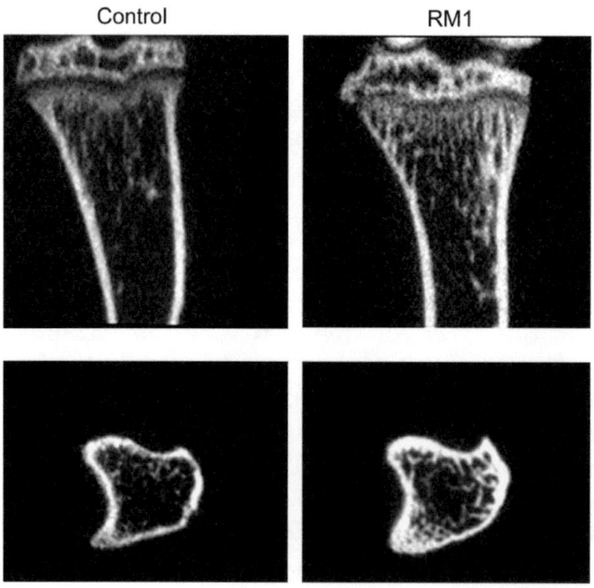

Fig. 1. Reconstructions of microCT scanned bones. Immunocompetent mice were injected with $4x10^5$ murine prostate cancer cells (RM1) or mock injected (Control). Both frontal (top) and transverse planes (bottom) are shown of the proximal tibia.

we found that BV/TV was increased 1.79 fold in mice bearing tumors (Figure 2A). In addition, BSA increased 1.58 fold, demonstrating an overall stimulation of bone formation (Figure 2A). Tb.Th was found to be 1.37 fold higher in mice bearing tumors, with a corresponding 0.72 fold decrease in Tb.Sp. Tb.N did not change significantly during tumor growth (Figure 2B). Thus, bone formation occurred through remodelling of the existing trabeculae and not *de novo* bone formation.

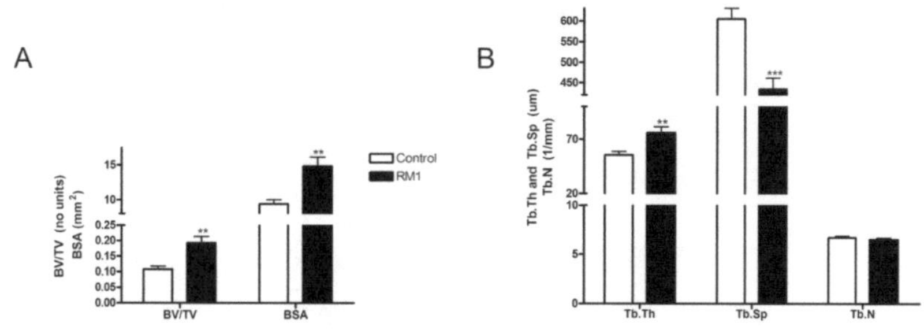

Fig. 2. Bone formation is enhanced in mice bearing prostate cancer tumors. Immunocompetent mice were injected with $4x10^5$ murine prostate cancer cells (RM1; black bars) or mock injected (Control; white bars). (A) MicroCT scanning was performed after 12 days of tumor growth and bone volume to total volume ratio (BV/TV) and bone surface area (BSA) were measured to assess overall volume changes. (B) Trabecular indices were analyzed by microCT and trabecular thickness (Tb.Th), trabecular spacing (Tb.Sp), and trabecular number (Tb.N) were quantified. Measurements are represented as mean ± S.E.M. ** represents $p<0.01$ and *** represents $p<0.001$ by Student's *t* test vs. control.

We next used a xenograft model to determine whether these findings were specific to RM1 cells. Injection of human prostate cancer cells subcutaneously in immunodeficient mice demonstrated similarly increased bone formation. MicroCT scanning was performed 4, 11, and 18 days after tumor implantation to assess changes in the bone architecture over time. Reconstructions exhibit the changes in trabecular structure between days 11 and 18 (Figure 3).

Quantification of changes in bone structural indices demonstrated that significant bone formation occurs between 4 and 11 days of tumor growth, followed by a compensatory decrease around day 18. BV/TV was 0.94 fold of control on day 4, 1.27 fold higher on day 11, and 0.46 fold lower on day 18 compared with mice without tumors (Figure 4A). Further, BSA values of injected mice compared with control were 1.05 fold on day 4, 1.11 fold on day 11, and 0.55 fold on day 18 (Figure 4B). Thus, the overall amount of bone increases between days 4 and 11, then begins to decrease by day 18.

To determine if the trabecular bone remodelling was responsible for these changes in BV and BSA, the structural indices of the trabecular bone were quantified. Tb.Th was increased 1.16 fold on day 11 and decreased 0.70 fold on day 18, while Tb.Sp demonstrated corresponding changes of 0.82 fold on day 11 and 2.87 fold on day 18 compared with control (Figure 5 A and B). Tb.N remained unchanged over the time course (Figure 5C). Thus, subcutaneous tumor growth stimulates bone formation initially, with later compensatory bone destruction as the enhanced osteoblast proliferation and function stimulates osteoclast activity.

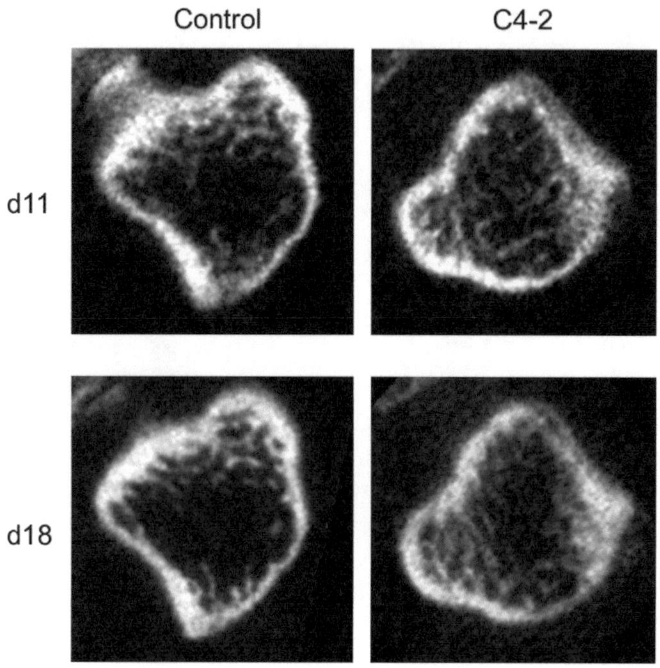

Fig. 3. Reconstructions of the microCT scanned bones. Immunodeficient mice were injected with $4x10^5$ human prostate cancer cells subcutaneously (C4-2) or mock injected (Control). Both frontal and transverse planes are shown of the proximal tibia from scans completed on days (d) 11 and 18.

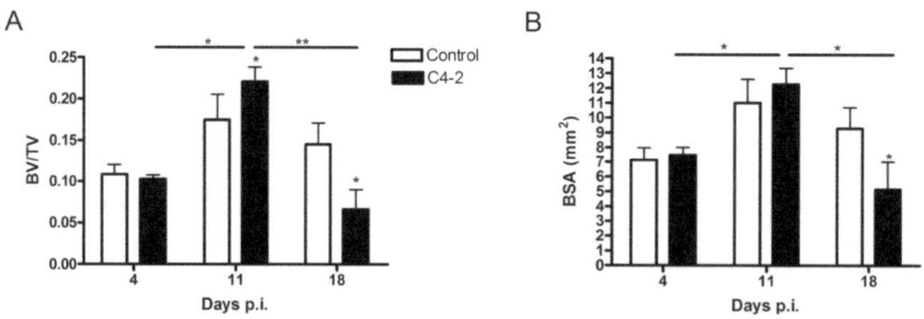

Fig. 4. Implantation of human prostate cancer in immunodeficient mice results in initial bone formation followed by bone resorption. Human prostate cancer cells ($4x10^5$ cells/side) (C4-2; black columns) were injected or a mock injection was performed (Control; white columns). MicroCT scanning was used to quantify bone volume to total volume ratio (BV/TV; A) or bone surface area (BSA; B). Measurements are represented as mean ± S.E.M. * represents $p<0.05$ and ** represents $p<0.01$ by one-way ANOVA (between time points) or Student's *t* test (vs. Control).

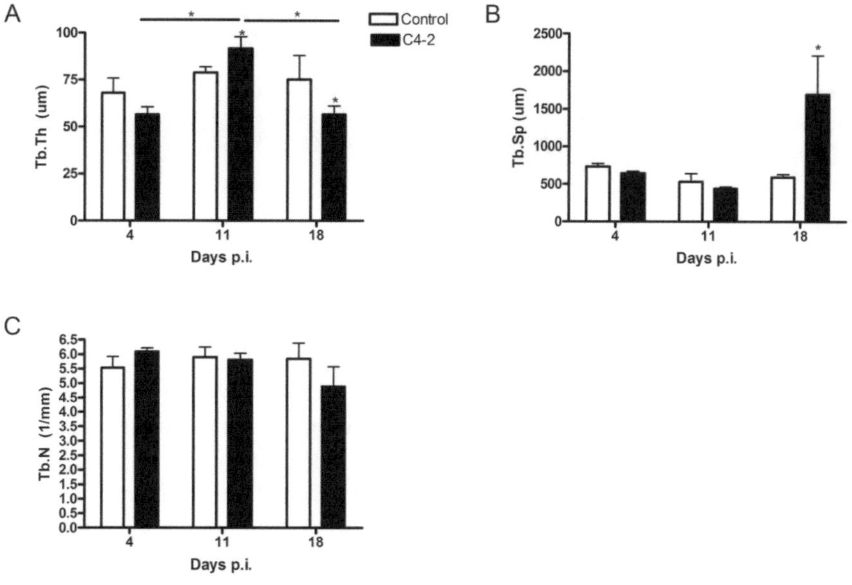

Fig. 5. Subcutaneous human tumor implantation stimulates changes in trabecular bone architecture. Human prostate cancer cells ($4x10^5$ cells/side) (C4-2; black columns) were injected or a mock injection was performed (Control; white columns). MicroCT scanning was used to quantify trabecular thickness (Tb.Th; A), trabecular spacing (Tb.Sp; B), and trabecular number (Tb.N; C). Measurements are represented as mean ± S.E.M. * represents $p<0.05$ by one-way ANOVA (between time points) or Student's *t* test (vs. Control).

Our data demonstrate that primary tumor growth stimulates bone formation, possibly followed later by compensatory bone resorption. This increase in bone formation is similar to that seen in prostate cancer patients (Kingsley et al., 2007). Stimulation of bone remodelling may result in the release of growth factors and cytokines capable of promoting tumor growth. Several cytokines known to be sequestered within the bone matrix or produced by osteoblasts, including transforming growth factor β1, receptor activator of NF-κB ligand, and osteopontin, are capable of promoting tumor growth. In addition, bone turnover may induce the release of bone marrow-progenitor cells into the circulation (Lymperi et al., 2011). We have shown that these progenitors are recruited into tumors supporting angiogenesis and continued tumor growth (Feng et al., 2011). The enhanced bone remodelling may also function to prepare the microenvironment for the future invasion of the metastatic tumor. We have previously shown that tumors secrete into the circulation several cytokines which may be promoting bone remodelling (Kerr et al., 2010), demonstrating a possible direct link between the tumor and the induced bone turnover. Thus, our studies demonstrate the importance of microCT as a tool to examine the bone structure in bone metastasis research.

4. Future of microCT in cancer bone metastasis research

The dominant microCT systems currently used are desktop microCT machines which focus mainly on the microstructural level. Newer machines using synchrotron radiation microCT and nanoCT provide higher resolution images and may provide more precise measurements of bone structure indices. Further, combining microCT with PET or bioluminescence will result in the improved imaging of tumors within the bone microenvironment. Improved imaging of both the bone and tumor at the cellular level promotes the use of these technologies in metastatic signaling and micrometastasis, as well as the testing of various therapeutic target efficacies.

4.1 NanoCT

While the dominant desktop microCT systems available provide resolutions between 5-100 µm, third-generation synchrotron radiation systems have resolutions below 1 µm. These resolutions down to 100 nm are called nanoCT and may allow for imaging on the cellular level including the canal network, osteocyte lacunae, and even single cells. In addition, these machines can be used in the visualization of microfractures (Muller, 2009; Stock, 2009). A recent study used nanoCT to examine osteocyte lacunae and the canalicular network (Dierolf et al., 2010). Analysis of scans from nanoCT machines will provide increased precision of measurements and improved quantification of early changes in the bone structure due to osteoporosis or therapeutic treatments. Until the development of nanoCT systems is completed and the systems become widely available, desktop microCT systems alone or in combination with other imaging systems will remain the main tool for analysis of the bone structure.

4.2 Combined imaging techniques

A recent trend in microCT imaging has been the development of PET-CTs, which allow simultaneous PET and CT scanning. Using this machine, overlays of low resolution tumors with high resolution microCT scans can be produced (Schambach et al., 2010). Further, fusion of bioluminescent imaging with microCT would allow for improved visualization of tumor cells along the bone and of local changes in bone cells and architecture. Bioluminescent imaging requires the use of luciferase reporters to be expressed by the tumor cells and results in a strong signal without any requirement for external illumination. In addition, fluorescent proteins or dots can be introduced to cells prior to implantation (de Boer et al., 2006; Henriquez et al., 2007). The use of bioluminescent imaging with microCT was recently used to measure the kinetics of intraosseous tumor growth, resultant bone destruction, and correlations between the two over time (Fritz et al., 2007). In addition, luciferase can be introduced to osteoblasts or osteoclasts to monitor their activity, proliferation, and migration along the bone during metastatic tumor growth or in response to pre-metastatic signals from a primary tumor. Finally, luciferase activity can be used to monitor inflammation, angiogenesis, apoptosis, or signal transduction in metastatic tumors within the bone microenvironment and their association with altered bone architecture (de Boer et al., 2006). PET-CT or bioluminescent imaging, when combined with microCT, will permit visualization of micrometastases and metastatic soft tumors in the bone microenvironment.

4.3 Metastatic signaling

MicroCT scanning can also be used to study the proteins and signaling cascades involved in inducing bone changes during the metastatic process. The mechanisms of primary cancer metastasis to bone are still being elucidated, although several proteins and signaling cascades have been shown to play important roles in bone metastasis. For example, the $\alpha_v\beta_3$ integrin on prostate cancer cells is necessary for the progression of metastatic growth in bone. Further, this integrin is responsible for increases in bone formation caused by metastatic prostate cancer visualized by microCT scanning (McCabe et al., 2007). Building upon this study, the importance of extracellular proteins recognized by the $\alpha_v\beta_3$ integrin in prostate cancer progression has been studied using microCT and transgenic mice (McCabe et al., 2011). Using transgenic mice or cancer cells with proteins over-expressed or knocked-down, the signals regulating the metastasis of prostate cancer to bone can be examined using microCT to repeatedly and non-invasively study the bone structure.

4.4 Treatment efficacies

The efficacy of therapeutics can be measured using *ex vivo* microCT scanning of human biopsies or *in vivo* scanning of small animals. MicroCT imaging alone can be used on biopsies or animals to determine the effectiveness of drugs in altering the bone microenvironment. Therapies aimed at improving bone density or trabecular thickness can easily be measured and may be used in studies of osteoporosis and osteogenesis imperfecta. MicroCT scanning of biopsies can also be used to assess changes in primary osteosarcoma tumor structure and size. For metastatic soft tumors, a combination of microCT and optical imaging techniques are most useful in analyzing therapeutic effectiveness on shrinking tumors and maintaining the bone architecture. This non-invasive testing allows for the continuous monitoring of tumors during their growth or remission (Henriquez et al., 2007). MicroCT scanning has been used to study the effectiveness of treatments designed to slow down the progression of osteolysis during bone metastasis progression. In a small animal model, zolendronic acid treatment decreased bone resorption as shown by microCT scanning (Johnson et al., 2011). In another study, an osteoprotegrin-producing adenovirus was demonstrated to result in increased BV/TV and connectivity and thus, was shown to protect against metastatic bone loss (Chanda et al., 2008). Further, the main symptom resulting from bone metastases is pain, which is the major factor responsible for decreased quality of life. Intraosseous tumor implantation and microCT scanning were used to study the correlation of bone pain with bone destruction in a rat model (Dore-Savard et al., 2010). This model can be used in the future to examine the effectiveness of therapeutics targeting bone pain. In summary, microCT imaging can be used to determine the efficacy of treatments in altering the bone architecture in a variety of diseases.

5. Conclusion

The development of microCT scanners provided a means for analyzing the bone structure and mineralization level non-destructively. MicroCT alone provides quantitative and qualitative scanning at a high sensitivity and micrometer resolution, with newer imaging systems providing even nanometer resolutions. These machines have allowed for extensive research on bone and bone metastasis to be completed. Current studies are using microCT scanning to elucidate the mechanisms behind cancer metastasis and to determine the effectiveness of treatments. Using the basic procedures and considerations when planning microCT scanning experiments discussed, consistency and precision can be achieved in repeated scans of small animals. The data presented here establish the usefulness of microCT scanning to measure pre-metastatic bone changes. Our data demonstrate that primary tumors communicate with the bone microenvironment prior to metastasis stimulating bone formation in two tumor models. Using microCT imaging alone or in combination with other methodologies will permit continued examination of the metastatic process. Combined imaging techniques and advances in microCT systems will allow for continued research on metastatic signaling, metastatic tumor development and progression, and therapeutic efficacies. Thus, microCT has been come an essential tool in bone metastasis research.

6. Acknowledgment

We would like to thank Dr. Amit Vasanji, who developed the software and analysis techniques for our microCT analysis, and Rick Rozic for technical assistance with the microCT scanner. We also thank Miroslava Tischenko for her assistance with the mouse colony. B.A.K. was supported by a Ruth L. Kirschstein NRSA award (F32 CA142133) from the NIH/NCI. This study was supported by research funding from the NIH/NCI grant (CA126847) to T.V.B.

7. References

Adams, C. S., V. Antoci, Jr., G. Harrison, P. Patal, T. A. Freeman, I. M. Shapiro, J. Parvizi, N. J. Hickok, S. Radin & P. Ducheyne. (2009). Controlled release of vancomycin from thin sol-gel films on implant surfaces successfully controls osteomyelitis. *J Orthop Res*, Vol. 27, No. 6, pp. 701-709. ISSN 1554-527X

Bouxsein, M. L., S. K. Boyd, B. A. Christiansen, R. E. Guldberg, K. J. Jepsen & R. Muller. (2010). Guidelines for assessment of bone microstructure in rodents using micro-computed tomography. *J Bone Miner Res*, Vol. 25, No. 7, pp. 1468-1486. ISSN 1523-4681

Chanda, D., T. Isayeva, S. Kumar, G. P. Siegal, A. A. Szafran, K. R. Zinn, V. V. Reddy & S. Ponnazhagan. (2008). Systemic osteoprotegerin gene therapy restores tumor-induced bone loss in a therapeutic model of breast cancer bone metastasis. *Mol Ther*, Vol. 16, No. 5, pp. 871-878. ISSN 1525-0024

Chappard, D., H. Libouban, E. Legrand, N. Ifrah, C. Masson, M. F. Basle & M. Audran. (2010). Computed microtomography of bone specimens for rapid analysis of bone changes associated with malignancy. *Anat Rec (Hoboken)*, Vol. 293, No. 7, pp. 1125-1133. ISSN 1932-8494

de Boer, J., C. van Blitterswijk & C. Lowik. (2006). Bioluminescent imaging: emerging technology for non-invasive imaging of bone tissue engineering. *Biomaterials*, Vol. 27, No. 9, pp. 1851-1858. ISSN 0142-9612

Delahunty, K. M., L. G. Horton, H. F. Coombs, 3rd, K. L. Shultz, K. L. Svenson, M. A. Marion, M. F. Holick, W. G. Beamer & C. J. Rosen. (2009). Gender- and compartment-specific bone loss in C57BL/6J mice: correlation to season? *J Clin Densitom*, Vol. 12, No. 1, pp. 89-94. ISSN 1094-6950

Dierolf, M., A. Menzel, P. Thibault, P. Schneider, C. M. Kewish, R. Wepf, O. Bunk & F. Pfeiffer. (2010). Ptychographic X-ray computed tomography at the nanoscale. *Nature*, Vol. 467, pp. 436-9. ISSN 0028-0836

Dore-Savard, L., V. Otis, K. Belleville, M. Lemire, M. Archambault, L. Tremblay, J. F. Beaudoin, N. Beaudet, R. Lecomte, M. Lepage, L. Gendron & P. Sarret. (2010). Behavioral, medical imaging and histopathological features of a new rat model of bone cancer pain. *PLoS One*, Vol. 5, No. 10, pp. e13774. ISSN 1932-6203

Feng, W., M. Madajka, B. A. Kerr, G. H. Mahabeleshwar, S. W. Whiteheart & T. V. Byzova. (2011). A novel role for platelet secretion in angiogenesis: mediating bone marrow-derived cell mobilization and homing. *Blood*, Vol. 117, No. 14, pp. 3893-902. ISSN 1528-0020

Fowler, J. A., G. R. Mundy, S. T. Lwin, C. C. Lynch & C. M. Edwards. (2009). A murine model of myeloma that allows genetic manipulation of the host microenvironment. *Dis Model Mech*, Vol. 2, No. 11-12, pp. 604-611. ISSN 1754-8411

Freeman, T. A., P. Patel, J. Parvizi, V. Antoci, Jr. & I. M. Shapiro. (2009). Micro-CT analysis with multiple thresholds allows detection of bone formation and resorption during ultrasound-treated fracture healing. *J Orthop Res*, Vol. 27, No. 5, pp. 673-679. ISSN 1554-527X

Fritz, V., P. Louis-Plence, F. Apparailly, D. Noel, R. Voide, A. Pillon, J. C. Nicolas, R. Muller & C. Jorgensen. (2007). Micro-CT combined with bioluminescence imaging: a dynamic approach to detect early tumor-bone interaction in a tumor osteolysis murine model. *Bone*, Vol. 40, No. 4, pp. 1032-1040. ISSN 8756-3282

Genant, H. K., K. Engelke & S. Prevrhal. (2008). Advanced CT bone imaging in osteoporosis. *Rheumatology (Oxford)*, Vol. 47 Suppl 4, pp. iv9-16. ISSN 1462-0332

Gielkens, P. F., J. Schortinghuis, J. R. de Jong, M. C. Huysmans, M. B. Leeuwen, G. M. Raghoebar, R. R. Bos & B. Stegenga. (2008). A comparison of micro-CT, microradiography and histomorphometry in bone research. *Arch Oral Biol*, Vol. 53, No. 6, pp. 558-566. ISSN 0003-9969

Gomes, R. R., Jr., P. Buttke, E. M. Paul & R. A. Sikes. (2009). Osteosclerotic prostate cancer metastasis to murine bone are enhanced with increased bone formation. *Clin Exp Metastasis*, Vol. 26, No. 7, pp. 641-651. ISSN 1573-7276

Henriquez, N. V., P. G. van Overveld, I. Que, J. T. Buijs, R. Bachelier, E. L. Kaijzel, C. W. Lowik, P. Clezardin & G. van der Pluijm. (2007). Advances in optical imaging and novel model systems for cancer metastasis research. *Clin Exp Metastasis*, Vol. 24, No. 8, pp. 699-705. ISSN 0262-0898

Hildebrand, T., A. Laib, R. Muller, J. Dequeker & P. Ruegsegger. (1999). Direct three-dimensional morphometric analysis of human cancellous bone: microstructural data from spine, femur, iliac crest, and calcaneus. *J Bone Miner Res*, Vol. 14, No. 7, pp. 1167-1174. ISSN 0884-0431

Jiang, Y., J. Zhao, D. L. White & H. K. Genant. (2000). Micro CT and Micro MR imaging of 3D architecture of animal skeleton. *J Musculoskelet Neuronal Interact*, Vol. 1, No. 1, pp. 45-51. ISSN 1108-7161

Johnson, L. C., R. W. Johnson, S. A. Munoz, G. R. Mundy, T. E. Peterson & J. A. Sterling. (2011). Longitudinal live animal microCT allows for quantitative analysis of tumor-induced bone destruction. *Bone*, pp. ISSN 1873-2763

Jones, J. R., R. C. Atwood, G. Poologasundarampillai, S. Yue & P. D. Lee. (2009). Quantifying the 3D macrostructure of tissue scaffolds. *J Mater Sci Mater Med*, Vol. 20, No. 2, pp. 463-471. ISSN 0957-4530

Kerr, B. A., R. Miocinovic, A. K. Smith, E. A. Klein & T. V. Byzova. (2010). Comparison of tumor and microenvironment secretomes in plasma and in platelets during prostate cancer growth in a xenograft model. *Neoplasia*, Vol. 12, No. 5, pp. 388-396. ISSN 1476-5586

Kingsley, L. A., P. G. Fournier, J. M. Chirgwin & T. A. Guise. (2007). Molecular biology of bone metastasis. *Mol Cancer Ther*, Vol. 6, No. 10, pp. 2609-2617. ISSN 1535-7163

Kurth, A. A. & R. Muller. (2001). The effect of an osteolytic tumor on the three-dimensional trabecular bone morphology in an animal model. *Skeletal Radiol*, Vol. 30, No. 2, pp. 94-98. ISSN 0364-2348

Laib, A., O. Barou, L. Vico, M. H. Lafage-Proust, C. Alexandre & P. Rugsegger. (2000). 3D micro-computed tomography of trabecular and cortical bone architecture with application to a rat model of immobilisation osteoporosis. *Med Biol Eng Comput*, Vol. 38, No. 3, pp. 326-332. ISSN 0140-0118

Langheinrich, A. C., C. Stolle, M. Kampschulte, D. Lommel, W. S. Rau & B. Bassaly. (2008). Diagnostic value of ex-vivo three-dimensional micro-computed tomography imaging of primary nonhematopoietic human bone tumors: osteosarcoma versus chondrosarcoma. *Acta Radiol*, Vol. 49, No. 8, pp. 940-948. ISSN 1600-0455

Lymperi, S., A. Ersek, F. Ferraro, F. Dazzi & N. J. Horwood. (2011). Inhibition of osteoclast function reduces hematopoietic stem cell numbers in vivo. *Blood*, Vol. 117, No. 5, pp. 1540-1549. ISSN 1528-0020

Martin-Badosa, E., A. Elmoutaouakkil, S. Nuzzo, D. Amblard, L. Vico & F. Peyrin. (2003). A method for the automatic characterization of bone architecture in 3D mice microtomographic images. *Comput Med Imaging Graph*, Vol. 27, No. 6, pp. 447-458. ISSN 0895-6111

Mayer-Kuckuk, P. & A. L. Boskey. (2006). Molecular imaging promotes progress in orthopedic research. *Bone*, Vol. 39, No. 5, pp. 965-977. ISSN 8756-3282

McCabe, N. P., S. De, A. Vasanji, J. Brainard & T. V. Byzova. (2007). Prostate cancer specific integrin alphavbeta3 modulates bone metastatic growth and tissue remodeling. *Oncogene*, Vol. 26, No. 42, pp. 6238-6243. ISSN 0950-9232

McCabe, N. P., M. Madajka, A. Vasanji & T. V. Byzova. (2008). Intraosseous injection of RM1 murine prostate cancer cells promotes rapid osteolysis and periosteal bone deposition. *Clin Exp Metastasis*, Vol. 25, No. 5, pp. 581-590. ISSN 0262-0898

McCabe, N. P., B. A. Kerr, M. Madajka, A. Vasanji & T. V. Byzova. (2011). Augmented Osteolysis in SPARC-Deficient Mice with Bone-Residing Prostate Cancer. *Neoplasia*, Vol. 13, No. 1, pp. 31-39. ISSN 1476-5586

Muller, R. (2009). Hierarchical microimaging of bone structure and function. *Nat Rev Rheumatol*, Vol. 5, No. 7, pp. 373-381. ISSN 1759-4804

Nishiyama, K. K., G. M. Campbell, R. J. Klinck & S. K. Boyd. (2010). Reproducibility of bone micro-architecture measurements in rodents by in vivo micro-computed tomography is maximized with three-dimensional image registration. *Bone*, Vol. 46, No. 1, pp. 155-161. ISSN 1873-2763

Paulus, M. J., S. S. Gleason, S. J. Kennel, P. R. Hunsicker & D. K. Johnson. (2000). High resolution X-ray computed tomography: an emerging tool for small animal cancer research. *Neoplasia*, Vol. 2, No. 1-2, pp. 62-70. ISSN 1522-8002

Paulus, M. J., S. S. Gleason, M. E. Easterly & C. J. Foltz. (2001). A review of high-resolution X-ray computed tomography and other imaging modalities for small animal research. *Lab Anim (NY)*, Vol. 30, No. 3, pp. 36-45. ISSN 0093-7355

Postnov, A. A., H. Rozemuller, V. Verwey, H. Lokhorst, N. De Clerck & A. C. Martens. (2009). Correlation of high-resolution X-ray micro-computed tomography with bioluminescence imaging of multiple myeloma growth in a xenograft mouse model. *Calcif Tissue Int*, Vol. 85, No. 5, pp. 434-443. ISSN 1432-0827

Ravoori, M., A. J. Czaplinska, C. Sikes, L. Han, E. M. Johnson, W. Qiao, C. Ng, D. D. Cody, W. A. Murphy, K. A. Do, N. M. Navone & V. Kundra. (2010). Quantification of mineralized bone response to prostate cancer by noninvasive in vivo microCT and non-destructive ex vivo microCT and DXA in a mouse model. *PLoS One*, Vol. 5, No. 3, pp. e9854. ISSN 1932-6203

Reynolds, D. G., S. Shaikh, M. O. Papuga, A. L. Lerner, R. J. O'Keefe, E. M. Schwarz & H. A. Awad. (2009). muCT-based measurement of cortical bone graft-to-host union. *J Bone Miner Res*, Vol. 24, No. 5, pp. 899-907. ISSN 1523-4681

Rolf, Z., H. Astrid, S. Franziska, R. Heinrich, K. C. James, S. Helmut & B. Christoph. (2010). High Resolution X-Ray Tomography- 3D Imaging for Tissue Engineering Applications, In: *Tissue Engineering*, D. Eberli. pp. 337-358, InTech. ISBN 978-953-307-079-7, Vienna, Austria

Rosol, T. J., S. H. Tannehill-Gregg, B. E. LeRoy, S. Mandl & C. H. Contag. (2003). Animal models of bone metastasis. *Cancer*, Vol. 97, No. 3 Suppl, pp. 748-757. ISSN 0008-543X

Ruegsegger, P., B. Koller & R. Muller. (1996). A microtomographic system for the nondestructive evaluation of bone architecture. *Calcif Tissue Int*, Vol. 58, No. 1, pp. 24-29. ISSN 0171-967X

Schambach, S. J., S. Bag, L. Schilling, C. Groden & M. A. Brockmann. (2010). Application of micro-CT in small animal imaging. *Methods*, Vol. 50, No. 1, pp. 2-13. ISSN 1095-9130

Singh, A. S. & W. D. Figg. (2005). In vivo models of prostate cancer metastasis to bone. *J Urol*, Vol. 174, No. 3, pp. 820-826. ISSN 0022-5347

Sone, T., T. Tamada, Y. Jo, H. Miyoshi & M. Fukunaga. (2004). Analysis of three-dimensional microarchitecture and degree of mineralization in bone metastases from prostate cancer using synchrotron microcomputed tomography. *Bone*, Vol. 35, No. 2, pp. 432-438. ISSN 8756-3282

Stock, S. R. (2009). *MicroComputed Tomography: Methodology and Applications* CRC Press, ISBN 978-1-4200-5876-5, Boca Raton

Stoico, R., S. Tassani, E. Perilli, F. Baruffaldi & M. Viceconti. (2010). Quality control protocol for in vitro micro-computed tomography. *J Microsc*, Vol. 238, No. 2, pp. 162-172. ISSN 1365-2818

Thorpe, M. P., R. J. Valentine, C. J. Moulton, A. J. Johnson, E. M. Evans & D. K. Layman. (2010). Breast tumors induced by N-methyl-N-nitrosourea are damaging to bone strength, structure and mineralization in the absence of metastasis in rats. *J Bone Miner Res*, pp. ISSN 1523-4681

Wazen, R. M., L. P. Lefebvre, E. Baril & A. Nanci. (2010). Initial evaluation of bone ingrowth into a novel porous titanium coating. *J Biomed Mater Res B Appl Biomater*, Vol. 94, No. 1, pp. 64-71. ISSN 1552-4981

Yang, S. Y., H. Yu, J. E. Krygier, P. H. Wooley & M. P. Mott. (2007). High VEGF with rapid growth and early metastasis in a mouse osteosarcoma model. *Sarcoma*, Vol. 2007, pp. 95628. ISSN 1357-714X

14

CT Imaging of Hepatic Arteries

Luca Saba
Department of Science of the Images, Policlinico Universitario
University of Cagliari
Italy

The reason why the water in wells becomes colder in summer is that the earth is then rarefied by the heat, and releases into the air all the heat-particles it happens to have. So, the more the earth is drained of heat, the colder becomes the moisture that is concealed in the ground. On the other hand, when all the earth condenses and contracts and congeals with the cold, then, of course, as it contracts, it squeezes out into the wells whatever heat it holds.
Lucretius, poet (99 B.C.-55 B.C.) Rome

1. Introduction

The knowledge and reliable depiction of celiac trunk vascularization and hepatic arteries is extremely important in several condition like surgery in the hepato-biliary pancreatic area, as well as in interventional radiological treatments[1,2]. In particular, in the setting of liver transplantation a frequently used approach is the split liver from living donors. This kind of procedure is complex and an exact knowledge of the arterial anatomy is necessary to plan the best resection approach and to minimize the risk of mortality[3,4]. Similarly, an accurate depiction of hepatic arterial variants can also help in ensuring a safe operation in treating isolated liver tumors, performing partial hepatectomy.
The patterns of arterial blood supply to the liver are variable. *Nelson et al*[5] reported a typical scheme, in which the liver receives its total inflow from the hepatic branch of the celiac trunk, that occurs in 25-75% of cases (**Figure 1**). In the variant configurations, the liver receives arterial flow through branches coming from the superior mesenteric artery, left gastric artery, abdominal aorta or other visceral branches. Moreover, these vessels may be replaced, representing the primary arterial blood supply to the liver, or accessory, occurring in addition to the normal arterial supply.
Both in the early and in the most recent literature in this subject[6,7,8,9], authors made an effort to compare the several types of variation in order to obtain a single scheme for the most common variants.
Digital Subtraction Angiography (DSA), despite its invasive nature, was regarded as the method of choice for hepatic artery evaluation[10,11] until the introduction of Multi-Detector-Row CT Angiography (MDCTA), which is now considered to be an extremely reliable and non-invasive method in the analysis of hepatic vasculature[12,13]. Modern MDCT scanners acquire their dataset with isotropic sub-millimetric voxels and are capable of visualizing even small vessels like the Adamkiewicz artery[14].

With the introduction of MDCT indications have expanded to include assessment of hepatic arteries by replacing the use of Digital Subtraction Angiography (DSA)[15,16]. Combined with patient- and scanner-adjusted CT data acquisition and contrast medium application strategies, an accurate, retrospective and reliable evaluation of the hepatic artery configuration is possible even in routinely MDCTA exams performed for other indications.
In the analysis of MDCTA, it is possible to use several post-processing methods to visualize the arteries. The most frequently used are Maximum Intensity Projection (MIP), Multi Planar Reconstruction (CPR), Curved Planar Reconstruction (CPR) and Volume Rendering (VR)[17,18,19]. With the more recent workstations, these post-processing images are obtained in real-time, such that the processing time, which was a problem some years ago, is no longer an issue. However, the time taken for the radiologist to visualize datasets using all the different post-processing techniques may be important. For this reason it is important to determine the most reliable post-processing technique(s) for visualizing the vessels.

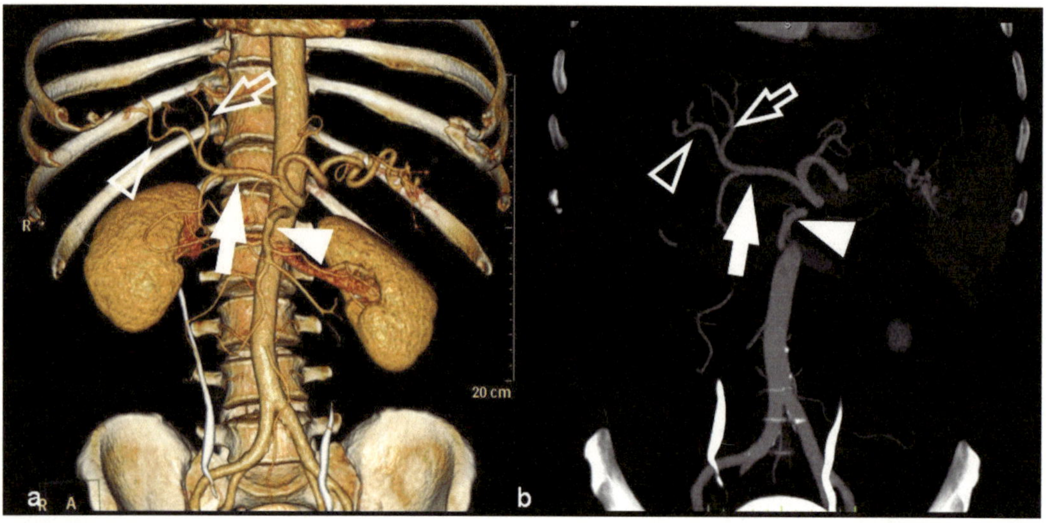

Fig. 1. MDCTA volume rendered (a) and Maximum Intensity Projection (b) images of a Michels type I configuration. In the panel a,b is visible the common hepatic artery (white arrow), the right hepatic artery (open white arrowhead), the left hepatic artery (white open arrow) and the superior mesenteric artery (white arrowhead).

2. Normal anatomy and variants

The anatomy of hepatic artery and its variants, have been extensively described in the literature[9,20,21,22,23] and nowadays the most frequently used is the Michels's classification[9] even if Michel's description is an anatomical classification having nowadays less relevance to modern surgical practice than in the past. Michels described 10 types of configuration for hepatic arteries vasculature, by including the normal anatomy in type 1 and gathering all other types of variants in types 2 -10.
In the conventional anatomy, -**type I** (**Figure 2**) according to Michels classification- the main hepatic artery arises from coeliac artery, gives off the gastroduodenal artery and the proper hepatic artery. The proper hepatic artery continues as the right hepatic artery after giving off the left hepatic artery and then the right hepatic artery splits into its anterior and posterior

branches. The left hepatic artery splits into branches which feed segments II and III. Segment IV is fed by the branch or branches originating from the right, left, or by the proper hepatic artery. The frequency of occurrence of normal hepatic arterial anatomy ranges between 55%-76%.

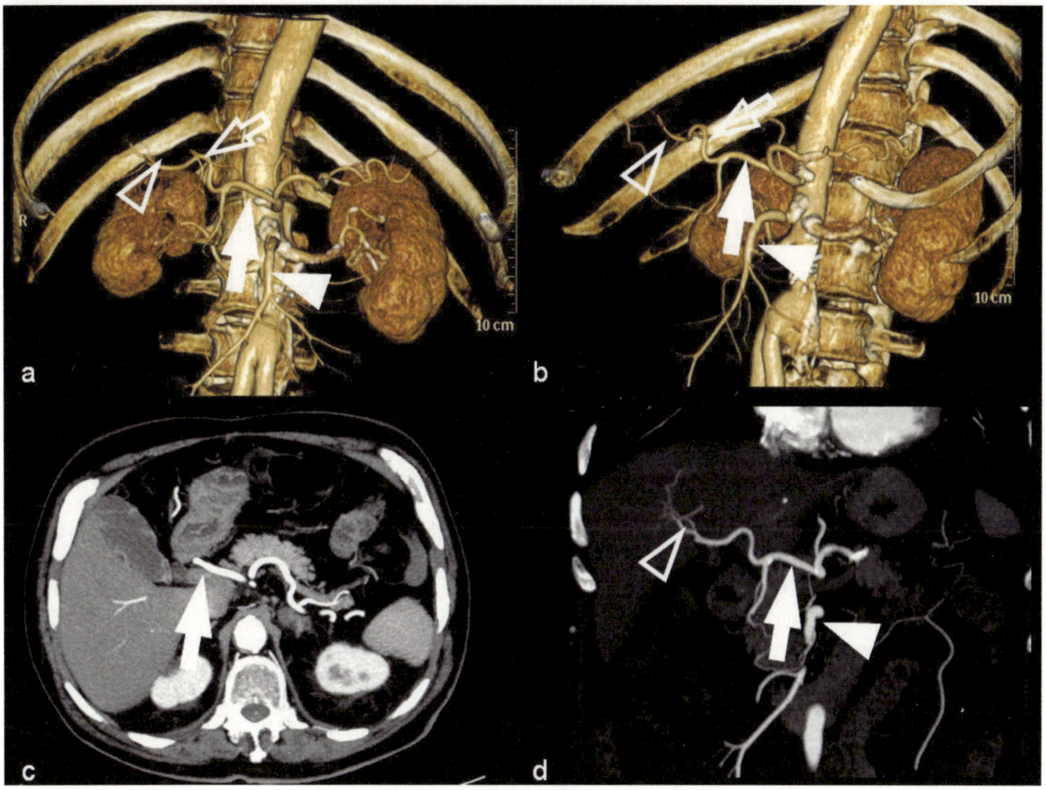

Fig. 2. MDCTA volume rendered (a,b) and Maximum Intensity Projection (c,d) images of a Michels type I configuration. It is visible the common hepatic artery (white arrow), the right hepatic artery (open white arrowhead), the left hepatic artery (white open arrow) and the superior mesenteric artery (white arrowhead).

In the **type II** of Michels variant (replaced left hepatic artery) the left hepatic artery (LHA) originates from the left gastric artery (LGA) (**Figure 3**). The frequency of occurrence of this type of variants is 10%.
In the **type III** of Michels variant (replaced right hepatic artery) the right hepatic artery (RHA) starts from the superior mesenteric artery (SMA) (**Figure 4**) . This case occurs in 11% of the patients.
Type IV of Michels variant identifies a situation where variant II and variant III cohexist: it is a combination of replaced right and replaced left hepatic artery: the RHA originated from SMA and the LHA originated from the GHA. This variant is uncommon and its incidence in population is near 1%.
In the **type V** of Michels variants (accessory left hepatic artery), the left lobe is fed by both the left hepatic artery originating from the proper hepatic artery and the accessory left hepatic artery originating from the LGA; the incidence of this variant is 8%.

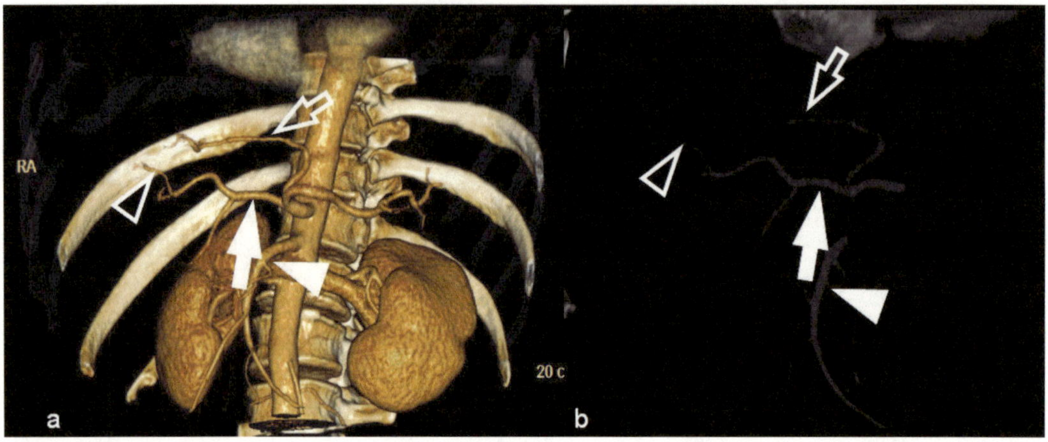

Fig. 3. MDCTA volume rendered (a) and Maximum Intensity Projection (b) images of a Michels type II configuration, where the left hepatic artery origins from the left gastric artery. It is visible the common hepatic artery (white arrow), the right hepatic artery (open white arrowhead), the left hepatic artery (white open arrow) and the superior mesenteric artery (white arrowhead).

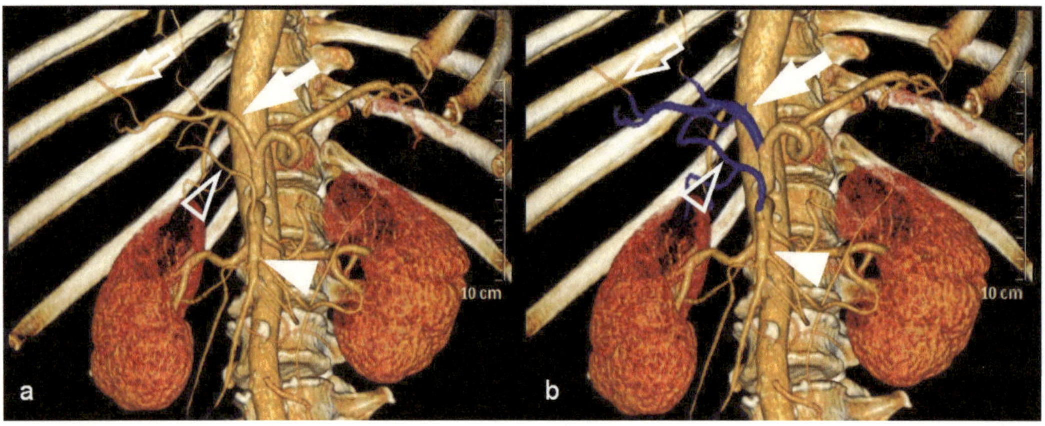

Fig. 4. MDCTA volume rendered (a,b) images of a Michels type III configuration where the right hepatic artery origins from the superior mesenteric artery. It is visible the common hepatic artery (white arrow), the right hepatic artery (open white arrowhead), the left hepatic artery (white open arrow) and the superior mesenteric artery (white arrowhead).

In the **type VI** of Michels variant (accessory right hepatic artery) the right lobe is fed by both the RHA originating from the proper hepatic artery and the accessory RHA deriving from the SMA (incidence 7%).

In the **type VII** of Michels variant, the left lobe is fed by both the left hepatic artery (LHA) originating from the proper hepatic artery and the accessory left hepatic artery originating from the left gastric artery; the right lobe is fed by both the right hepatic artery originating from the proper hepatic artery and the accessory right hepatic artery starting from the superior mesenteric artery; this variant is uncommon with an incidence of 1 %.

In the **type VIII** of Michels variant, the replaced RHA originates from the superior mesenteric artery and the accessory LHA originates from the left gastric artery (VIIIa) or a replaced LHA is accompanied by the presence of accessory RHA (VIIIb); this variant occurs in 2% of our study population.
In the **type IX** of Michels variant the main hepatic artery originates from the superior mesenteric artery (incidence1%) whereas the **type X** of Michels variant shows that the main hepatic artery originates from the left gastric artery (this is an extremely uncommon variant, less that 0.2% of cases).
It is also possible to find other anatomical variants, not included in Michel's classification, as replaced RHA that originates directly from aorta, or the main hepatic artery directly beginning from aorta or from the SMA (**Figure 5**).
Even the anatomy of the artery (or arteries) that feed the segment IV may be of interest, because of their crucial position in the surgical procedures. The arterial supply for segment IV may be quite variable. It is possible to observe single, double and triple supply for segment IV, originating from right, left, and proper hepatic artery. Usually segment IV artery originates form the left hepatic artery in 64-75% of patients and from the right hepatic artery in 25%[24,25,26]. In case of living donor liver transplantation (LDLT) the arterial supply for segment IV, must be carefully preserved to prevent remnant liver failure when the right lobe is removed during the harvest[27].

3. MDCTA technical parameters

MDCTA acquisition parameters as section thickness, increment, pitch, kV and mAs can markedly change according to the employed CT scanner and on the number of available channels; with MDCT scanners at present, up to 256 simultaneous helices are acquired and the system performance has greatly increased. Usually arterial enhancement is provided by the intravenous administration in an antecubital vein of 80-100 (depending of iodine concentration) ml non ionic iodinated contrast material, at an injection speed variable from 3 to 6 mL/sec. We usually use a 5 or 6 mL/sec flow rate.
The contrast material volume should be always defined according to the number of detector-rows of the scanner. *Kamel and colleagues*[28] suggested that the use of high flow rate (5 ml\sec) in the study of hepatic vasculature produces optimal results and we agree with their observations. By using high flow rates it is possible to obtain high e fast opacification of the hepatic arteries.
It is important to remember that the presence of reduced scan time (8 seconds in 64-row scanner to cover 50 cm) requires a reduced volume of contrast material injection. Although aortic CTA studies can be performed with a lower total iodine dose, liver CTA requires a total iodine dose of 45 g in order to produce a correct imaging. Hence, with a 300 mgI/mL concentration, 150 mL is injected at 5 mL/sec, whereas with 370 mgI/mL iodine concentration, it is possible to inject the 45-g iodine dose with a volume of 120 mL injecting it at a rate of 4 mL/sec. We usually used 370 mgI/mL iodine concentration because this determines higher HU hepatic arteries values than the use of 300 mgI/mL iodine concentration.
A contrast material bolus may be followed by a saline bolus in order to reduce streak artefacts due to beam hardening. An antecubital vein is usually chosen, but also other sites may be used: if this situation occurs it is opportune to calculate the delay time again, which indicates delay in seconds between the starting of injection of i.v. contrast material and MDCTA acquisition.

For timing of image acquisition it is necessary to use the bolus tracking technique because it allows customization of scan delay for individuals with reduced cardiac output. In particular, a fixed scanning delay cannot be recommended in patients with cardiovascular disorders: with short acquisition times in fact , it is possible to completely miss the bolus if the delay time is not properly chosen.

For hepatic CTA, bolus-tracking scans that monitor aortic attenuation are acquired every 2 seconds beginning at 10 seconds after start of injection, and imaging is triggered at aortic enhancement of 150 HU. In our experience, the targeted arterial density during CTA of hepatic vasculature, is 300 to 450 HU: with this range values it is possible to obtain optimal post-processing images.

In our Institute CT of hepatic arteries are currently performed with a 16-detector-row scanner and the **arterial phase scans** are performed with the following parameters: a voltage of 120 kV, a tube current of 280-330 mA, collimation 16 x 0.625 mm, field of view of 32–36 cm]: 80–110 mL of a contrast medium were injected into a cubital vein, using a power injector at a flow rate of 5 mL/s and an 18-gauge intravenous catheter in order to obtain a constant iodine delivery rate (2 gI\sec). A bolus tracking technique is used to determine the correct timing of the scan. Dynamic monitoring scanning began 6 seconds after the beginning of the intravenous injection of contrast material. The trigger threshold inside the ROI was set at + 60 HU above the baseline. The delay between the acquisition of each monitoring scan is 1 second. When the threshold was reached, the patient was instructed not to breathe and after an interval of 4 seconds the scan started in the cranio-caudal direction.

4. Post processing techniques

The introduction and widespread availability of 16-section multi-detector row CT technology and, more recently, 64/128/256-section and dual source scanners, has greatly advanced the role of MDCTA in clinical practice. The success of CT angiography depends on a number of critical steps, including the correct timing of data acquisition, the timed delivery of iodinated contrast material and the selection of appropriate scanning parameters. The reconstruction of CT angiographic datasets may result in 1000–5000 images per examination. The large size of the dataset sometimes makes it impractical to extract all the information using standard two-dimensional techniques and makes clear the importance of post-processing techniques. Moreover, post-processing techniques allow to assess the three-dimensional relationship of the arteries to each other or the surrounding organs in a more "surgical view". To obtain high quality post-processed images it is necessary to use data set with thin slice thickness; isotropic voxels provide the best results. Several post-processing techniques may be used to evaluate the hepatic arteries: MPR (Multi Planar reconstruction), CPR (Curved Planar Reconstruction), MIP (Maximum Intensity projection) and VR (Volume Rendering). All of these tools show strengths and pitfalls regarding quantification but it is important to underline that all of them are based upon post processing procedures of the CT data.

Maximum Intensity Projection (MIP) is commonly used as a three-dimensional post-processing method to depict volumetric vascular data sets acquired with Computed Tomography. To produce MIPs, a viewing angle is chosen to define the projection plane, then parallel rays are cast from the projection plane through the stack of reconstructed sections that make up data volume, and the maximum intensity encountered along each ray is placed into the projection plane to create the MIP. It is possible to use different types of

MIP as thin-thick slab MIP or curved MIP. In the Maximum Intensity Projection (MIP) image, only the voxel with highest CT number is displayed depending on the voxel position along the projecting ray40. MIP may generate high quality DSA-like images and it provides an overview of the target vessel but, on the other hand, it shows lower sensitivity in case of dense calcification since it may obscure contrast material in the lumen. MIP allows the visualization of smaller branch vessels with less work than is required for volume rendering and it is widely used in the study of the hepatic vasculature.

Multi-Planar Reconstruction (MPR) is a post-processing technique widely used in the vascular studies. This technique is very simple and, in particular by using near isotropic CT data set, can produce high defined sagittal, coronal and oblique visual plane. MPR creates views in arbitrary plane without loss of information. Multiplanar reformatted images are created starting from the retrospectively reconstructed axial images (deriving from projection data) and resulted image may be oriented in every spatial direction. Moreover, by using 32-256 slice scanner producing isotropic voxels, spatial resolution is similar to the original source images. Usually, the use of MPR in the study of hepatic arteries does not produce acceptable results because of the tortuosity and spatial orientation of hepatic arteries.

Curved Planar Reformation (CPR). CPR is a flexible multi-planar reformatting method that works along the course of the target artery and can be performed using an axial image as a reference to define the course of the desired reformation. This technique has been shown to be useful in displaying both renal arteries and intra-cerebral vessels. In this procedure axial sections are stacked to generate an imaging volume and a reformatting algorithm is applied to the arbitrarily rotated imaging volume. On each image within these contiguous reference images, the course of the target vessel is traced by a series of mouse clicks. Then, along the defined curved line, a single-voxel-thick plane, orthogonal to the reference plane, is extruded through the entire dataset. At the end of the procedure the resulting "curved plane" is flattened and displayed as a 2D, composite sagittal image representing the target vessel. An important issue concerning the use of the CPR is that vascular images depend on the course of the curved plane selected in fact CPR creates images in an arbitrary plane and while the vessel of interest is exquisitely displayed, the neighboring anatomy becomes distorted.

Volume rendering (VR) started to become common in the late 1980s. In the VR CT numbers that make up the image are assigned to be either visible or invisible, to be displayed in varying colours and often to be displayed with varying opacity levels (transparency). VR is an advanced computer intensive rendering algorithm and it incorporates all the CT raw data into a resulting image producing high quality three dimensional pictures. VR always accurately depicts 3D relationships, while MIP may do not. Moreover VR enables a color display, which improves image quality and visualization of hepatic arteries. Unlike MIP, VR does not require slab editing since the bones do not interfere with visualization of the vasculature.

The use of post-processed images play an important role in the interpretation of MDCTA vascular images. MIP is an optimal choice in all situations except in case of vessel tortuosity and when there is not a perfect arterial phase: in fact presence of tortuosity and venous phase may produce superimposition with consequent suboptimal image quality. Superimposition can prevent radiologist from correctly detect and qualify a vessel. VR allows to evaluate vessel tortuosity and it avoid arterial\venous superimposition by depicting 3D relationship. Nowadays, VR and MIP reconstructions are obtained in real-time and the "time consuming" problem is avoided. Saba et al[29] demonstrated that MIP and VR methods showed optimal inter- and intra-observer agreement and the highest quality scores and therefore should be used preferentially as post-processing techniques to study the hepatic arteries when using MDCTA.

5. Conclusion

MDCTA allows to precisely analyze hepatic arteries configuration. The presence of hepatic arterial variant is a condition with an high prevalence. Arterial patterns should be identified with precision because these are important in the planning and performance of all radiological and surgical procedures in the liver as well as in the upper abdomen.

6. References

[1] Marcos A, Fisher RA, Ham JM, Shiffman ML, Sanyal AJ, Luketic VA, Sterling RK, Posner MP Right lobe living donor liver transplantation. Transplantation 1999;68: 798-803.

[2] Park KM, Lee SG, Lee YJ, Hwang S, Nam CW, Choi KM, Nam CH, Choi DN, Kim KH, Choi KT, Ko KS, Min PC (1999). Adult-to-adult living donor liver transplantation at Asian Medical Center, Seoul, Korea. Transplant Proc 31: 456-8.

[3] Chen YS, Chen CL, Liu PP, Chiang YC (1996) Preoperative evaluation of donors for living related liver transplantation. Transplant Proc 28:2415-2416.

[4] Imamura H, Makuuchi M, Sakamoto Y, Sugawara Y, Sano K, Nakayama A, Kawasaki S, Takayama T (2000) Anatomical keys and pitfalls in living donor liver transplantation. J Hepatobiliary Pancreat Surg 7: 380-94.

[5] Nelson TM, Pollak R, Jonasson O, Abcarian H (1988) Anatomic variants of the celiac, superior mesenteric and inferior mesenteric arteries and their clinical relevance. Clin Anat 1:75-91.

[6] Adachi, B. (1928) Anatomieder Japaner I. Das Arteriensystem der Japaner. BandII. Kaiserlish-Japanischen Universitatzu Kyoto. Maruzen Publishing Co. Kyoto; 20–71.

[7] Hiatt JR, Gabbay J, Busuttil RW (1994) Surgical anatomy of the hepatic arteries in 1000 cases. Ann Surg 220:50–52.

[8] Michels, NA (1955) Blood Supply and Anatomy of the Upper Abdominal Organs with a Descriptive Atlas. JB Lippincot Co., Philadelphia, Montreal, pp3–137.

[9] Michels, NA (1966). Newer anatomy of the liver and its variant blood supply and collateral circulation. Am J Surg. 112:337–347.

[10] Marcos A, Fisher RA, Ham JM, et al. Right lobe living donor liver transplantation. Transplantation 1999; 68:798–803.

[11] Cheng YF, Huang TL, Lee TY, Chen TY, Chen CL. Overview of imaging in living related donor hepatic transplantation. Transplant Proc 1996; 28:2412–2414.

[12] Saba L, Mallarini G. Multidetector row CT angiography in the evaluation of the hepatic artery and its anatomical variants. Clin Radiol 2008;63:312-21.

[13] De Cecco CN, Ferrari R, Rengo M, Paolantonio P, Vecchietti F, Laghi A.Anatomic variations of the hepatic arteries in 250 patients studied with 64-row CT angiography. Eur Radiol. 2009;19:2765-70.

[14] Nakayama Y, Awai K, Yanaga Y, Nakaura T, Funama Y, Hirai T, Yamashita Y. Optimal contrast medium injection protocols for the depiction of the Adamkiewicz artery using 64-detector CT angiography. Clin Radiol. 2008;63:880-7.

[15] Coşkun M, Kayahan EM, Ozbek O, Cakir B, Dalgiç A, Haberal M (2005) Imaging of hepatic arterial anatomy for depicting vascular variations in living related liver transplant donor candidates with multidetector computed tomography: comparison with conventional angiography. Transplant Proc 37:1070-3.

[16] Zhuang ZG, Qian LJ, Gong HX, Zhou Y, Chai WM, Li QG, Xu JR (2008) Multidetector computed tomography angiography in the evaluation of potential living donors for liver transplantation: single-center experience in China. Transplant Proc. 40:2466-77.

[17] Fishman EK, Ney DR, Heath DG, Corl FM, Horton KM, Johnson PT. Volume rendering versus maximum intensity projection in CT angiography: what works best, when, and why. Radiographics. 2006;26:905-22.

[18] FishmanEK, Drebin B, Magid D, et al. Volumetric rendering techniques: applications for three-dimensional imaging of the hip. Radiology 1987; 163: 737–738.

[19] Raman R, Napel S, Rubin GD. Curved-Slab Maximum Intensity Projection: Method and Evaluation. Radiology 2003;229:255-260.

[20] Haller A. Icones Anatomicae in quibus praecipae partes corporis humani delineate proponuntur et arteriarum potissimum historia continetur. Gottingen. Vandenhoeck, 1756: VIII 270.

[21] Tiedemann F. Tabularum arteriarum corporus humani. In: Koerpers, Carlsruhe, Muller CF, eds. Abbildungen der Pulsadern des menschlichen, 1822: 1-250.

[22] Adachi B. Arterien system der Japaner. Kyoto: Kerkyusha, Tokyo Press, 1928: Band II 46-60.

[23] Flint ER. Abnormalities of the right hepatic, cystic and gastroduodenal arteries and of the bile ducts. Brit J Surg, 1923; 10: 509-19.

[24] Saylisoy S, Atasoy C, Ersoz S, et al Multislice CT angiography in the evaluation of hepatic vascular anatomy in potential right lobe donors. Diagn Interv Radiol 2005;11:51-59.

[25] Covey AM, Brody LA, Maluccio MA. Variant hepatic arterial anatomy revisited: digital subtraction angiography performed in 600 patients. Radiology 2002;224:542-547.

[26] Kapoor V, Brancatelli G, Federle MP, et al. Multidetector CT arteriography with volumetric three-dimensional rendering to evaluate patients with metastatic colorectal disease. AJR Am J Roentegenol 2003;181:455-463.

[27] Williams RS, Alisa AA, Karani JB, Muiesan P, Rela SM, Heaton ND. Adult-to-adult living donor liver transplant: UK experience. Eur J Gastroenterol Hepatol 2003;15: 7-14.

[28] Kamel JR, Kruskal JB, Pomfret EA et al. Impact of multidetector CT on donor selection and surgical planning before living adult right lobe liver transplantation. AJR Am J Roentgenol 2001; 176:193-200.

[29] Saba L, Sanfilippo R, Anzidei M, Montisci R, Pascalis L, Mallarini G. Comparison between post-processing techniques in the analysis of hepatic arteries using multi-detector-row computed tomography angiography. J Comput Assist Tomogr 2011; 35: 174-80.

15

CT Imaging to Assess the Left Atrial Appendage Anatomy: Clinical Implications

Pasquale Santangeli, Luigi Di Biase,
Rodney Horton, J. David Burkhardt and Andrea Natale
*Texas Cardiac Arrhythmia Institute, St. David's Medical Center, Austin (TX)
USA*

1. Introduction

The left atrial appendage (LAA) is a highly complex anatomical structure distinct from the rest of the left atrium from an embryologic, anatomic, and pathophysiologic standpoint. While the LAA is a remnant of the embryonic left atrium, the remaining of the left atrial cavity derives from an outgrowth of the pulmonary veins. From a pathophysiologic perspective, the LAA is not just an embryologic remnant. Rather, it plays a significant role in the thromboembolic risk associated with atrial fibrillation, and is a demonstrated trigger site of atrial tachyarrhythmias. Moreover, LAA regulates normal cardiac physiology through functional receptors that influence heart rate, and secretes natriuretic peptides in response to change in left atrial pressure. In recent years, the study of LAA anatomy and its relationship with surrounding structures has gained increasing interest, as transcatheter techniques of LAA exclusion and radiofrequency ablation of left atrial tachyarrhythmias have been increasingly implemented.
Multidetector computerized tomography (CT), with its capability to distinguish among small density differences in structures attenuation, is emerging as the noninvasive reference test to image the LAA and define its anatomy and topographic relationships.
This chapter will review the role of CT to image the LAA, discussing the clinical implications different LAA morphologies detected at CT imaging.

2. Anatomy and physiology of the LAA

The LAA originates from primordial atrial tissue and is a remnant of the embryonic left atrium. The LAA lies in the left atrioventricular sulcus atop the proximal portion of the left circumflex artery; posteriorly it has a close relationship with the left superior pulmonary vein, with a distance between the ostia of these two structures (i.e., ridge) varying from 5.8 to 23.7 mm (Su et al., 2008). Another structure that have relationship with the epicardial lateral aspect of the LAA is the left phrenic nerve, which risks to be damaged when the LAA is approached during epicardial procedures (Sanchez-Quintana et al., 2005).
The shape of the LAA has significant variability. Anatomical studies have described the LAA as a long, narrow, tubular, and hooked structure (Kitzman et al., 1988, Sharma et al., 1988). Significant age- and sex-related differences in macroscopic anatomy have also been reported (Veinot et al., 1997).

In more than two-thirds of cases, the LAA consists of two or more lobes, which are usually located in different planes. This has important clinical implications when the LAA is studied to rule out intracavitary thrombus. Indeed, failure to image all the lobes or incomplete visualization of a lobe may account for under- or over-diagnosis of LAA thrombosis. The lobes extend toward the atrioventricular groove and the basal surface of the left ventricle.

The ostium of the LAA is typically elliptical, with a long diameter ranging from 10 to 24.1 mm and a short diameter ranging from 5.2 to 19.5 mm (Su et al., 2008). The length of the LAA ranges from 20 to 45 mm (Veinot et al., 1997), and the average distance between the ostium and the point at which the LAA change its orientation is 7 to 12 mm (Su et al., 2008).

The LAA is lined by a single layer of endothelium and contains pectinate muscles with a course perpendicular to its long axis. The thickness of the pectinate muscles is variable, and areas with deficient myocardium have been described on the anterolateral wall close to the mitral valve (Su et al., 2008), at an average distance of 4 mm from the LAA ostium. In these areas, the LAA may reach a minimum thickness of 0.5 mm, and particular care should be taken to avoid perforation during invasive procedures.

From a physiologic perspective, the LAA is not just an embryologic remnant.

It contains functional stretch-sensitive receptors that influence heart rate, and secretes natriuretic peptides in response to change in atrial pressure. A quantitative analysis of atrial natriuretic peptides (ANP) contained in excised LAAs revealed a content of approximately 30% of all cardiac ANP (Chapeau et al., 1985). Experimental studies have demonstrated that infusion of fluid in the LAA result in increased heart rate, diuresis and natriuresis; this further supports a significant role of the LAA in regulating normal cardiac physiology (Kappagoda et al., 1972a, Kappagoda et al., 1972b).

The LAA has a distinct pattern of contraction, and shortens to a greater extent than the rest of the left atrium. The pattern of normal blood flow in the LAA has been extensively studied with transesophageal echocardiography (Garcia-Fernandez et al., 1992, Pollick &Taylor, 1991). The LAA empties with a typical biphasic pattern; with a first passive phase that occurs in protodiastole and a second active phase that occurs during left atrial contraction. Therefore, pathophysiological changes leading to either decreased diastolic performance of the left ventricle or absence of left atrial contraction (or both), may lead to incomplete emptying of the LAA and thrombus formation.

3. Role of the LAA in cardiac pathophysiology

The LAA is the site most commonly associated with thrombus formation in patients with atrial fibrillation. The reasons why during atrial fibrillation thrombus occurs most frequently in the LAA and spare other regions, including the right atrial appendage, are incompletely understood. Transesophageal echocardiography studies have reported that up to 98-100% of atrial thrombi occurring during atrial fibrillation derive from the LAA (Leung et al., 1994, Manning et al., 1994). The variants of LAA structure and function have been studied in relation to thrombus formation and stroke.

The LAA size is associated with increased thromboembolic risk (Somerville &Chambers, 1964). Studies with transesophageal echocardiography have reported occurrence of spontaneous echocontrast and smoke-like effect most likely in patients with larger LAA (Pollick &Taylor, 1991). Thus far, no data have linked different shapes of the LAA to the thromboembolic risk of patients with atrial fibrillation.

The hemodynamic function of the LAA is also important in relation to the thromboembolic risk of patients with atrial fibrillation. To this regard, three LAA flow patterns have been described: type I characterized by a regular biphasic emptying pattern, and occurring in sinus rhythm; type II characterized by a saw-tooth emptying pattern, and occurring in some patients with atrial fibrillation; type III without any active emptying pattern and typically occurring during atrial fibrillation. The latter pattern is associated with the highest incidence of spontaneous echocontrast and thrombus (Garcia-Fernandez et al., 1992).
The arrhythmogenic role of the LAA in triggering atrial tachyarrhythmias is a matter of increasing interest (Di Biase et al., 2010b, Miyazaki et al., 2011, Takahashi et al., 2005). Our group has recently reported that up to one third of patients presenting for repeat catheter ablation of atrial fibrillation actually have the LAA as the triggering site for atrial fibrillation (Di Biase et al., 2010b).

4. CT imaging of the LAA: Clinical implications

4.1 CT imaging to diagnose LAA thrombosis

Transesophageal echocardiography is the imaging modality of choice to diagnose LAA thrombosis. Studies of comparison with intraoperative observations have disclosed a sensitivity and specificity of transesophageal echocardiography of 100% and 99%, respectively, with a positive and negative predictive values of 86% and 100% (Manning et al., 1995). However, transesophageal echocardiography is semi-invasive. Multidetector cardiac CT is emerging as a powerful diagnostic tool to detect LAA thrombosis (Kim et al., 2007, Patel et al., 2008, Shapiro et al., 2007, Singh et al., 2009, Tang et al., 2008, Tani et al., 2003).
Tani et al. evaluated the usefulness of CT for detecting LAA thrombi in patients with chronic atrial fibrillation as compared to transesophageal echocardiography (Tani et al., 2003). In this study, 96 patients with chronic atrial fibrillation underwent CT scan either in the standard supine position (71 cases) or in the prone position (25 cases). A LAA filling defects, defined as a clearly circumscribed area with lack of contrast enhancement in the LAA, was diagnosed in 13 (18%) patients undergoing CT in the supine position, and in 4 (16%) of those undergoing CT in the prone position. Transesophageal echocardiography confirmed LAA thrombi in 9/13 patients in whom CT was performed in the supine position, and in 4/4 of those who undergo CT in the prone position. In conclusion, CT was demonstrated to high sensitivity and specificity to diagnose LAA thrombosis, especially when it was performed in the prone position.
Shapiro et al. have compared the diagnostic performance of CT with that of transesophageal echocardiography to diagnose LAA thrombosis or spontaneous echocontrast (Shapiro et al., 2007). Overall, 43 patients were included in the study; of these, 10 (23%) had evidence of LAA thrombosis at transesophageal echocardiography, while 11 (26%) patients had spontaneous echocontrast without LAA thrombus. Cardiac CT failed to detect 3 of 10 thrombi (sensitivity, 70%; negative predictive value, 90%) and misclassified 6 of 33 filling defects (specificity, 82%; positive predictive value, 54%). Interestingly, in each of the 6 false-positive computer tomographic cases, the TEE revealed spontaneous echo contrast.
The role of CT to rule out LAA thrombosis has been also extensively evaluated in patients undergoing atrial fibrillation ablation (Table 1). These patients frequently undergo both transesophageal echocardiography to exclude thrombus and CT to define pulmonary vein anatomy.

Study	N. Pts	Prevalence LAA thromb.	Sens.	Spec.	PPV	NPV
Kim et al. 2007	223	15 (6.7%)	93%	85%	31%	99%
Tang et al. 2008	170	11 (6.5%)	36%	94%	29%	96%
Singh et al. 2009	51	2 (3.9%)	100%	96%	50%	100%
Martinez et al. 2009	402	9 (2.2%)	100%	92%	23%	100%

N. = number; Pts = patients; Thromb. : thrombosis; Sens. = sensitivity; Spec. = specificity; PPV = positive predictive value; NPV = negative predictive value.

Table 1. Diagnostic accuracy of LAA filling defects on CT in diagnosing LAA thrombosis (assessed by transesophageal echocardiography) in selected studies of atrial fibrillation ablation.

Kim et al. have evaluated the accuracy of CT detect LAA filling defects in patients undergoing pulmonary vein antrum isolation (Kim et al., 2007). Overall, 223 patients were included in the study. CT identified LAA filling defects with a sensitivity, specificity, positive and negative predictive values of 93%, 85%, 31% and 99% respectively, as compared to TEE (Kim et al., 2007).

These results have been recently confirmed by Martinez et al. in a cohort of 402 patients (Martinez et al., 2009). Overall, 362 patients (91%) had no evidence of a filling defect by CT or left atrial spontaneous echo contrast or thrombus by transesophageal echocardiography. In 40 patients, a LAA filling defect was detected by CT, which was confirmed as thrombus in 9 patients. The estimated sensitivity and specificity were 100% and 92%, respectively, with a positive and negative predictive values of 23% and 100%, respectively. Notably, in the Martinez's paper, most patients (91%) actually had no evidence of any LAA filling defect at CT or thrombosis at transesophageal echocardiography.

In fact, the incidence of LAA thrombosis in patients undergoing catheter ablation of AF has been reported low also by our group in a previous study (Khan et al., 2008). We assessed the incidence of LAA thrombosis in a prospective study including 1,221 patients undergoing pulmonary vein antrum isolation. All patients received a CT before the ablation procedure; 601 received a transesophageal echocardiography and all patients who had LAA filling defects at CT received also a transesophageal echocardiography to confirm the presence of LAA thrombosis. Overall, 9 patients had LAA filling defects on CT scan, but only 3 of these had LAA thrombosis on transesophageal echocardiography. Notably, 2 of these patients had chronic atrial fibrillation with an average left ventricular ejection fraction of 48%, and 1 patient had paroxysmal atrial fibrillation with severe left ventricular dysfunction (ejection fraction = 25%). These data support that patients with paroxysmal atrial fibrillation and normal left ventricular ejection fraction have very low incidence of LAA thrombosis, and CT alone is likely to be sufficient in these patients to reliably rule out LAA thrombosis (Khan et al., 2008).

The introduction of atrial fibrillation ablation under therapeutic warfarin has significantly changed the scenario of pre-procedural screening for LAA thrombosis (Di Biase et al., 2010a). We have recently reported that when ablation is performed without therapeutic warfarin discontinuation and patients had at least 4 weeks of international normalized ratio consistently >2, even pre-procedural transesophageal echocardiography can be avoided, as already it is the common practice for electrical cardioversion of persistent atrial fibrillation (Fuster et al., 2011).

4.2 CT imaging for transcatheter LAA exclusion

Percutaneous transcatheter exclusion of the LAA is an important strategy to virtually eliminate the thromboembolic risk of atrial fibrillation and avoid the need for long-term oral anticoagulant therapy. This technique has been developed as an alternative to surgical ligation or amputation, which have been demonstrated very effective in reducing the risk of thromboembolism associated with atrial fibrillation. Three devices have been specifically designed for percutaneous LAA exclusion: the Percutaneous LAA Transcatheter Occlusion (PLAATO; ev3, MN, USA), the WATCHMAN® LAA device (Atritech Inc., MN, USA) and the AMPLATZER® Cardiac Plug (AGA Medical, MN, USA). The effectiveness and safety of LAA exclusion with the WATCHMAN® device has been demonstrated in a large international trial (Figure 1). The PLAATO has been withdrawn from the market in 2006. At that time most of the published reports suggested acceptable efficacy and safety profiles; the formal reason provided by the company for the withdrawal of the device was the over-large financial investment projected to obtain clinical approval (Ostermayer et al., 2005). The AMPLATZER® device is currently undergoing active investigation in a prospective trial (NCT01118299); this device has several important differences with the WATCHMAN® and may be useful for different subsets of patients (Table 2).

Specification	AMPLATZER®	WATCHMAN®
Manufacturer	AGA Medical, MN, USA	Atritech Inc., MN, USA
FDA Approval	No	No
CE-Mark	Yes	Yes
Sizes	8 sizes (16 mm to 30 mm)	5 sizes (21 mm to 33 mm)
Delivery sheath size	9-13 French	12 French
Transesophageal echo guidance	Recommended	Recommended
Device retrieval	Possible before release	Possible before release
Oral anticoagulants	Not necessary	Recommended at least 45 days
Initial dual antiplatelet therapy	Yes	Yes (after oral anticoagulant)
Long-term antiplatelet therapy	No	Recommended

Table 2. Characteristics of commercially available percutaneous occlusion devices for the LAA.

Percutaneous LAA exclusion is most reasonably indicated for patients with significant risk of thromboembolic complications (i.e., $CHADS_2$ score ≥2) who are unable to tolerate anticoagulants because of increased risk of bleeding complications or poor compliance.

An accurate imaging assessment of the LAA and its relationship with surrounding structures is of utmost importance for percutaneous LAA exclusion. As mentioned, the LAA is closely associated with the left aortic sinus and, therefore, with the ostium of the left coronary artery. Particular care should be exercised when choosing the size of a LAA occlusion device, since oversizing the device may result in compression of the left circumflex artery.

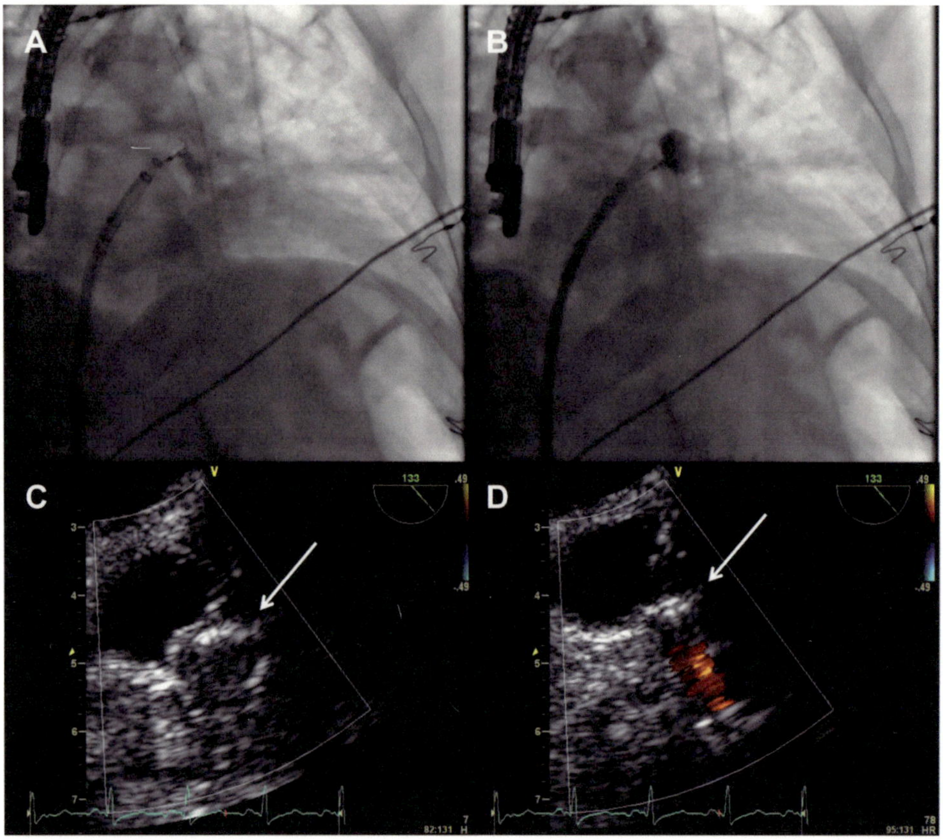

Fig. 1. Placement of a WATCHMAN® left atrial appendage exclusion device. Panels A and B show transcatheter deployment (Panel A) and contrast injection (Panel B) in the left atrial appendage, without evidence of contrast leaking. The correct positioning of the device is confirmed by real-time transesophageal echocardiography (Panels C and D), which confirms absence of leaking by Color Doppler study (Panel D).

With regard to the shape of the LAA, it is important to remark that the ostium of this structure is typically elliptical, while all available occluders have a round shape. This may well account for incomplete sealing of the orifice and leakage from the LAA. More than two-thirds of the LAA have two or more lobes originating from a common opening; usually different lobes are positioned in different anatomical planes. The distance between the LAA orifice and the point at which the LAA first deviates from its original course (LAA neck) range from 7 to 12 mm; this distance is very important for a correct device deployment (Su et al., 2008).

A correct imaging assessment of the LAA is crucial to plan for LAA device closure. Transesophageal echocardiography is required to define the size and shape of the LAA; the ostium, neck, and depth of the LAA. The zone of device landing is usually the junction between the proximal third and the medial third of the LAA, and can be easily assessed with transesophageal echocardiography.

Cardiac CT is of valuable aid in evaluating the shape of the LAA and in defining its relationships with surrounding critical structures.

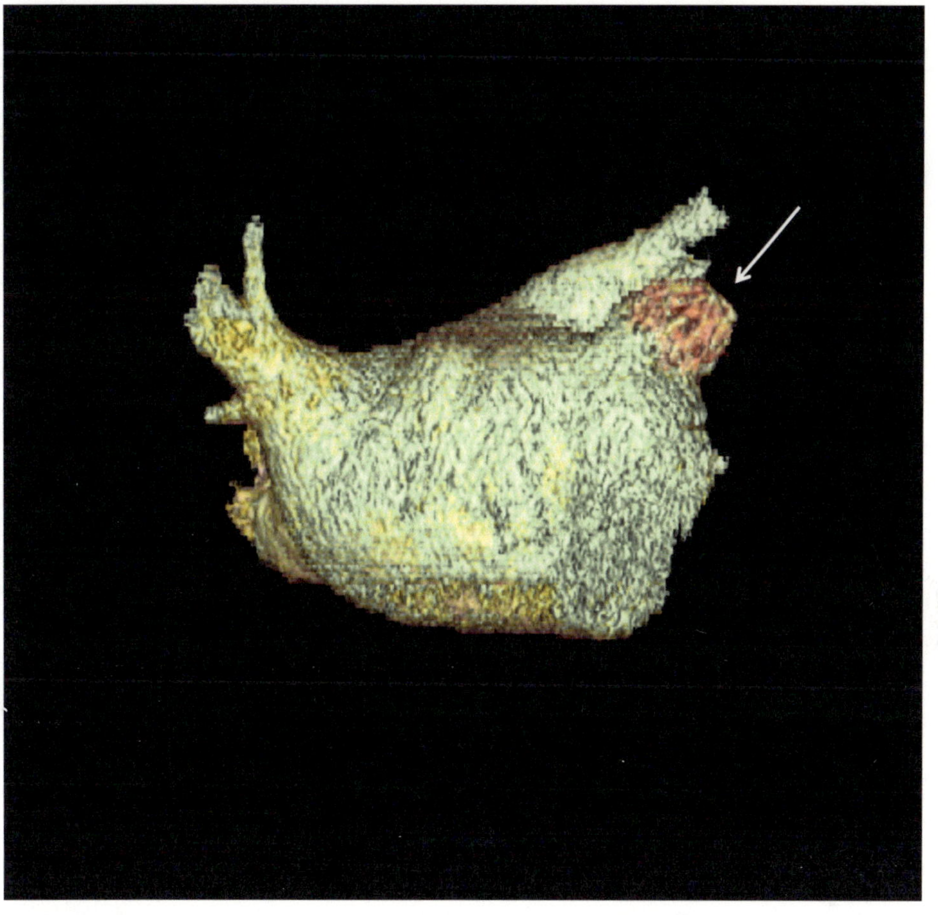

Fig. 2. Antero-posterior CT imaging of the left atrium after WATCHMAN® device placement (Arrow).

As mentioned, the ostium of the LAA is in close proximity to both the left superior pulmonary vein and the left aortic sinus, from which the left coronary artery arises. CT studies have demonstrated that the LAA ostium can be located at different levels relative to the left superior pulmonary vein ostium, namely, above the left superior pulmonary vein, in the same plane, or underneath it.

In the latter case, the LAA is in the closest contact with the circumflex coronary artery (Su et al., 2008). In this case, particular care should be taken with implantation of percutaneous LAA exclusion devices or with radiofrequency catheter ablation, since damage to the circumflex artery can occur.

In a recent study, our group investigated the LAA morphology in 612 patients, evaluating the reproducibility of different measurement methods for determining the size of the LAA orifice in different cardiac phases.

In particular, the LAA morphology, the relationship with the left pulmonary veins, the LAA volume, number of lobes, the angle of the first LAA bend, the distance from the first bend to the LAA orifice, and the distance between the LAA orifice and the septum were studied on three-dimensional CT images (Wang et al., 2010).

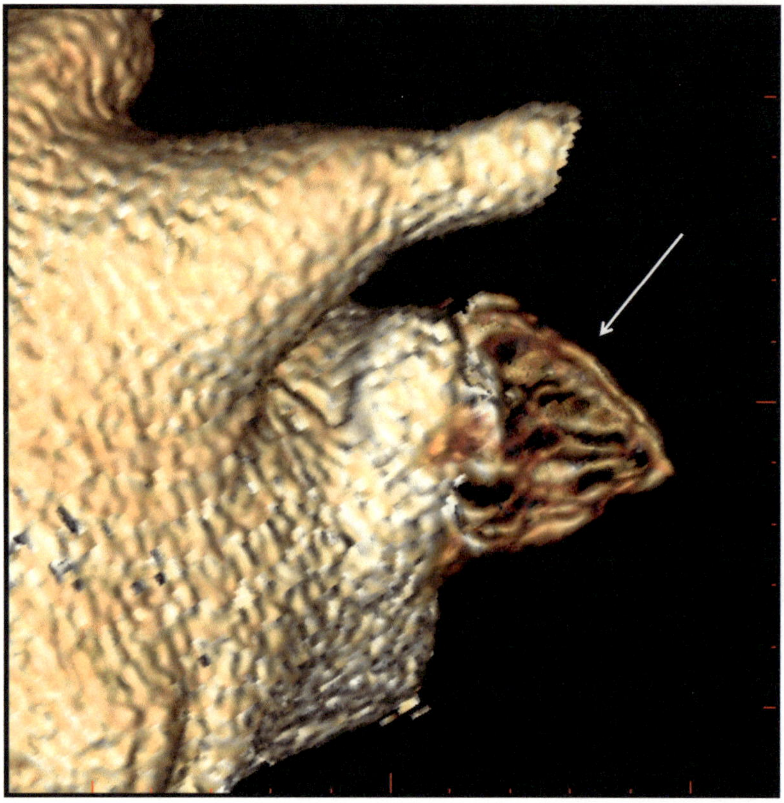

Fig. 3. CT detail of the WATCHMAN® device correctly positioned in the left atrial appendage.

The LAA morphology was initially classified on the basis of the presence of an obvious bend, giving to the LAA an appearance similar to a chicken wing (18.3% of cases).

In the absence of an obvious bend, the LAA was classified as: 1) windsock shaped (46.7%), with 1 dominant lobe; 2) cauliflower shaped (29.1%), that has limited overall length with more complex internal characteristics; 3) cactus shaped (5.9%), with a dominant central lobe and secondary lobes extending from the central lobe in both superior and inferior directions (Figure 4).

The approximate LAA length, defined as length of the primary lobe only from the LAA orifice to the LAA apex was 45.8 ± 12.1 mm and the LAA volume was 8.8 ± 5.6 mL. An obvious bend in the primary lobe was seen in 73.2% of patients, with an angle of the first bend of 97.6 ± 20.3 degrees.

Analysis of the LAA ostium showed a round shape only in 5.7% of cases, with the majority of LAA presenting an elliptical shape (68.9%). The diameters of the ostium in the horizontal, coronal, and sagittal plane were 18.5 ± 4.9 mm, 20.6 ± 4.4 mm, and 17.0 ± 4.0 mm. Long- and short-axis diameters were 25.4 ± 5.5 mm and 16.8 ± 4.5 mm, respectively. Interestingly, these diameters showed minimal changes during different phases of the cardiac cycle in sinus rhythm (maximal change 1 to 2 mm), while no change was observed during atrial fibrillation.

Our study shed additional light on the complex anatomy of the LAA, which is crucial for a correct positioning of LAA occlusion devices. Those factors may include the distance between the fossa ovalis where the transseptal access is obtained to the base of the LAA, the LAA shape, its anatomic relationships with the left pulmonary veins, the distance between the ostium and the first bend, and the shape and dimension of the LA orifice.

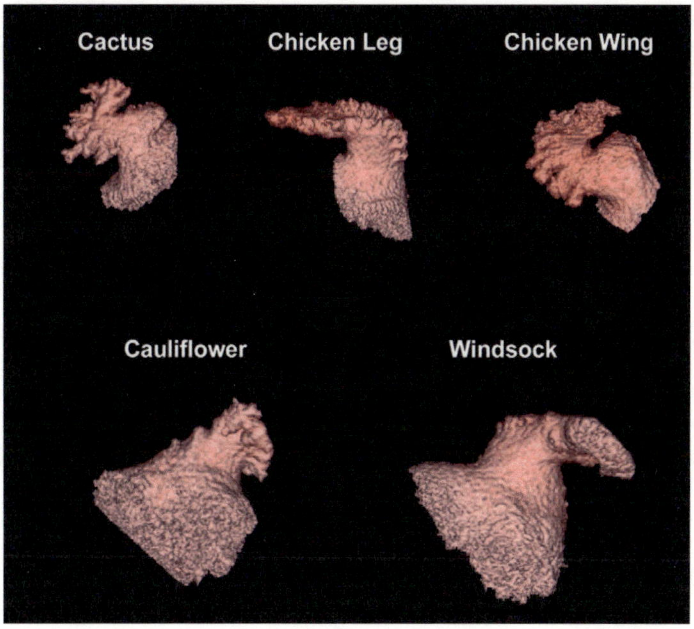

Fig. 4. Different shapes of the left atrial appendage as assessed by cardiac CT imaging.

5. Conclusions

CT is an accurate tool to non-invasively detect LAA thrombosis. Moreover, it allows an accurate assessment of the LAA anatomy. Different parameters such as the morphology and diameter of the LAA orifice, the shape of the LAA, and the angle of the LAA bend can be accurately defined by CT. All these parameters are crucial for a correct positioning of LAA occlusion devices.

6. References

Chapeau, C., Gutkowska, J., Schiller, P. W., Milne, R. W., Thibault, G., Garcia, R., Genest, J. & Cantin, M. (1985). Localization of immunoreactive synthetic atrial natriuretic factor (ANF) in the heart of various animal species, *J Histochem Cytochem*, Vol. 33, No. 6, (Jun), pp. (541-50), 0022-1554 (Print) 0022-1554 (Linking)

Di Biase, L., Burkhardt, J. D., Mohanty, P., Sanchez, J., Horton, R., Gallinghouse, G. J., Lakkireddy, D., Verma, A., Khaykin, Y., Hongo, R., Hao, S., Beheiry, S., Pelargonio, G., Dello Russo, A., Casella, M., Santarelli, P., Santangeli, P., Wang, P., Al-Ahmad, A., Patel, D., Themistoclakis, S., Bonso, A., Rossillo, A., Corrado, A., Raviele, A., Cummings, J. E., Schweikert, R. A., Lewis, W. R. & Natale, A. (2010a). Periprocedural stroke and management of major bleeding complications in patients undergoing catheter ablation of atrial fibrillation: the impact of periprocedural therapeutic international normalized ratio, *Circulation*, Vol. 121, No. 23, (Jun 15), pp. (2550-6), 1524-4539 (Electronic) 0009-7322 (Linking)

Di Biase, L., Burkhardt, J. D., Mohanty, P., Sanchez, J., Mohanty, S., Horton, R., Gallinghouse, G. J., Bailey, S. M., Zagrodzky, J. D., Santangeli, P., Hao, S., Hongo, R., Beheiry, S., Themistoclakis, S., Bonso, A., Rossillo, A., Corrado, A., Raviele, A., Al-Ahmad, A., Wang, P., Cummings, J. E., Schweikert, R. A., Pelargonio, G., Dello Russo, A., Casella, M., Santarelli, P., Lewis, W. R. & Natale, A. (2010b). Left atrial appendage: an underrecognized trigger site of atrial fibrillation, *Circulation*, Vol. 122, No. 2, (Jul 13), pp. (109-18), 1524-4539 (Electronic) 0009-7322 (Linking)

Fuster, V., Ryden, L. E., Cannom, D. S., Crijns, H. J., Curtis, A. B., Ellenbogen, K. A., Halperin, J. L., Kay, G. N., Le Huezey, J. Y., Lowe, J. E., Olsson, S. B., Prystowsky, E. N., Tamargo, J. L., Wann, L. S., Smith, S. C., Jr. & Priori, S. G. (2011). 2011 ACCF/AHA/HRS Focused Updates Incorporated Into the ACC/AHA/ESC 2006 Guidelines for the Management of Patients With Atrial Fibrillation: A Report of the American College of Cardiology Foundation/American Heart Association Task Force on Practice Guidelines, *Circulation*, Vol. 123, No. 10, (Mar 15), pp. (e269-367), 1524-4539 (Electronic) 0009-7322 (Linking)

Garcia-Fernandez, M. A., Torrecilla, E. G., San Roman, D., Azevedo, J., Bueno, H., Moreno, M. M. & Delcan, J. L. (1992). Left atrial appendage Doppler flow patterns: implications on thrombus formation, *Am Heart J*, Vol. 124, No. 4, (Oct), pp. (955-61), 0002-8703 (Print) 0002-8703 (Linking)

Kappagoda, C. T., Linden, R. J. & Saunders, D. A. (1972a). The effect on heart rate of distending the atrial appendages in the dog, *J Physiol*, Vol. 225, No. 3, (Sep), pp. (705-19), 0022-3751 (Print) 0022-3751 (Linking)

Kappagoda, C. T., Linden, R. J. & Snow, H. M. (1972b). The effect of distending the atrial appendages on urine flow in the dog, *J Physiol*, Vol. 227, No. 1, (Dec), pp. (233-42), 0022-3751 (Print) 0022-3751 (Linking)

Khan, M. N., Usmani, A., Noor, S., Elayi, S., Ching, C. K., Di Biase, L., Patel, D., Burkhardt, J. D., Cummings, J., Schweikert, R., Saliba, W. & Natale, A. (2008). Low incidence of left atrial or left atrial appendage thrombus in patients with paroxysmal atrial fibrillation and normal EF who present for pulmonary vein antrum isolation procedure, *J Cardiovasc Electrophysiol*, Vol. 19, No. 4, (Apr), pp. (356-8), 1540-8167 (Electronic) 1045-3873 (Linking)

Kim, Y. Y., Klein, A. L., Halliburton, S. S., Popovic, Z. B., Kuzmiak, S. A., Sola, S., Garcia, M. J., Schoenhagen, P., Natale, A. & Desai, M. Y. (2007). Left atrial appendage filling defects identified by multidetector computed tomography in patients undergoing radiofrequency pulmonary vein antral isolation: a comparison with transesophageal echocardiography, *Am Heart J*, Vol. 154, No. 6, (Dec), pp. (1199-205), 1097-6744 (Electronic) 0002-8703 (Linking)

Kitzman, D. W., Scholz, D. G., Hagen, P. T., Ilstrup, D. M. & Edwards, W. D. (1988). Age-related changes in normal human hearts during the first 10 decades of life. Part II (Maturity): A quantitative anatomic study of 765 specimens from subjects 20 to 99 years old, *Mayo Clin Proc*, Vol. 63, No. 2, (Feb), pp. (137-46), 0025-6196 (Print) 0025-6196 (Linking)

Leung, D. Y., Black, I. W., Cranney, G. B., Hopkins, A. P. & Walsh, W. F. (1994). Prognostic implications of left atrial spontaneous echo contrast in nonvalvular atrial fibrillation, *J Am Coll Cardiol*, Vol. 24, No. 3, (Sep), pp. (755-62), 0735-1097 (Print) 0735-1097 (Linking)

Manning, W. J., Silverman, D. I., Katz, S. E., Riley, M. F., Come, P. C., Doherty, R. M., Munson, J. T. & Douglas, P. S. (1994). Impaired left atrial mechanical function after cardioversion: relation to the duration of atrial fibrillation, *J Am Coll Cardiol*, Vol. 23, No. 7, (Jun), pp. (1535-40), 0735-1097 (Print) 0735-1097 (Linking)

Manning, W. J., Weintraub, R. M., Waksmonski, C. A., Haering, J. M., Rooney, P. S., Maslow, A. D., Johnson, R. G. & Douglas, P. S. (1995). Accuracy of transesophageal echocardiography for identifying left atrial thrombi. A prospective, intraoperative study, *Ann Intern Med*, Vol. 123, No. 11, (Dec 1), pp. (817-22), 0003-4819 (Print) 0003-4819 (Linking)

Martinez, M. W., Kirsch, J., Williamson, E. E., Syed, I. S., Feng, D., Ommen, S., Packer, D. L. & Brady, P. A. (2009). Utility of nongated multidetector computed tomography for detection of left atrial thrombus in patients undergoing catheter ablation of atrial fibrillation, *JACC Cardiovasc Imaging*, Vol. 2, No. 1, (Jan), pp. (69-76), 1876-7591 (Electronic)

Miyazaki, S., Shah, A. J., Wilton, S. B. & Haissaguerre, M. (2011). Is The Left Atrial Appendage Electrically Silent?, *Heart Rhythm*, Vol. No. (Feb 23), pp. 1556-3871 (Electronic) 1547-5271 (Linking)

Ostermayer, S. H., Reisman, M., Kramer, P. H., Matthews, R. V., Gray, W. A., Block, P. C., Omran, H., Bartorelli, A. L., Della Bella, P., Di Mario, C., Pappone, C., Casale, P. N., Moses, J. W., Poppas, A., Williams, D. O., Meier, B., Skanes, A., Teirstein, P. S., Lesh, M. D., Nakai, T., Bayard, Y., Billinger, K., Trepels, T., Krumsdorf, U. & Sievert, H. (2005). Percutaneous left atrial appendage transcatheter occlusion (PLAATO system) to prevent stroke in high-risk patients with non-rheumatic atrial fibrillation: results from the international multi-center feasibility trials, *J Am Coll Cardiol*, Vol. 46, No. 1, (Jul 5), pp. (9-14), 0735-1097 (Print) 0735-1097 (Linking)

Patel, A., Au, E., Donegan, K., Kim, R. J., Lin, F. Y., Stein, K. M., Markowitz, S. M., Iwai, S., Weinsaft, J. W., Min, J. K. & Lerman, B. B. (2008). Multidetector row computed tomography for identification of left atrial appendage filling defects in patients undergoing pulmonary vein isolation for treatment of atrial fibrillation: comparison with transesophageal echocardiography, *Heart Rhythm*, Vol. 5, No. 2, (Feb), pp. (253-60), 1547-5271 (Print) 1547-5271 (Linking)

Pollick, C. & Taylor, D. (1991). Assessment of left atrial appendage function by transesophageal echocardiography. Implications for the development of thrombus, *Circulation*, Vol. 84, No. 1, (Jul), pp. (223-31), 0009-7322 (Print) 0009-7322 (Linking)

Sanchez-Quintana, D., Cabrera, J. A., Climent, V., Farre, J., Weiglein, A. & Ho, S. Y. (2005). How close are the phrenic nerves to cardiac structures? Implications for cardiac interventionalists, *J Cardiovasc Electrophysiol*, Vol. 16, No. 3, (Mar), pp. (309-13), 1045-3873 (Print) 1045-3873 (Linking)

Shapiro, M. D., Neilan, T. G., Jassal, D. S., Samy, B., Nasir, K., Hoffmann, U., Sarwar, A., Butler, J., Brady, T. J. & Cury, R. C. (2007). Multidetector computed tomography for the detection of left atrial appendage thrombus: a comparative study with transesophageal echocardiography, *J Comput Assist Tomogr*, Vol. 31, No. 6, (Nov-Dec), pp. (905-9), 0363-8715 (Print) 0363-8715 (Linking)

Sharma, S., Devine, W., Anderson, R. H. & Zuberbuhler, J. R. (1988). The determination of atrial arrangement by examination of appendage morphology in 1842 heart specimens, *Br Heart J*, Vol. 60, No. 3, (Sep), pp. (227-31), 0007-0769 (Print) 0007-0769 (Linking)

Singh, N. K., Nallamothu, N., Zuck, V. P. & Issa, Z. F. (2009). Left atrial appendage filling defects on 64-slice multidetector computed tomography in patients undergoing pulmonary vein isolation: predictors and comparison to transesophageal echocardiography, *J Comput Assist Tomogr*, Vol. 33, No. 6, (Nov-Dec), pp. (946-51), 1532-3145 (Electronic) 0363-8715 (Linking)

Somerville, W. & Chambers, R. J. (1964). Systemic Embolism in Mitral Stenosis: Relation to the Size of the Left Atrial Appendix, *Br Med J*, Vol. 2, No. 5418, (Nov 7), pp. (1167-9), 0007-1447 (Print) 0007-1447 (Linking)

Su, P., McCarthy, K. P. & Ho, S. Y. (2008). Occluding the left atrial appendage: anatomical considerations, *Heart*, Vol. 94, No. 9, (Sep), pp. (1166-70), 1468-201X (Electronic) 1355-6037 (Linking)

Takahashi, Y., Sanders, P., Rotter, M. & Haissaguerre, M. (2005). Disconnection of the left atrial appendage for elimination of foci maintaining atrial fibrillation, *J Cardiovasc Electrophysiol*, Vol. 16, No. 8, (Aug), pp. (917-9), 1045-3873 (Print) 1045-3873 (Linking)

Tang, R. B., Dong, J. Z., Zhang, Z. Q., Li, Z. A., Liu, X. P., Kang, J. P., Yu, R. H., Long de, Y. & Ma, C. S. (2008). Comparison of contrast enhanced 64-slice computed tomography and transesophageal echocardiography in detection of left atrial thrombus in patients with atrial fibrillation, *J Interv Card Electrophysiol*, Vol. 22, No. 3, (Sep), pp. (199-203), 1383-875X (Print) 1383-875X (Linking)

Tani, T., Yamakami, S., Matsushita, T., Okamoto, M., Toyama, J., Suzuki, S., Fukutomi, T. & Itoh, M. (2003). Usefulness of electron beam tomography in the prone position for detecting atrial thrombi in chronic atrial fibrillation, *J Comput Assist Tomogr*, Vol. 27, No. 1, (Jan-Feb), pp. (78-84), 0363-8715 (Print) 0363-8715 (Linking)

Veinot, J. P., Harrity, P. J., Gentile, F., Khandheria, B. K., Bailey, K. R., Eickholt, J. T., Seward, J. B., Tajik, A. J. & Edwards, W. D. (1997). Anatomy of the normal left atrial appendage: a quantitative study of age-related changes in 500 autopsy hearts: implications for echocardiographic examination, *Circulation*, Vol. 96, No. 9, (Nov 4), pp. (3112-5), 0009-7322 (Print) 0009-7322 (Linking)

Wang, Y., Di Biase, L., Horton, R. P., Nguyen, T., Morhanty, P. & Natale, A. (2010). Left atrial appendage studied by computed tomography to help planning for appendage closure device placement, *J Cardiovasc Electrophysiol*, Vol. 21, No. 9, (Sep), pp. (973-82), 1540-8167 (Electronic) 1045-3873 (Linking)

Part 3

CT-PET and Radiation Dose

16

Integrated PET/CT in the Staging of NSCLC

Walter De Wever
University Hospitals – Leuven
Belgium

1. Introduction

Lung cancer is a common disease with approximately 3-million new cases per year worldwide and is the leading cause of cancer-related death in many countries. Eighty percent of the lung cancers are non-small cell lung cancers (NSCLC) and 20% are small cell lung cancers (SCLC) [1]. The imaging diagnostic assessment of patients with lung cancer includes morphological imaging modalities such as chest X-ray, Computed Tomography (CT) and Magnetic Resonance (MR) as well as metabolic imaging modalities such as nuclear medicine procedures, including Positron Emission Tomography (PET) and PET/CT. Staging a patient with lung cancer implies an accurate determination of the size of the tumor, the potential infiltration of the tumor into the adjacent structures, the involvement of hilar and mediastinal lymph nodes and the detection of distant metastases. Till recently, CT was the routine imaging procedure for staging patients with NSCLC. The success of CT is related to the very detailed imaging information of the localization and extent of the tumor, the presence of enlarged lymph nodes and the presence of metastatic disease [2]. PET has more recently been introduced in tumor staging and it has been used successfully for detection of primary tumors, metastases, early tumor recurrence, and for the detection of metastatic lymph nodes [3, 4]. This imaging modality possesses a greater sensitivity for detection of malignancy though it is inhibited by relatively poor spatial resolution and anatomical localization of disease. Combining detailed anatomical information obtained by CT with metabolic information from PET seems logical, therefore. Integrated PET/CT is the most recent approach to post hoc image fusion. It combines these image modalities into one scanner that acquires accurately aligned anatomical and metabolical images in the same scanning session [1].

2. Evaluation of a solitary pulmonary nodule

Lung lesions detected in a chest radiograph, incidentally or by systematic investigation, need a definite confirmation of diagnosis. The key point is the evaluation of malignancy in peripheral lung nodules. A solitary pulmonary nodule (SPN) is defined as a focal round or oval lung lesion with a diameter smaller than 3 cm, completely surrounded by normal lung tissue, not associated with atelectasis or adenopathies. Lung lesions greater than 3 cm are classified as masses [5]. Non-invasive evaluation of SPN is usually performed by different imaging procedures including CT, MR, PET and PET/CT. CT is considered to be an excellent tool for the detection and localization of SPNs with a good sensitivity (96%, range 91–98%) but a poor specificity (50%, range 41–58%) [6]. CT provides data regarding the nodule shapes, borders and density [7]. Central or concentric calcifications, round shape or a morphologic stability over 2 years are features of benignancy. On the contrary, non-demarcated borders, calcifications with eccentric appearance or spiculated pattern, a doubling time of <10 month and cavitation or pseudocavitation are features of malignancy [8, 9]. Contrast enhanced CT can be used to characterize SPN. Enhancement of the pulmonary nodule with 15 Hounsfield Units (HU) has a sensitivity and specificity of 98% and 58% in the detection of malignancy, respectively and the absence of lung nodule enhancement is strongly predictive of a benign diagnosis (negative predictive value of 96.5%) [10].

Several studies showed that PET had similar sensitivity (92–95%) but superior specificity (72–83%) as compared to CT for the characterization of SPN [11, 12]. In one of the largest published studies (450 patients) with lung nodules evaluated with PET, Gould et al. reported a high PET sensitivity (94.2%) and specificity (83.3%) [12]. Lower sensitivity (91.7%) but similar specificity (82.3%) was observed by Fletcher et al. in a population of 344 patients [13]. Malignant lesions with a size of more than 10 mm in diameter are detected with a sensitivity of 96% [14]. Gupta et al. showed that PET using Fluor-Deoxy-Glucose (FDG) as tracer, is highly accurate in differentiating malignant from benign solitary pulmonary nodules for sizes from 6 to 30 mm when radiographic findings are indeterminate [15]. An important contribution of two more recent meta-analyses [16, 17] is the assessment of the performance of FDG-PET in small lung nodules. Nomori et al. demonstrated that the sensitivity clearly decreases for malignant lung lesions of less than 10 mm in diameter [18]. For technical reasons, the lower limit has to be set in dependence from the spatial resolution and will be around 6–10 mm according to the most common PET scanners used. Thus, FDG-PET is not indicated for the evaluation of solitary pulmonary nodules of less than 6–10 mm. The meta-analysis of Ung et al. mentioned that the accuracy for the characterization of lung lesions by FDG-PET depends on the amount of tumoral FDG uptake given as Standardized Uptake Value (SUV) [16]. Grgic et al. reported that it is possible to estimate the individual risk for malignancy considering the SUVmax of a given nodule and clinically relevant information [19]. The authors reported that the mean SUVmax of malignant SPNs was higher than benign lesions (SUVmax 9.7 ± 5.5 vs. 2.6 ± 2.5; $P < 0.01$).

False positive FDG-PET findings are represented by lung inflammatory conditions such as pneumonia, pyogenic abscesses, aspergillosis, granulomatous diseases (tuberculosis, sarcoidosis, histoplasmosis, Wegener's granulomatosis) [20]. False negative findings on PET images can be the result of small lesion size (<1 cm) or tumor types characterized by low glucose metabolism (such as Neuro Endocrine Tumors (NET), Broncho Alveolar Cell Carcinomas (BAC) or pulmonary carcinoids [21, 22].

The widespread introduction in clinical practice of FDG PET/CT has allowed a more accurate assessment of SNPs. With integrated PET/CT, additional certainty to the presence or absence of FDG uptake in the pulmonary nodule can be achieved because morphologic CT criteria and metabolical PET criteria are available simultaneously [23]. Kim et al. reported a sensitivity of 97% and a specificity of 85% for the detection of SPNs, concluding that the combination of the anatomical and metabolic images preserves the sensitivity of the CT and the specificity of the PET scan, but improves significantly the overall accuracy [24, 25].

3. Assessment of T stage

The most significant improvement in staging results with combined PET/CT compared with PET alone relates to T staging. This superiority is attributed entirely to the CT component of the examination [26]. The major benefit of PET/CT lies in the direct link between the information on metabolic changes of structures and the highly detailed anatomic CT information of these structures. Recent published studies showed that PET/CT is the best noninvasive imaging technique for correct prediction of T-stage: PET/CT correctly predicts the T-stage in +/_ 82% of cases, in comparison with 55, 68 and 76% for PET, CT and visual correlation of PET and CT, respectively [20]. Halpern et al.[27] demonstrated an accuracy rate of 97% with PET/CT compared with 67% with PET only. Another study by Cerfolio et al. [28] showed that PET/CT more accurately predicted T status (70% of cases) than did PET alone (47%). Lardinois et al. described accuracy rates for T staging with PET/CT and CT as 88% and 58%, respectively [29]. Pauls et al. found that the advantages of integrated PET/CT also depend on the histological T-stage of the primary tumor [30]. Changes of the therapeutic strategy due to PET/CT are especially seen in T3 and T4 tumors.

It has been demonstrated that integrated PET/CT is a useful tool for the detection of tumor invasion into the chest wall [1, 29, 31]. Due to the exact anatomic correlation to the FDG uptake, the delineation of the primary tumor can be defined precisely. Integrated PET/CT provides important information on mediastinal infiltration as well. In addition, PET can be helpful in evaluating the cause of pleural effusions [29] (figure 1). One of the most important attributes of PET/CT is the ability to distinguish between tumor and distal atelectasis (figure 2). This is particularly important for the planning of radiotherapy in patients with lung cancer associated with atelectasis [23]. Table 1 summarizes the most important studies concerning T-staging with PET/CT.

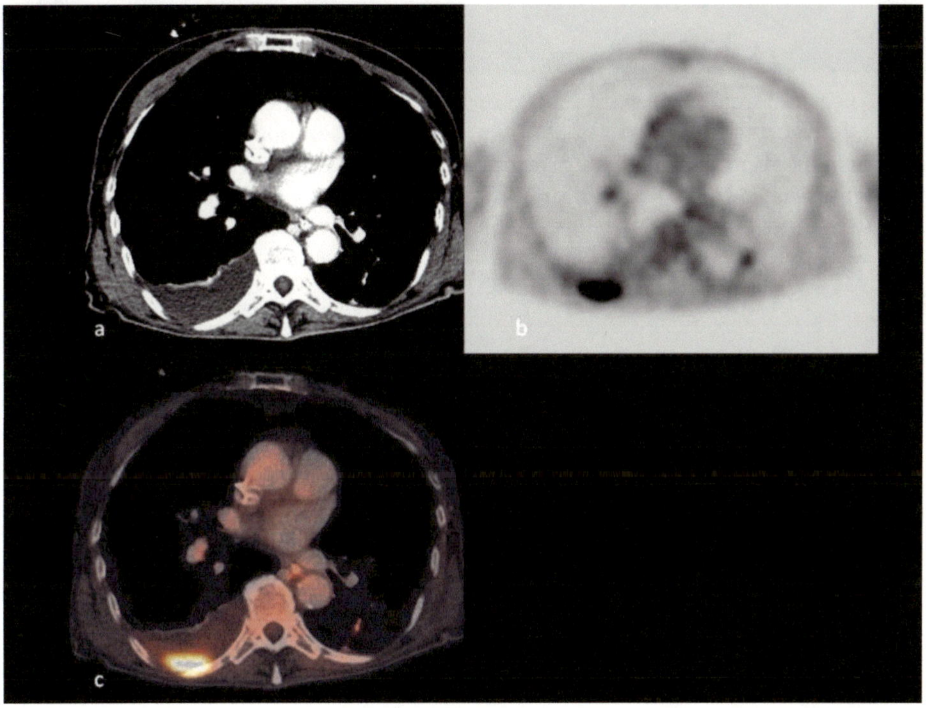

Fig. 1. A 74-year-old woman with an abdominal tumor. CT showed a pleural effusion in the right hemi-thorax (fig 1a). CT could not demonstrate contrast-captated pleural lesions suspect for pleural metastases. PET demonstrates FDG-uptake in the dorsal part of the right hemi-thorax (fig 1b). Integrated PET/CT localizes this FDG-uptake in the pleura, indicating pleural metastases. This was confirmed after pleuroscopy.

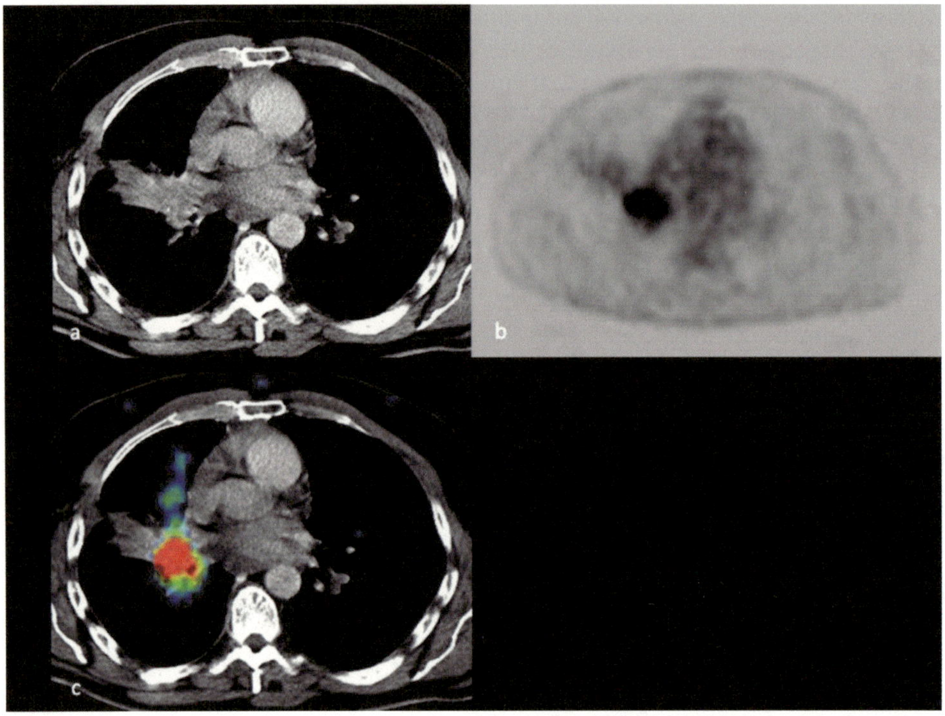

Fig. 2. A 57-year-old man with a central tumor in the right lung. CT demonstrates a central mass with a retro-obstructive consolidation in the right upper lobe (fig 2a). PET demonstrates FDG uptake in the right hilar region corresponding with the central tumor (fig 2b). Integrated PET/CT demonstrates the central tumor in the right lung and can delineate the tumor from the surrounding retro-obstructive consolidation in the right upper lobe (fig 2c).

Author	Year	Number of Subjects	Accuracy (%)
T staging			
Lardinois [29]	2003	40	88
Antoch [31]	2003	27	94
Cerfolio [28]	2004	129	70
Shim [41]	2005	106	86
Halpern [27]	2005	36	97
De Wever [1]	2007	50	86
Average		388	87

Table 1. Accuracy of PET/CT in T staging

4. Assessment of N stage

The accuracy of CT for the prediction of intrathoracic nodal spread of tumor remains limited and the more recently developed CT systems do not change this [7]. Lymph node size (diameter >10 mm in short axis) is used as the only criterion to determine metastatic disease. Different studies with CT have shown a marked heterogeneity in the results, going from 52% to 69% for sensitivity and from 69% to 82% for specificity [32].

Over the past years, several studies have found that FDG-PET has a significantly higher sensitivity and specificity than CT in the detection of tumoral involvement of mediastinal lymph nodes[33-35]. Meta-analyses have confirmed sensitivities ranging between 79–85% and specificities between 89–92% [36-38]. The clinical importance of FDG-PET lies in the high negative predictive value in lymph node staging, which has been estimated as >90% in several studies [39]. Some studies have demonstrated that the accuracy of PET imaging in the mediastinum is dependent on the size of lymph nodes. PET scanning is more sensitive but less specific when CT imaging identifies enlarged nodes. A median sensitivity and specificity of PET scans of 100 and 78%, respectively, in patients with enlarged lymph nodes has been reported [40]. It has been concluded that PET scanning is very accurate in identifying malignant lymph nodes when lymph nodes are enlarged. Conversely, PET scanning is less sensitive but more specific in patients with normal-sized mediastinal nodes on CT. It has been shown that CT of the mediastinum is falsely negative in about 20% of patients with normal-sized malignant lymph nodes. Gould et al. reported a median sensitivity and specificity in these patients of 82 and 93%, respectively [38]. There is an ongoing controversy whether a negative PET scan can be used to obviate further invasive mediastinal staging in patients with enlarged lymph nodes on CT. Microscopic foci of metastases cannot be detected with any imaging modality. In our institution, in patients with negative PET scan but with enlarged mediastinal lymph nodes on CT further evaluation by EBUS or mediastinoscopy will be performed.

PET/CT result in improvement of nodal staging compared with PET alone due to ability to reveal the exact location of metastatic lymph nodes [26]. Accurate anatomic correlation is of benefit for exact localization of a solitary lymph node metastasis and thus allows exact classification as N1 or N2 disease. PET/CT is also important when identifying supraclavicular N3 disease [26]. Initial studies demonstrated a pooled average sensitivity, specificity, positive predictive value, negative predictive value and accuracy of PET/CT of 73%, 80%, 78%, 91% and 87%, respectively. Shim and colleagues [41] demonstrated accuracy rate for PET/CT and CT in N disease of 84% and 69%, respectively. In a recent study by Kim et al.[42] the overall sensitivity, specificity and accuracy of PET/CT for mediastinal nodal staging were 61%, 96% and 86%, respectively Another study by Yi et al. [43] reported that in T1 stage NSCLC, contrast-enhanced helical dynamic CT better predicts mediastinal nodal metastasis than PET/CT, whereas PET/CT shows perfect specificity and higher accuracy than helical dynamic CT [26]. Table 2 summarizes the most important studies concerning N stage with PET/CT. The benefit of PET/CT compared with PET for nodal staging appears to lie in an increase in specificity and positive predictive value, and the benefit in accuracy of PET/CT is due to the appropriate assignment of focally increased FDG uptake. This emphasizes the importance of anatomic information in conjunction with PET imaging for appropriate PET image interpretation.

False-negative results can occur when the cancer involvement of the mediastinal nodes is low (micro metastases). Because of limitations in spatial resolution of PET, it is often not possible to distinguish between a central tumor and hilar lymph nodes or adjacent mediastinal lymph nodes. Additionally, differentiation between malignant lymph node and residual brown fat or inflammatory lymph nodes can be challenging [44]. Therefore, mediastinal staging with mediastinoscopy or endo-bronchial ultrasonography or endo-eosophageal ultrasonography remains the standard for mediastinal staging, even if not all mediastinal lymph nodes can be accessed with each technique alone [45] (figures 3-5). On the other hand, previous or concomitant inflammatory and infectious conditions even as granulomatous diseases are mainly responsible for false-positive results of PET/CT.

Author	Year	Number of Subjects	Sensitivity (%)	Specificity (%)	PPV (%)	NPV (%)	Accuracy (%)
N Staging							
Lardinois [29]	2003	40					81
Cerfolio [28]	2004	129	77-92				78
Shim [41]	2005	106	85				84
Halpern [27]	2005	36					78
Kim [59]	2006	150	47	100	100	87	88
De Wever [1]	2007	50					80
Yi [43]	2007	143	56	100	100	88	90
Lee	2007	126	86	81	56	95	82
Melek [60]	2008	170	74	73	55	87	74
Yang [61]	2008	122					85
Billé [62]	2009	159	45	94	67	88	85
Average		1231					82

PPV: Positive Predictive Value
NPV: Negative Predictive Value

Table 2. Accuracy of PET/CT in N staging

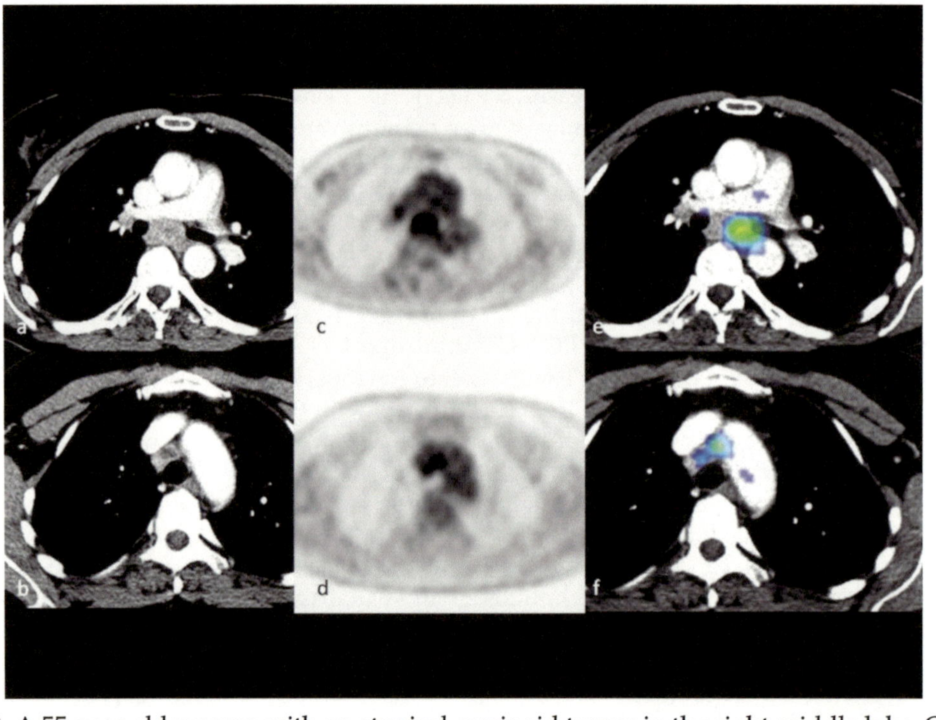

Fig. 3. A 55-year-old woman with an atypical carcinoid tumor in the right middle lobe. CT showed enlarged lymph nodes in the subcarinal (fig 3a) and right paratracheal (fig 3b) region. These lymph nodes are FDG positive on PET (fig 3 c,d). PET/CT (fig 3e,f) confirmed the correlation of these findings. On histopathology these nodes were metastatic lymph nodes.

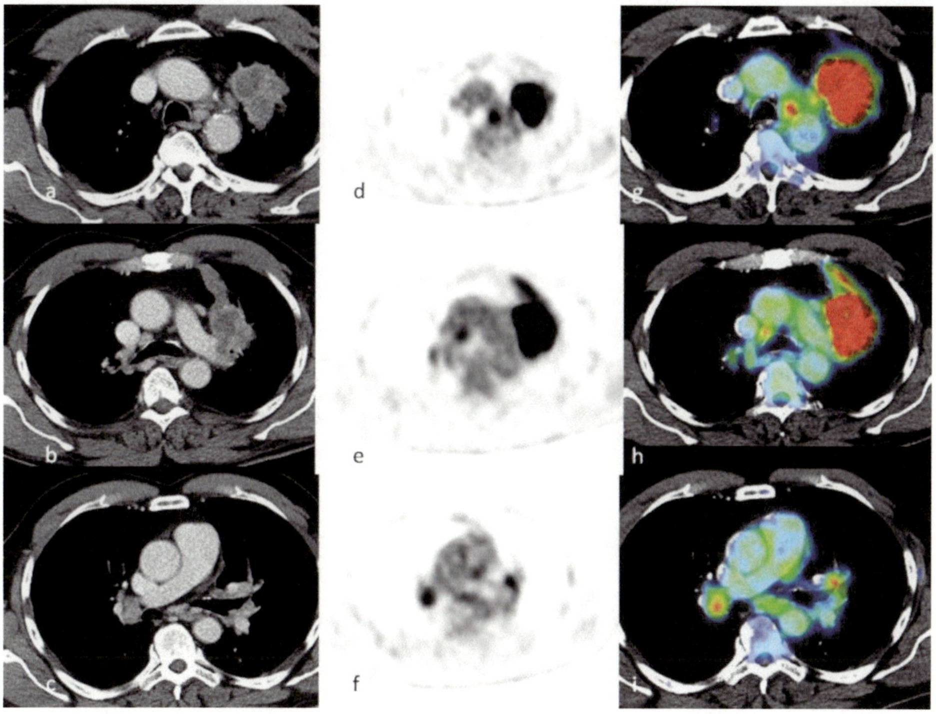

Fig. 4. A 60-year-old man with a spinocellular carcinoma in the left upper lobe. CT demonstrates the tumor in the left upper lobe (fig 4a), even as an enlarged lymph node in the right hilum (fig 4c) and not enlarged mediastinal lymph nodes (fig 4b) . PET and PET/CT (fig 4d-i) demonstrate FDG uptake on the tumor and the lymph nodes visible on CT. Histopathology examination of these lymph nodes could not demonstrate metastatic disease. These were false positive lymph nodes.

5. Assessment of M stage

The observation of distant metastases in patients with NSCLC has major implications for management and prognosis. In total, 40% of patients with NSCLC have distant metastases at presentation, most commonly in the adrenal glands, bones, liver or brain [46, 47]. After radical treatment for seemingly localized disease, 20% of these patients develop an early distant relapse, probably due to systemic micro-metastases that were present at the time of initial staging [48].

In general, a routine search for disease beyond the chest and the upper abdomen in asymptomatic patients is not undertaken with CT and so a staging CT for lung cancer is usually done caudally from the thoracic inlet to the inferior edge of the liver, including the adrenal glands. Many reports suggest that FDG-PET is more sensitive than CT in the diagnosis of extrathoracic metastases. Sensitivity rates of 88–100% have been reported in characterizing adrenal masses detected on CT in patients with lung and other primary cancers [49, 50]. Similarly, in a small series, figures of 100% sensitivity and specificity have been recorded in the detection of liver metastases from NSCLC with PET [51]. PET is also

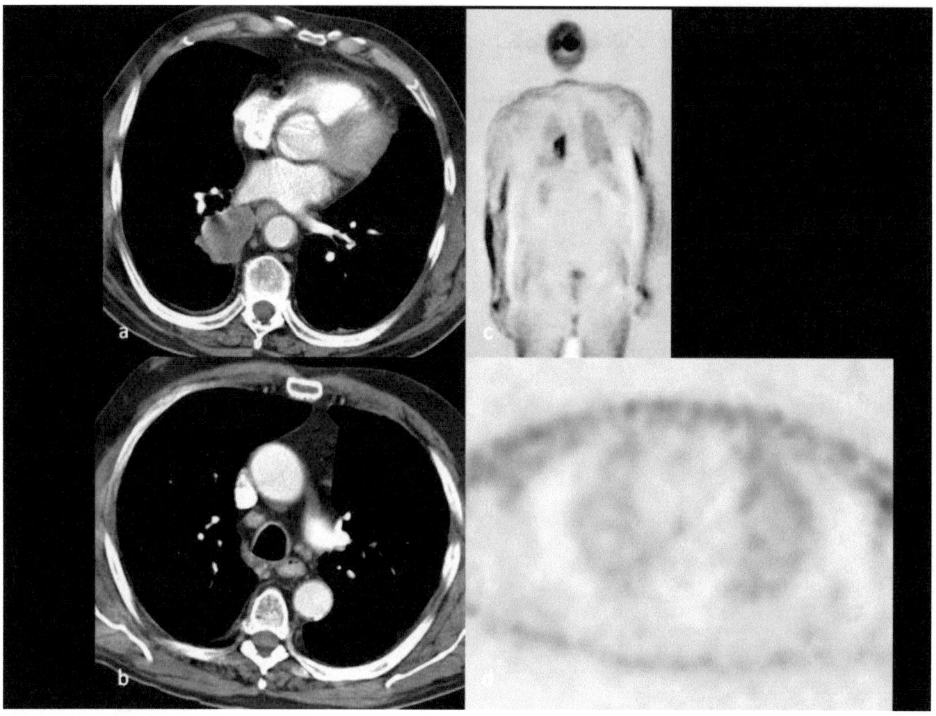

Fig. 5. A 88-year-old man with a spinocellular carcinoma of the right lower lobe. CT demonstrates a central tumor in the right lower lobe (fig 5a) and an enlarged lymph node in the right paratracheal region (fig 5b). PET (fig 5c-d) showed FDG-uptake on the tumor, but could not demonstrate FDG uptake on the CT-enlarged lymph node. Histopathological examination showed a metastatic lymph node in the right paratracheal region.

stated to be more specific than, and equally sensitive as, bone scintigraphy in the detection of bone metastases [52]. However, PET is less useful in recognizing brain metastases, owing to high levels of glucose uptake within normal brain tissue. The significance of isolated areas of avid FDG uptake, without anatomical reference, is uncertain and exclusion of malignancy by PET requires caution in the case of small lesions (<1 cm) [39].

The advantage of integrated PET/CT imaging is the ability to exactly locate a focal abnormality on PET images. PET/CT was found to be the best noninvasive imaging technique in evaluating distant metastases in several studies [20]. Cerfolio et al. [28] proved that PET/CT predicts the metastatic disease better than PET alone: 92% *versus* 87% correctly predicted. PET/CT and PET, respectively, correctly predicted 100% *versus* 86% of bone metastases, 80% *versus* 100% of the chest wall or pleural metastases, 100% *versus* 100% of the liver metastases, 66% *versus* 66% of the adrenal metastases and 100% *versus* 50% of the gastrointestinal metastases. PET/CT identified one brain metastasis while PET missed this metastasis.

6. Restaging and tumor recurrence

Patients with stage IIIA lung cancer and in whom neoadjuvant treatment results in "downstaging" may be candidates for potentially curative surgery. While PET is very good

in the initial nodal staging of lung cancer, PET alone has limited accuracy for mediastinal restaging after chemotherapy [53]. Furthermore, the results of remediastinoscopy are disappointing. De Leyn et al. used surgical findings as the gold standard for comparing the accuracy of PET/CT for N-staging with that of remediastinoscopy after neoadjuvant therapy. In this setting, PET/CT was more accurate than remediastinoscopy (83% versus 60%; $p<0.05$) and significantly more accurate than PET or CT alone [54].
Progression of disease may occur as intrathoracic recurrence or metastases. The differentiation of recurrent lung cancer and post-therapeutic changes remains a problem for radiological imaging. Both processes can appear identical on CT images, which present a challenge to the use of this modality in the post-treatment patient with lung cancer. Conversely scar and fibrosis are, by definition, dead tissue and should not result in any FDG uptake, which makes PET or PET/CT ideal for this indication. A high accuracy of F-18 FDG-PET or PET/CT in distinguishing recurrent disease from benign treatment effects has been reported [55-57]. PET has been shown to have a sensitivity of 98%-100% for the differentiation of tumor from post-treatment changes in the lung [26].
Concerning restaging following extensive surgery or radiation, it is common to have some degree of scarring within the remaining lung parenchyma. Serial CT is typically used to follow these patients up. With PET and PET/CT, most of these patients can be evaluated more accurately and earlier than with other imaging modalities. Much of the FDG uptake due to inflammation from surgery resolves relatively quickly. Therapy changes after radiation therapy resolves typically within 6 weeks, and these patients can be reevaluated at this time for residual or recurrent tumor. Patients should be evaluated a minimum of 2 months after completion of therapy. Otherwise, post-therapeutic healing processes or radiation pneumonitis may result in false positive findings [23].

7. Radiation treatment and PET/CT

In recent years, many of the radiation therapy planning systems have been upgraded to be able to incorporate both CT and PET data sets. Many also have the ability to fuse the two data sets by using the planning software. Some preliminary studies have shown that radiation portals and tumor volumes change up to 50% of the time when both PET and CT data sets are considered compared with the traditional CT planning method [58]. This anatomic and functional plan has the biggest effect when there are portions of a tumor that may not be visible or are not included on CT images alone. With both the anatomic and metabolic data, radiation oncologists are able to define viable tumor volume more accurately, as well as minimize the amount of exposure to normal tissue.[26]

8. Conclusion

Integrated PET/CT is the best imaging technique for T-staging; it is better than CT alone, PET alone and visual correlation of PET and CT. With integrated PET/CT, tumors can be better delineated from surrounding structures, such as chest wall, mediastinum or surrounding atelectasis, which is important in the exclusion of T3 or T4 stage. For N-(re)staging, integrated PET/CT increases the specificity and positive predictive value, owing to the combination of metabolic and anatomic information. For M-staging, the additional value of integrated PET/CT is related to the availability of a whole-body CT and the better localization of FDG-hotspots. The CT part of the integrated PET/CT is often able to detect and diagnose metastatic disease, obviating specific diagnostic CT examinations while the additional FDG hotspots detected with PET are better characterized when the CT information is used. However, there are still many indeterminate lesions that need histopathological proof, and integrated PET/CT can be helpful in guiding these interventional procedures.

9. References

[1] De Wever W, Ceyssens S, Mortelmans L, Stroobants S, Marchal G, Bogaert J, Verschakelen JA. Additional value of PET-CT in the staging of lung cancer: comparison with CT alone, PET alone and visual correlation of PET and CT. *Eur Radiol* 2007: 17(1): 23-32.

[2] Hany TF, Steinert HC, Goerres GW, Buck A, von Schulthess GK. PET diagnostic accuracy: improvement with in-line PET-CT system: initial results. *Radiology* 2002: 225(2): 575-581.

[3] Scott WJ, Gobar LS, Terry JD, Dewan NA, Sunderland JJ. Mediastinal lymph node staging of non-small-cell lung cancer: a prospective comparison of computed tomography and positron emission tomography. *J Thorac Cardiovasc Surg* 1996: 111(3): 642-648.

[4] Weder W, Schmid RA, Bruchhaus H, Hillinger S, von Schulthess GK, Steinert HC. Detection of extrathoracic metastases by positron emission tomography in lung cancer. *Ann Thorac Surg* 1998: 66(3): 886-892; discussion 892-883.

[5] Tan BB, Flaherty KR, Kazerooni EA, Iannettoni MD. The solitary pulmonary nodule. *Chest* 2003: 123(1 Suppl): 89S-96S.

[6] Swensen SJ, Jett JR, Hartman TE, Midthun DE, Sloan JA, Sykes AM, Aughenbaugh GL, Clemens MA. Lung cancer screening with CT: Mayo Clinic experience. *Radiology* 2003: 226(3): 756-761.

[7] Verschakelen JA, De Wever W, Bogaert J. Role of computed tomography in lung cancer staging. *Curr Opin Pulm Med* 2004: 10(4): 248-255.

[8] Gurney JW, Lyddon DM, McKay JA. Determining the likelihood of malignancy in solitary pulmonary nodules with Bayesian analysis. Part II. Application. *Radiology* 1993: 186(2): 415-422.

[9] Seemann MD, Seemann O, Luboldt W, Bonel H, Sittek H, Dienemann H, Staebler A. Differentiation of malignant from benign solitary pulmonary lesions using chest radiography, spiral CT and HRCT. *Lung Cancer* 2000: 29(2): 105-124.

[10] Swensen SJ, Viggiano RW, Midthun DE, Muller NL, Sherrick A, Yamashita K, Naidich DP, Patz EF, Hartman TE, Muhm JR, Weaver AL. Lung nodule enhancement at CT: multicenter study. *Radiology* 2000: 214(1): 73-80.

[11] Divisi D, Di Tommaso S, Di Leonardo G, Brianzoni E, De Vico A, Crisci R. 18-fluorine fluorodeoxyglucose positron emission tomography with computerized tomography versus computerized tomography alone for the management of solitary lung nodules with diameters inferior to 1.5 cm. *Thorac Cardiovasc Surg*: 58(7): 422-426.

[12] Gould MK, Maclean CC, Kuschner WG, Rydzak CE, Owens DK. Accuracy of positron emission tomography for diagnosis of pulmonary nodules and mass lesions: a meta-analysis. *JAMA* 2001: 285(7): 914-924.

[13] Fletcher JW, Kymes SM, Gould M, Alazraki N, Coleman RE, Lowe VJ, Marn C, Segall G, Thet LA, Lee K. A comparison of the diagnostic accuracy of 18F-FDG PET and CT in the characterization of solitary pulmonary nodules. *J Nucl Med* 2008: 49(2): 179-185.

[14] Hellwig D, Baum RP, Kirsch C. FDG-PET, PET/CT and conventional nuclear medicine procedures in the evaluation of lung cancer: a systematic review. *Nuklearmedizin* 2009: 48(2): 59-69, quiz N58-59.

[15] Gupta NC, Maloof J, Gunel E. Probability of malignancy in solitary pulmonary nodules using fluorine-18-FDG and PET. *J Nucl Med* 1996: 37(6): 943-948.

[16] Ung YC, Maziak DE, Vanderveen JA, Smith CA, Gulenchyn K, Lacchetti C, Evans WK. 18Fluorodeoxyglucose positron emission tomography in the diagnosis and staging of lung cancer: a systematic review. *J Natl Cancer Inst* 2007: 99(23): 1753-1767.

[17] Wahidi MM, Govert JA, Goudar RK, Gould MK, McCrory DC. Evidence for the treatment of patients with pulmonary nodules: when is it lung cancer?: ACCP evidence-based clinical practice guidelines (2nd edition). *Chest* 2007: 132(3 Suppl): 94S-107S.

[18] Nomori H, Watanabe K, Ohtsuka T, Naruke T, Suemasu K, Uno K. Evaluation of F-18 fluorodeoxyglucose (FDG) PET scanning for pulmonary nodules less than 3 cm in diameter, with special reference to the CT images. *Lung Cancer* 2004: 45(1): 19-27.

[19] Grgic A, Yuksel Y, Groschel A, Schafers HJ, Sybrecht GW, Kirsch CM, Hellwig D. Risk stratification of solitary pulmonary nodules by means of PET using (18)F-fluorodeoxyglucose and SUV quantification. *Eur J Nucl Med Mol Imaging*: 37(6): 1087-1094.

[20] De Wever W, Stroobants S, Coolen J, Verschakelen JA. Integrated PET/CT in the staging of nonsmall cell lung cancer: technical aspects and clinical integration. *Eur Respir J* 2009: 33(1): 201-212.

[21] Erasmus JJ, McAdams HP, Patz EF, Jr., Coleman RE, Ahuja V, Goodman PC. Evaluation of primary pulmonary carcinoid tumors using FDG PET. *AJR Am J Roentgenol* 1998: 170(5): 1369-1373.

[22] Higashi K, Ueda Y, Seki H, Yuasa K, Oguchi M, Noguchi T, Taniguchi M, Tonami H, Okimura T, Yamamoto I. Fluorine-18-FDG PET imaging is negative in bronchioloalveolar lung carcinoma. *J Nucl Med* 1998: 39(6): 1016-1020.

[23] Steinert HC. PET and PET-CT of lung cancer. *Methods Mol Biol*: 727: 33-51.

[24] Kim SK, Allen-Auerbach M, Goldin J, Fueger BJ, Dahlbom M, Brown M, Czernin J, Schiepers C. Accuracy of PET/CT in characterization of solitary pulmonary lesions. *J Nucl Med* 2007: 48(2): 214-220.

[25] Martins Rde C, Almeida SA, Siciliano AA, Landesmann MC, Silva FB, Franco CA, Fonseca LM. [Value of [18F]-FDG-PET/CT as a predictor of cancer in solitary pulmonary nodule]. *J Bras Pneumol* 2008: 34(7): 473-480.

[26] Mattar EH. Integrated PET/CT in imaging of non-small cell lung cancer. *J Egypt Natl Canc Inst* 2007: 19(4): 263-274.

[27] Halpern BS, Schiepers C, Weber WA, Crawford TL, Fueger BJ, Phelps ME, Czernin J. Presurgical staging of non-small cell lung cancer: positron emission tomography, integrated positron emission tomography/CT, and software image fusion. *Chest* 2005: 128(4): 2289-2297.

[28] Cerfolio RJ, Ojha B, Bryant AS, Raghuveer V, Mountz JM, Bartolucci AA. The accuracy of integrated PET-CT compared with dedicated PET alone for the staging of patients with nonsmall cell lung cancer. *Ann Thorac Surg* 2004: 78(3): 1017-1023; discussion 1017-1023.

[29] Lardinois D, Weder W, Hany TF, Kamel EM, Korom S, Seifert B, von Schulthess GK, Steinert HC. Staging of non-small-cell lung cancer with integrated positron-emission tomography and computed tomography. *N Engl J Med* 2003: 348(25): 2500-2507.

[30] Pauls S, Buck AK, Hohl K, Halter G, Hetzel M, Blumstein NM, Mottaghy FM, Glatting G, Kruger S, Sunder-Plassmann L, Moller P, Hombach V, Brambs HJ, Reske SN. Improved non-invasive T-Staging in non-small cell lung cancer by integrated 18F-FDG PET/CT. *Nuklearmedizin* 2007: 46(1): 9-14; quiz N11-12.

[31] Antoch G, Stattaus J, Nemat AT, Marnitz S, Beyer T, Kuehl H, Bockisch A, Debatin JF, Freudenberg LS. Non-small cell lung cancer: dual-modality PET/CT in preoperative staging. *Radiology* 2003: 229(2): 526-533.

[32] Dillemans B, Deneffe G, Verschakelen J, Decramer M. Value of computed tomography and mediastinoscopy in preoperative evaluation of mediastinal nodes in non-small cell lung cancer. A study of 569 patients. *Eur J Cardiothorac Surg* 1994: 8(1): 37-42.

[33] Pieterman RM, van Putten JW, Meuzelaar JJ, Mooyaart EL, Vaalburg W, Koeter GH, Fidler V, Pruim J, Groen HJ. Preoperative staging of non-small-cell lung cancer with positron-emission tomography. *N Engl J Med* 2000: 343(4): 254-261.

[34] Steinert HC, Hauser M, Allemann F, Engel H, Berthold T, von Schulthess GK, Weder W. Non-small cell lung cancer: nodal staging with FDG PET versus CT with correlative lymph node mapping and sampling. *Radiology* 1997: 202(2): 441-446.

[35] Vansteenkiste JF, Stroobants SG, De Leyn PR, Dupont PJ, Bogaert J, Maes A, Deneffe GJ, Nackaerts KL, Verschakelen JA, Lerut TE, Mortelmans LA, Demedts MG. Lymph node staging in non-small-cell lung cancer with FDG-PET scan: a prospective study on 690 lymph node stations from 68 patients. *J Clin Oncol* 1998: 16(6): 2142-2149.

[36] Birim O, Kappetein AP, Stijnen T, Bogers AJ. Meta-analysis of positron emission tomographic and computed tomographic imaging in detecting mediastinal lymph node metastases in nonsmall cell lung cancer. *Ann Thorac Surg* 2005: 79(1): 375-382.

[37] Dwamena BA, Sonnad SS, Angobaldo JO, Wahl RL. Metastases from non-small cell lung cancer: mediastinal staging in the 1990s--meta-analytic comparison of PET and CT. *Radiology* 1999: 213(2): 530-536.

[38] Gould MK, Kuschner WG, Rydzak CE, Maclean CC, Demas AN, Shigemitsu H, Chan JK, Owens DK. Test performance of positron emission tomography and computed tomography for mediastinal staging in patients with non-small-cell lung cancer: a meta-analysis. *Ann Intern Med* 2003: 139(11): 879-892.

[39] Schrevens L, Lorent N, Dooms C, Vansteenkiste J. The role of PET scan in diagnosis, staging, and management of non-small cell lung cancer. *Oncologist* 2004: 9(6): 633-643.

[40] Toloza EM, Harpole L, McCrory DC. Noninvasive staging of non-small cell lung cancer: a review of the current evidence. *Chest* 2003: 123(1 Suppl): 137S-146S.

[41] Shim SS, Lee KS, Kim BT, Chung MJ, Lee EJ, Han J, Choi JY, Kwon OJ, Shim YM, Kim S. Non-small cell lung cancer: prospective comparison of integrated FDG PET/CT and CT alone for preoperative staging. *Radiology* 2005: 236(3): 1011-1019.

[42] Kim YK, Lee KS, Kim BT, Choi JY, Kim H, Kwon OJ, Shim YM, Yi CA, Kim HY, Chung MJ. Mediastinal nodal staging of nonsmall cell lung cancer using integrated 18F-FDG PET/CT in a tuberculosis-endemic country: diagnostic efficacy in 674 patients. *Cancer* 2007: 109(6): 1068-1077.

[43] Yi CA, Lee KS, Kim BT, Shim SS, Chung MJ, Sung YM, Jeong SY. Efficacy of helical dynamic CT versus integrated PET/CT for detection of mediastinal nodal metastasis in non-small cell lung cancer. *AJR Am J Roentgenol* 2007: 188(2): 318-325.

[44] Truong MT, Erasmus JJ, Macapinlac HA, Marom EM, Mawlawi O, Gladish GW, Sabloff BS, Bruzzi JF, Munden RF. Integrated positron emission tomography/computed tomography in patients with non-small cell lung cancer: normal variants and pitfalls. *J Comput Assist Tomogr* 2005: 29(2): 205-209.

[45] Janssen-Heijnen ML, Coebergh JW. Trends in incidence and prognosis of the histological subtypes of lung cancer in North America, Australia, New Zealand and Europe. *Lung Cancer* 2001: 31(2-3): 123-137.

[46] De Wever W, Bruyeer E, Demaerel P, Wilms G, Coolen J, Verschakelen J. Staging of lung cancer. Do we need a diagnostic CT of the brain after an integrated PET/CT for the detection of brain metastases? *JBR-BTR*: 93(2): 71-76.

[47] Quint LE, Tummala S, Brisson LJ, Francis IR, Krupnick AS, Kazerooni EA, Iannettoni MD, Whyte RI, Orringer MB. Distribution of distant metastases from newly diagnosed non-small cell lung cancer. *Ann Thorac Surg* 1996: 62(1): 246-250.

[48] Pantel K, Izbicki J, Passlick B, Angstwurm M, Haussinger K, Thetter O, Riethmuller G. Frequency and prognostic significance of isolated tumour cells in bone marrow of patients with non-small-cell lung cancer without overt metastases. *Lancet* 1996: 347(9002): 649-653.

[49] Jana S, Zhang T, Milstein DM, Isasi CR, Blaufox MD. FDG-PET and CT characterization of adrenal lesions in cancer patients. *Eur J Nucl Med Mol Imaging* 2006: 33(1): 29-35.

[50] Kumar R, Xiu Y, Yu JQ, Takalkar A, El-Haddad G, Potenta S, Kung J, Zhuang H, Alavi A. 18F-FDG PET in evaluation of adrenal lesions in patients with lung cancer. *J Nucl Med* 2004: 45(12): 2058-2062.

[51] Marom EM, McAdams HP, Erasmus JJ, Goodman PC, Culhane DK, Coleman RE, Herndon JE, Patz EF, Jr. Staging non-small cell lung cancer with whole-body PET. *Radiology* 1999: 212(3): 803-809.

[52] Bury T, Barreto A, Daenen F, Barthelemy N, Ghaye B, Rigo P. Fluorine-18 deoxyglucose positron emission tomography for the detection of bone metastases in patients with non-small cell lung cancer. *Eur J Nucl Med* 1998: 25(9): 1244-1247.

[53] Hoekstra CJ, Stroobants SG, Smit EF, Vansteenkiste J, van Tinteren H, Postmus PE, Golding RP, Biesma B, Schramel FJ, van Zandwijk N, Lammertsma AA, Hoekstra OS. Prognostic relevance of response evaluation using [18F]-2-fluoro-2-deoxy-D-glucose positron emission tomography in patients with locally advanced non-small-cell lung cancer. *J Clin Oncol* 2005: 23(33): 8362-8370.

[54] De Leyn P, Stroobants S, De Wever W, Lerut T, Coosemans W, Decker G, Nafteux P, Van Raemdonck D, Mortelmans L, Nackaerts K, Vansteenkiste J. Prospective

comparative study of integrated positron emission tomography-computed tomography scan compared with remediastinoscopy in the assessment of residual mediastinal lymph node disease after induction chemotherapy for mediastinoscopy-proven stage IIIA-N2 Non-small-cell lung cancer: a Leuven Lung Cancer Group Study. *J Clin Oncol* 2006: 24(21): 3333-3339.

[55] Hicks RJ, Kalff V, MacManus MP, Ware RE, McKenzie AF, Matthews JP, Ball DL. The utility of (18)F-FDG PET for suspected recurrent non-small cell lung cancer after potentially curative therapy: impact on management and prognostic stratification. *J Nucl Med* 2001: 42(11): 1605-1613.

[56] Inoue T, Kim EE, Komaki R, Wong FC, Bassa P, Wong WH, Yang DJ, Endo K, Podoloff DA. Detecting recurrent or residual lung cancer with FDG-PET. *J Nucl Med* 1995: 36(5): 788-793.

[57] Keidar Z, Haim N, Guralnik L, Wollner M, Bar-Shalom R, Ben-Nun A, Israel O. PET/CT using 18F-FDG in suspected lung cancer recurrence: diagnostic value and impact on patient management. *J Nucl Med* 2004: 45(10): 1640-1646.

[58] Klopp AH, Chang JY, Tucker SL, Sulman EP, Balter PA, Liu HH, Bucci MK, Macapinlac HA, Komaki R, Cox JD. Intrathoracic patterns of failure for non-small-cell lung cancer with positron-emission tomography/computed tomography-defined target delineation. *Int J Radiat Oncol Biol Phys* 2007: 69(5): 1409-1416.

[59] Kim BT, Lee KS, Shim SS, Choi JY, Kwon OJ, Kim H, Shim YM, Kim J, Kim S. Stage T1 non-small cell lung cancer: preoperative mediastinal nodal staging with integrated FDG PET/CT--a prospective study. *Radiology* 2006: 241(2): 501-509.

[60] Melek H, Gunluoglu MZ, Demir A, Akin H, Olcmen A, Dincer SI. Role of positron emission tomography in mediastinal lymphatic staging of non-small cell lung cancer. *Eur J Cardiothorac Surg* 2008: 33(2): 294-299.

[61] Yang W, Fu Z, Yu J, Yuan S, Zhang B, Li D, Xing L, Zhao D, Mu D, Sun X, Fang Y, Huang Y, Li W. Value of PET/CT versus enhanced CT for locoregional lymph nodes in non-small cell lung cancer. *Lung Cancer* 2008: 61(1): 35-43.

[62] Bille A, Pelosi E, Skanjeti A, Arena V, Errico L, Borasio P, Mancini M, Ardissone F. Preoperative intrathoracic lymph node staging in patients with non-small-cell lung cancer: accuracy of integrated positron emission tomography and computed tomography. *Eur J Cardiothorac Surg* 2009: 36(3): 440-445.

17

Hybrid PET/CT and SPECT/CT Imaging

Thomas Leitha[1] and Anton Staudenherz[2]
[1]*Department of Nuclear Medicine, Danube Hospital, Vienna*
[2]*University Clinic of Nuclear Medicine, Vienna*
Austria

1. Introduction

1.1 Definition of nuclear medicine, molecular imaging and hybrid imaging

Nuclear Medicine uses radioactive probes commonly referred to as tracers for the diagnosis and treatment of diseases. Monitoring the metabolic fate of nanomolar amounts of radiolabeled substances by tracking their photon emission with SPECT (Single Photon Emission Tomography) and PET (Positron Emission Tomography) was the first widely practiced branch of Molecular Imaging (MI). MI is the visualization, characterization and measurement of biological processes at the molecular and cellular levels in humans and other living systems (Mankoff, 2007). Among the different techniques summarized in MI, tracer imaging in Nuclear Medicine has the highest molecular sensitivity, tracing substances in the 10E-3 to 10E-5 mol/l range. Conventional imaging with x-ray was primarily used as a snapshot of anatomy and depicts tissue by its physical characteristics (e.g., X-ray density). Contrast agents in CT are used to increase the visibility of vessels and organ surfaces. Functional information is at best limited to that of perfusion and permeability. This is one of the most significant differences between Radiology and Nuclear Medicine.

The advantage of functional imaging is that of increasing sensitivity because metabolic changes precede anatomical changes and can be detected long before structural changes appear. Functional imaging, however, has a low specificity in distinctly different pathologies (e.g., degenerative, inflammatory or malignant bone lesions) if they are visualized by unspecific common properties as hyperaemia, increased regional tracer permeability and osteoplastic metabolism. To overcome this and to increase specificity, highly specific probes (e.g., receptor imaging) have been developed. With minimal uptake outside the targeted tissues, specific probes offer little information about the surrounding tissues and consequently do not provide the topographical information needed by surgeons or therapy planning systems in radio oncology. The advantage of anatomical imaging by CT is its high anatomical resolution and usually good topographical information. On the other hand it is a poor predictor of the functional consequences of a finding (e.g., borderline stenosis in coronary CT angiography) and consequently a poor predictor of prognosis. Structural data do not necessarily correlate with the metabolic status of disease and they have a limited diagnostic sensitivity in cases with abnormal anatomy (e.g., scar versus residual tumour). Anatomic tumour response metrics (WHO criteria, Response Evaluation Criteria in Solid Tumours (RECIST)) are insufficient to predict therapy response, particularly in assessing the activity of newer cancer therapies that stabilize disease and may be substituted by quantitative approaches in functional imaging (PET Response Criteria in Solid Tumours; PERCIST (Wahl et al 2009)). An ideal non-invasive technique provides complementary information on topography and anatomy as well as on the functional behaviour of a lesion.

Less than one decade ago, primarily forced by the manufacturers, hybrid devices were brought into clinical routine. It took only a few years after the first description of a working prototype (Beyer et al., 2000) to replace stand-alone PET by PET/CT. A similar success story may be appreciated with SPECT/CT (Schillaci et al., 2005). However, the development of hybrid imaging in PET and SPECT followed different pathways. Whereas PET was always combined with a state-of-the-art CT system, the first SPECT/CT design was based on a low-current, slow revolving CT (see chapter 2). Both hybrid devices have been shown to improve diagnosis and risk stratification by combining anatomical and functional information (see chapters 4 and 5).

Nuclear Medicine interpretation benefits from CT in three ways:

Firstly, scintigraphic uptake can now be localized topographically and enables local interventions (e.g., surgery, radio therapy planning). Secondly, physiological and unphysiological tracer uptake can be better discriminated by visualizing the anatomical background (e.g. FDG uptake in brown adipose tissue). Thirdly, an often overlooked advantage is that the CT attenuation map shortens imaging protocols and possibly improves attenuation and scatter correction of PET and SPECT.

On the other hand, Nuclear Medicine may also improve CT interpretation, e.g. in the differential diagnosis of minimally enlarged mediastinal or retroperitoneal lymph nodes and in therapy monitoring.

1.2 Is hybrid imaging the final answer to all our needs?

The complementary information of anatomical and functional imaging has been used for decades to define, characterize, stage and monitor disease, but until recently the different modalities have been performed in sequence (e.g. screening for bone metastases by whole body bone scanning followed by planar radiographs and possibly MRI). Before hybrid systems (PET/CT, SPECT/CT) came into the market the findings of different modalities had to be independently viewed or (as discussed in chapter 3.) digitally fused. The coming of hybrid devices was welcomed by many with overwhelming optimism (von Schulthess et al., 2002), but a more thorough assessment of the matter surfaces several unsolved problems which will be addressed below. Sceptics may even say that we - driven by the market and our own curiosity - have opened Pandora's box.

1.3 What is the incremental benefit of simultaneous hybrid imaging to the sequential use of optimized imaging?

The most obvious answer to this question seems to be that patient positioning and movement is not an issue in simultaneous hybrid imaging but sime of these problems may have not been eliminated. Modern systems combine both modalities on a single gantry, but different detectors are still needed to image both signals and both studies are acquired sequentially. The problems of misalignment of both investigations are discussed in detail in 1.6.1. The strongest evidence for the clinical effectiveness of FDG-PET is in staging NSCLC, restaging HL, staging/restaging colorectal cancer and detection of solitary pulmonary nodule (Facey et al., 2007). Numerous studies with a heterogeneous design claimed that the incremental benefit of simultaneous hybrid imaging to sequential protocols is well over 10 % at least in oncology (Czernin et al., 2010, Delbecke et al., 2009).

1.4 Can the additional accuracy be utilized in clinical practice?

The cost-effectiveness of a PET plus CT strategy was shown as early as in the late 90s (Gambhir et al., 1996) for diagnosis and staging of lung cancer and numerous other indications followed. Nevertheless especially in follow-up investigations, it all comes down to this:

Does the additional information affect clinical decisions in a significant number of patients and do they benefit from the additional information provided by advanced imaging?

There is some evidence in oncology that hybrid imaging has changed patient management (Almuhaideb et al. 2001, Facey et al., 2007). In cardiology the addition of calcium scoring has been described to improve the results of myocardial perfusion SPECT (Mahmarian, 2007). Though sometimes quoted (Farid et al., 2009) data are scarce that hybrid imaging in neurology has an additional advantage to digital image fusion.

1.5 Is the additional radiation burden of multiple diagnostic CTs worthwhile?

In Nuclear Medicine imaging can be performed as whole body imaging or dual phase protocols without additional radiation exposure. In contrast, multi-phase CT protocols and larger scanning volumes inevitably increase the radiation burden of the patient. Routinely combining PET or SPECT with diagnostic whole body CT unnecessarily increases the radiation dose in some patients. "Low dose CT" (for a definition see 2.2.) appears to be a good compromise, but it may overlook minute pathologies that show no tracer uptake but could have been revealed by a diagnostic CT. Diagnostic CTs in radiology (in contrast to low-dose CTs in Nuclear Medicine) are routinely acquired during maximum inspiration, increasing the intrathoracic volume, moving the diaphragm downwards and changing the relative organ positions in comparison to the situation during the PET/SPECT acquisition. A mid expiratory position would be a good compromise but is difficult to reproduce voluntarily (Pan et al., 2005) and it has yet to be determined to what extent this hampers the diagnostic accuracy of the CT in the lung. A step wise approach should be ideal but this is very difficult to implement into the busy scheduling of diagnostic imaging when all too often the tentative diagnosis of the referrer is imprecise and it is hard to decide the necessary depth of the diagnostic protocol. Thus, at present many CTs will be duplicated in hybrid imaging.

1.6 Is the CT information fully utilized in the reconstruction of PET and SPECT imaging?

Until recently most reviews about hybrid imaging have focused on the clinical advantages due to the better anatomical allocation of PET/SPECT images, but at least in PET/CT the biggest advantage was that of improving image reconstruction by speeding the transmission scan. Coincidence imaging in PET and Single Photon imaging in SPECT imaging, though completely different in some of their physical basics, need several corrections to improve imaging and to allow quantification, with attenuation and scatter correction being the most important. Whereas these corrections are now regarded as mandatory in PET, they may gain importance in quantitative SPECT, but at present are only implemented in myocardial perfusion imaging and brain imaging. Initially both, PET and SPECT, used radioactive sources for transmission imaging, but attenuation maps generated from CT scans can be acquired much faster. However, three issues may hamper this approach: Misalignment, energy dependent attenuation and CT artefacts.

1.6.1 Misalignment

Misalignment of both studies cannot be avoided completely as different detectors are needed to image signals from radionuclides and x-ray tubes (Goetze & Wahl, 2007). Both studies are acquired sequentially and differ significantly in imaging duration thus causing head, whole-body and extremity motion, diaphragmatic motion with breathing and bowel motility (Figure 1). The different expiratory positions between CT and PET/SPECT have been addressed in 1.5.

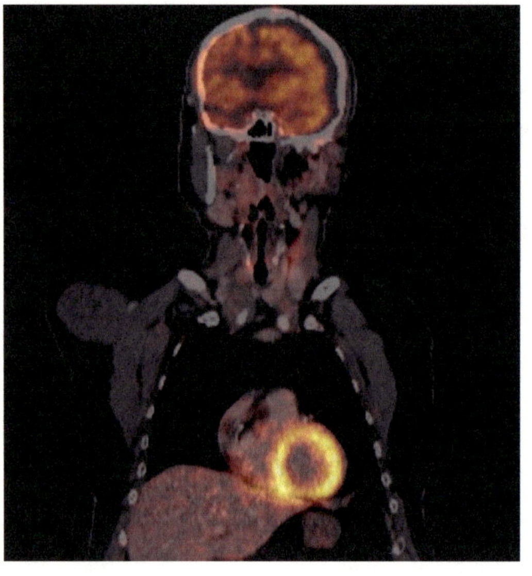

Fig. 1. FDG PET/CT with minimal head movement between both investigations

1.6.2 Energy dependent attenuation

The different energy spectrums of Nuclear Medicine tracers (PET monoenergetic 511-keV photons, SPECT mono- and multienergetic photons in a wide range of energies) and CT pose another challenge. The spectrum of photons energy from the anode of the x-ray tubes used in CT range from 0 keV up to peak energy used for the acquisition. Attenuation increases with lower energy this may cause artefacts, like beam-hardening effects. So, filtering of the beam is required. The resulting spectrum has a mean energy of about 70 keV. At the low energy level of some SPECT tracers (e.g., 68-80 keV (94.5%) Tl-201) and CT photons, interaction with body tissues takes place in part through photoelectric effects, whereas the high energy 511-keV annihilation photons used for PET are almost exclusively attenuated by Compton scattering. The attenuation coefficients need to be scaled appropriately in each energy window for the different materials (air, soft tissue, bone). This is more complex for SPECT than for PET, due to the wide range and sometimes multiplicity of energy windows of the used radioisotope. Before CT data can be used for attenuation correction in PET and SPECT, CT voxel sizes have to be downscaled due to the lower spatial resolution of those devices (Krishnasetty et al., 2008) and segmented according to the different materials. The used algorithms differ between different vendors and apparently have been set for optimized visual diagnosis and not quantitative requirements. The consequences for quantitative PET/CT have been summarized elsewhere (Weber et al., 2007). Until now quantitative SPECT was not a major issue but is rapidly emerging for diagnostic (fp-cit scan) imaging and dosimetry (Patton & Turkington, 2008).

1.6.3 CT artefacts

Attenuation artefacts (dental work, metallic implants) are other possible problems if CT is used for correction purposes in Nuclear Medicine imaging. Routine reconstruction for CT is filtered back projection and not iterative reconstruction and the first is especially susceptible to beam hardening artefacts if the patient does not fit into the field of view. This issue becomes more evident if low dose parameters are used and artefacts may hamper PET and SPECT reconstruction (Figure 2).

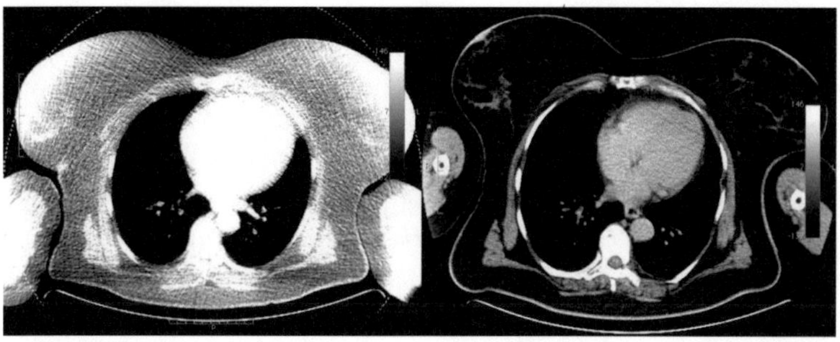

Fig. 2. Beam hardening artefacts in a large patient (height: 175 cm, body weight: 120 kg) at the edge of the field of view are evident in the image of the low dose CT (140 kV, 230 mAs) on the left and have disappeared in the image on the right after conventional CT parameters (140 kV, 300 mAs) have been applied.

This problem might be partially solved by using iterative reconstruction algorithm (Kinahan et al., 2003), but things get even more complicated if contrast media are involved in hybrid imaging (Büther et al., 2007). The different energy spectra of SPECT tracers pose an additional challenge to the reconstruction process if absolute quantification is aspired.

1.7 Do we need hybrid imaging in all situations?

Most likely not, but a more detailed analysis reveals a complex picture. Critics apparently have ample evidence of accusing our professions to succumb to a "the more the merrier" principle. We definitely have to provide evidence in which clinical situations hybrid imaging is warranted but then little is gained if a given diagnostic tool has shown to be the method of first choice in a certain situation, if this tool is not accessible: In most areas patient access to CT is much easier than to PET/CT or SPECT/CT thus many patients will already have a diagnostic CT before coming to Nuclear medicine imaging. This opens up the field for digital image fusion as described below (Chapter 3.).

2. From low dose to multi-slice CT

2.1 History and milestones

The origins of PET, SPECT and CT date back into the early 1970s. Burnham et al. (1972) developed a multi-crystal positron camera. Modern PET scanners are based on the work of

Phelps et al (1975), Ter-Pogossian et al. (1975) and Hoffmann et al (1976). Almost in parallel in the early 1970s Ambrose & Hounsfield (1973) introduced a computerized x-ray tube-based tomographic scanner providing images of tissue densities from acquired projections. In contrast to the evolution of SPECT/CT the first PET/CT scanner was developed as a combination of a then state-of-the-art spiral CT (Siemens *Somatom AR*) and a partial-slip-ring "poor man's PET" (*ECAT ART PET*) on a common rotational support within a single gantry with the PET components on the reverse side of the rotating support of the CT scanner. This design reduced the expensive detectors from 144 to 66 and brought the price tag down to below 1 Million US $. Townsend et al., (1998) published their combination SMART scanner providing sequential imaging using the table as shuttle using the advantage of having the patient in the same body position without changing. Almost a decade later the first prototype SPECT/CT system was developed (Lang et al., 1991). This prototype used the same high-purity germanium detector array for both x-ray and single-photon imaging. The same group (Hasegawa et al., 1993) developed a different design by combining a CT scanner with a commercial gamma camera but it was not until the millennium when a different design became the first commercially available SPECT/CT system. This was in part triggered by the fact that this manufacturer (then ELSCINT, now General Electrics) was the first who used a slip ring for its gamma camera gantry, allowing > 360° rotation. This design was based on low speed. low current CT (*Hawkeye*) that was explicitly developed for hybrid imaging with the *Infinia* gamma camera. At this time this was the logical approach as it provided sufficient topographic orientation and a transmission map for attenuation and scatter correction closely resembling the organ positions during the SPECT acquisition. The *Hawkeye* opened the market for SPECT-CT, but surprisingly or not in the end the market voted for other designs with MD CT scanners (Siemens, Philips). Siemens introduced the *Symbia* series in 2004 followed by Philips *Precidence.* Currently available SPECT/CT systems are: *Discovery NM/CT 670* (General Electric), *BrightView X/CT* (Philips) and the *Symbia T* series (Siemens). Today PET/CT systems are only available with diagnostic CT scanners. The CT system can be operated at reduced tube current if only used for attenuation correction. The latest development in the history of PET/CT appears to be the marketing of a "CT/PET". Siemens hides the fact that they are selling a PET/CT by naming it "molecular CT" (*Biograph mCT*). In 2008, the first hybrid PET/MRI system for humans was installed by Siemens (Pichler et al., 2008); but that is a completely different story.

2.2 Radiation exposure in hybrid imaging

Radionuclides used in PET and SPECT have a much lower photon flux and higher γ-rays energy in comparison to x-rays in CT. The effective dose caused by intravenously applied tracers in Nuclear Medicine is not only affected by the physical properties of the radionuclide but even more so by the biokinetics of the radiopharmaceuticals, thus in i.v. studies all organs are exposed to some extent. In contrast, the absorbed dose in CT is dependent on several operator dependent factors (mAs (directly proportional to radiation dose), kVp (not linearly proportional to dose), pitch (inversely related to dosage), slice thickness (smaller slices increase mAs), number of scans (multiplying radiation dose), scan time (faster scans lead to an increased scan area), scanning mode (step-based, spiral technique; single-slice, multi-slice) and proportional to the absorption coefficient of the irradiated tissue that is more or less limited to scanned body volume) (Bauhs et al., 2008).

Initially, attenuation correction for PET and SPECT was based on transmission scanning with radioactive sources (153-Gd for SPECT, 68-Ge for PET, respectively). Those sources exposed the patient to only low additional effective doses in the order of 0.1 to 0.2 mSv (Delbeke & Israel, 2010). Using CT as transmission source, especially in a diagnostic setting, the effective dose rises up to 100 times depending on the imaging protocols. A diagnostic CT of the chest, abdomen and pelvis will give an effective dose of about 13 mSv (140 kV, 340 mAs, 0,5 s rotation time and a pitch fo 17.5 cm/s). On the other hand 18-F FDG PET (370 MBq) causes an effective dose of about 11 mSv. The effective dose of SPECT varies, due to a wide range of different tracers. 99m-Tc (925 MBq) labelled white blood cell imaging is an investigation with one of the highest effective doses and delivers 18.5 mSv (Stabin et al., 1996) to the patient. In commonly applied protocols in Austria (Stemberger et al., 2011) the contribution of the CT to the average total body effective dose is 14 mSv in PET/CT and 1-3 mSv in SPECT/CT. Moving from diagnostic to "low dose" CT protocols lowers the effective dose considerably. Low dose CT is said to make up for only 10% to 15% of total effective dose in hybrid imaging, but some caution is advised: There is considerable confusion in the definition of the term "low dose" CT in hybrid imaging. Referring to the definition of the American College of Radiology (ACR) for Relative Radiation Level (RRL) values (Table 1), very few of the proposed protocols qualify for the definition of low radiation level.

Radiation Level	Effective Dose Range
None	0
Minimal	< 0.1 mSv
Low	0.1 - 1 mSv
Medium	1 - 10 mSv
High	> 10 mSv

Table 1. Modified according to the ACR Appropriateness Criteria

To put this into a clinical perspective, one has to address the issue how to quantify radiation risk: Basically, the effective dose does not reflect the individual risk but should be used to compare systems and to justify and optimize procedures. The individual risk is estimated by calculating mean doses of all organs and tissues in relation to age, sex and organ specific risk coefficients (ICRP 2007). The primary risk associated with radiation exposure in diagnostic imaging is the risk to develop cancer and this appears to be comparatively high. The seventh National Academy of Science report on Biological Effects of Ionizing Radiation estimated that a single dose of 10 mSv produces a lifetime risk of developing a solid cancer or leukemia of 1 in 1000 (BEIR VII 2006). This, however, has to be appreciated in the light of the chance of 1 in 4 dying from cancer in the developed countries. The most important way to reduce radiation dose in hybrid systems is to optimize the CT protocols. Most companies recommend protocols for optimal visual image quality but the question remains to what extent CT parameters can be modified to reduce dose without losing adequate information for attenuation correction, quantification and diagnostic information. Neuwirth et al., (2010) using a Siemens Biograph 64 PET/CT scanner showed that the attenuation correction of PET is not hampered even if the lowest possible CT parameters (80 keV, 28 mAs) are used. It goes without saying that those CT images contribute little diagnostic information. At present we lack sufficient data to quantify the diagnostic trade off between "low dose" and "diagnostic" CT. To this point we have only discussed the contribution of the x-ray tube and radiopharmaceutical to the effective dose of the patient. Often neglected is the contribution of the scout scan or topogram used to determine scan limits before acquisition starts to total radiation exposition. A recent study (Moore et al., 2010) showed that the additional dose contributed by the topogram can be minimized (25 μGy) but in clinical routine it may be as high as 10 to 20% of the diagnostic CT scan depending on exposure time, region length, mA and voltage (O'Daniel et al., 2005). In principle, the topogram could be easily substituted in hybrid systems by the emission data of PET or SPECT but this option is still not available in all current hybrid designs as most are basically two devices glued together working independently.

3. From digital Image fusion to hybrid imaging

Before the advent of hybrid devices several steps had to be taken to allow digital image fusion of CT and Nuclear Medicine techniques. Whereas Nuclear Medicine imaging became digital very early in its development, digital radiology emerged not before the late 80s. The second requirement was an interchangeable image format for both modalities. Initially images in Nuclear Medicine were stored in company proprietary formats. With several intermediate steps (e.g. interfile), the current definition of the DICOM standard (http://medical.nema.org/) allows handling, storing, printing, and transmitting of most study types in medical imaging. Nowadays accepted as natural law (Moore's law), the gigantic boost in computer power was mandatory to implement sophisticated iterative reconstruction and fusion algorithms in clinical routine. Often overlooked, but sufficient in some clinical situations, even simple manual fusion has an incremental diagnostic impact over the separate analysis (Nakamoto et al., 2008). However, if image-guided interventions or sophisticated dosimetry is needed, digital fusion is a necessity. Numerous algorithms have been described to retrospectively align 3-dimensional data acquired by stand-alone modalities to common spatial coordinates (Slomka, 2004). Two basic approaches (internal landmarks or external fiducials) can and have been used to fuse tomographic images (Kramer et al., 1991; Kessler, 2006). Whereas external markers with individualized masks are routine procedures in radio oncology, they require considerable logistics, can only be used for small volumes and neglect information about internal organ displacements. Internal landmarks have the advantage of correcting for different organ positions and can be used even if the first study was acquired without the knowledge of a later image fusion but require substantial user interference which is prone to errors and may lack reproducibility. Basically all the used algorithms can be separated into feature or volume based approaches. The first align the two image sets according to extracted image features (e.g. anatomic landmarks, organ surfaces ...) the latter maximize measures of similarity between images. Another important difference between these algorithms is if they are linear or nonlinear. Linear image fusion subjects all coordinates to the same extent of translation, rotation and scaling to be fused with the second study. This is perfect for the brain but insufficient for the non-rigid complex geometry of thoracic volumes. In contrast, nonlinear techniques are capable of fusing different intrathoracic volumes and to some extent different patient positioning but fail to correct for internal organ displacement, namely the liver. It has been reported that integrated PET/CT devices provided additional information in approximately 6–7% of all lesions. However, in this report (Reinarzt et al., 2004) abnormal CT findings in the absence of increased 18F-FDG uptake were excluded, thus have not strictly investigated the additional benefit of the combined devices. Available evidence for the incremental diagnostic utility of hybrid imaging in comparison to visual or digital fusion will be discussed below, but it is safe to predict that digital image fusion will continue to play an important role in patients with a previously performed diagnostic CT or MR.

4. Current state of clinical PET/CT

A recent survey showed PET is most frequently used in oncology (87%) followed by neurology (5%), radiation therapy planning and cardiology (4%), respectively. I.v. or oral contrast was used at 52% of the sites in up to 25% of patients but only 62% of the sites provided a fully integrated PET/CT report (Beyer et al., 2011). As stand alone PET systems have disappeared the clinical question is not if CT is used but to what extent (dose, contrast enhancement) it is performed as a diagnostic CT (Coleman et al., 2005).

4.1 Oncology

The utility of FDG PET in oncology has been recently summarized (Facey et al., 2007, Fletcher et al., 2008). PET/CT systems were not explicitly addressed due to the paucity of published data. Data for other PET tracers are not summarized here because of an even more limited database. Despite being the standard of care, there has been uncertainty about whether or not improved diagnostic accuracy translates into improved management of patients. The strongest evidence for the cost-effectiveness of PET is still in the staging of non-small cell lung cancer, but a recently performed analysis of FDG PET in oncology found only four studies (Mansueto et al., 2009, Lejeune et al., 2005, Krug et al., 2010, Yen et al., 2009) that based their findings explicitly on PET/CT (Langer, 2010). The following overview tries to suggest clinical setting where growing evidence exists that the initial use of a diagnostic CT or if no access to hybrid imaging is possible, image fusion between CT and PET has to be aspired.

4.1.1 Head neck cancer

Accurate T and N staging requires contrast enhanced CT and PET and both investigations are complementary. Reactive lymph nodes in CT can be identified if FDG uptake is very low and necrotic lymph node metastases can be diagnosed in CT that are false negative in PET due to a low FDG uptake (Schöder et al., 2004, Jeong et al., 2004). However, as 40% of cervical metastases are below one centimeter in diameter not even PET/CT can confirm N0 necks thus opening up the field for sentinel imaging (Hyde et al., 2003), possibly performed as SPECT/CT (see 5.1.3). Therapy monitoring should not be performed earlier than one month after therapy, due to a > 30% rate of false negatives (Rogers et al., 2004, Engles et al., 2006). Restaging with FDG PET is more sensitive than CT/MR (Klabbers et al., 2003) but we lack data if PET/CT could further improve diagnosis.

4.1.2 Lung cancer

The sensitivity of integrated FDG PET/CT for mediastinal lymph node staging is low. PET/CT is superior to PET or CT alone, and visual correlation of both techniques separately. In particular, it improves T3 and T4 staging and delineation of tumours associated with atelectasis (Gámez et al., 2006). When positive mediastinal lymph nodes are detected, invasive mediastinal staging has been advised. On the other hand, the specificity is high: patients with negative integrated FDG PET-CT can be operated upon without invasive mediastinal staging (Perigauda et al., 2009). Evidence accumulates that in patients with locally advanced NSCLC, quantitative analysis of a routine whole-body FDG PET/CT studies predicts tumour response to therapy (Eschmann et al., 2007).

4.1.3 Esophageal cancer

Endoscopic ultrasound (EUS) is superior to PET/CT for T staging and in identifying locoregional nodes but PET/CT has a high sensitivity and specificity for M staging. EUS and PET/CT independently affects treatment decisions, indicating complimentary and necessary roles in the staging (Walker et al., 2011). PET/CT is not sufficiently reliable in the individual patient for monitoring of treatment response but effective in detecting recurrent disease (Weber et al., 2001, Munden et al., 2006, Bruzzi et al., 2007, Kim et al., 2009).

4.1.4 Colorectal cancer

PET/CT is recognised in the preoperative evaluation of apparently limited metastatic disease, detection of disease recurrence, clarification of equivocal lesions, investigation of rising tumour markers, and incidental detection of occult primary colonic tumours (Chowdhury et al., 2010). Transrectal ultrasound and MRI provide much better anatomic resolution and are of greater value for T staging. The sensitivity for regional N staging is low (Kantorva et al., 2003). Yet, in a study of patients with low rectal cancers, FDG-PET/CT altered treatment plans in 38% of patients largely through the detection of unsuspected inguinal adenopathy (Gearhart et al., 2006). PET for diagnosis and staging does not generate additional survival effectiveness compared with CT alone but cost savings associated with its use and the improvement of therapeutic management (Lejeune et al., 2005).

4.1.5 Hepatic metastases

Size is a limiting factor and the additional value of PET/CT is not yet fully established (Wiering et al., 2008).

4.1.6 Breast cancer

The present evidence does not support the routine use of PET or PET-CT for the assessment of the clinically negative axilla but is superior to conventional staging for detecting internal mammary chain nodes (Cooper et al., 2011, Segaert et al., 2010). FDG-PET/CT changes the clinical management in 50% of breast cancer patients with elevated tumour markers and negative or equivocal conventional imaging modalities (Filippi et al., 2011). Several studies aimed to use PET/CT to monitor therapy response, yet lack sufficient validation (Groheux et al., 2011). PET/CT showed clear advantage over CT and PET alone for the diagnosis of breast cancer recurrence (Pennant et al., 2010).

4.1.7 Melanoma

The combination of PET and CT had a higher sensitivity than either technique alone in staging high risk-patients with potentially respectable cancer (Strobel et al., 2007). Integrating PET-CT in the management of patients with high risk MM appears to be less costly and more accurate by avoiding futile thoracotomies in one of five patients as well as by providing a small survival benefit at 10 years (Krug et al., 2010).

4.1.8 Lymphoma

PET/CT improves baseline staging compared with conventional staging with CT alone (Freudenberg et al., 2004) and has been extensively reviewed in this field (Cronin et al., 2010). PET/CT scanning had a significant predictive value for disease progression and survival of DLBCL in post-rituximab treatment; it might be the single most important determinant of clinical outcome in patients with the same IPI risk (Yang et al., 2011). Nevertheless it is still not proven that the use of interim FDG PET can improve patient outcomes (Hutchings et al., 2009).

4.1.9 Ovarian cancer

FDG PET/CT is not recommended for primary ovarian cancer detection but is the best technique for lesion detection and treatment follow-up (Veena et al., 2010). It alters management in close to 60% of patients, detects more sites of disease than abdominal and pelvic CT and is superior in the detection of nodal, peritoneal and subcapsular liver disease (Fulham et al., 2009).

4.1.10 Gastrointestinal stromal tumors (GIST)

PET/CT is the method of choice for staging of GIST because some lesions have only a weak FDG uptake. PET/CT was also successfully used for monitoring of imatinib therapy because tumour shrinkage is minimal even in histological successful therapy (Antoch et al., 2004).

4.1.11 Radiotherapy planning

Nine experts and three IAEA staff evaluated the use of PET in radiotherapy planning and considered integrated PET/CT as the best available approach in non-small cell lung cancer, head and neck cancers, lymphoma and in esophageal cancers, with promising preliminary data in many other cancers (MacManus et al., 2009, Paulino et al., 2003).

4.1.12 Thyroid cancer

FDG PET/CT is capable to detect disease in patients with differentiated thyroid carcinoma with elevated Tg levels and negative radioiodine scan and the localization of disease in patients with medullary thyroid cancer and elevated serum calcitonin levels (Basu et al., 2011). 124 Iodine PET/CT may serve a role in obtaining lesional dosimetry of I-131 therapy (Abraham & Schöder, 2011).

4.1.13 Prostate cancer

The role of PET in prostate cancer has not been established yet, but due to the limited anatomical information provided by the used tracers, notably radiolabeled choline, PET/CT will be mandatory for local therapy planning.

4.2 Neurology

We lack evidence that attenuation and scatter correction in the brain is significantly improved by CT in contrast to conventional correction. It might however be useful for image landmarking in image fusion with MR.

4.3 Cardiology

Although the introduction of hybrid PET/CT technology offers the exciting possibility of assessing the extent of anatomic CAD (CT coronary angiography) and its functional consequences (ischemic burden) in the same setting, there are technical challenges in the implementation of CT-based transmission imaging for attenuation correction (DiCarli et al., 2007). The clinical potential of PET/CT for the characterization of cardiovascular diseases has been reviewed recently (Schwaiger et al., 2010) and is apparently used in clinical routine with increasing frequency (Heller et al., 2009).

5. Current state of clinical SPECT/CT

Whereas the PET market has entirely focused on hybrid designs, it is still possible to buy stand alone SPECT systems, but in view of the commercial success of integrated PET/CT scanners, there is an increasing interest in SPECT/CT systems (Buck et al., 2008). World wide market sales according to an industry source are in the range of 75% SPECT and 25% SPECT/CT with a continuing increase of hybrid devices.

5.1 Oncology

The role of hybrid imaging in oncology has been recently reviewed (Chowdhury & Scarsbrook, 2008).

5.1.1 131-I thyroid cancer

Planar 131-I whole body scan is hampered by many pitfalls (Leitha & Staudenherz, 2003). SPECT/CT improves the differentiation between physiologic and pathologic uptake of whole body iodine scan (Kohlfürst et al. 2009) and changes the therapeutic approach in a significant group of patients (Yamamoto et al., 2003). The unique contribution of a diagnostic CT in addition to the information of the 131-I scan is the detection of non-iodine-avid nodular lung disease, lymph node metastases and lytic bone lesions. It remains to be determined to what extent these findings improve patient management.

5.1.2 Neuroendocrine tumors, neural crest tumors

Low dose CT improves image interpretation by providing a better anatomic localization of SPECT-detected lesions in 41 percent of the patients primarily by improving the discrimination between physiological and pathological tracer uptake (Even-Sapir et al., 2001). Pfannenberg et al., (2003) pointed out that "The problem of false-negative SPECT results cannot be solved by SPECT/CT because of inherent low resolution and lack of oral and intravenous contrast of the low-dose CT component. SPECT/CT is better than SPECT or CT alone but cannot replace high-end CT. Therefore a high end CT component should be implemented in the SPECT/CT device to allow for combined acquisition of high-quality contrast-enhanced CT in addition to SPECT." I-123 mIBG SPECT/CT had a sensitivity (93%) similar to that (99%) achieved by PET/CT with C-11-HED as a tracer (Franzius et al., 2006). A significant impact of SPECT/CT on therapeutic management was also demonstrated by Hillel et al., (2006) in neuroendocrine tumors. The addition of clinically relevant information for 40% of patients by SPECT/CT compared with SPECT was described by Gabriel et al., (2005). Co-registration with CT improves dose calculations in planning radionuclide therapy (Tang et al., 2001).

5.1.3 Lymphoscintigraphy

SPECT detects nodes missed on planar scintigraphy but stand-alone SPECT lacks anatomical landmarks. Pilot studies suggested incremental diagnostic efficacy in many cancers, including melanoma (Even-Sapir et al., 2003), head neck cancer (Wagner et al., 2007), cervical cancer (Zhang et al., 2006), invasive bladder cancer (Sherif et al., 2006), breast cancer (Gallowitsch et al., 2007) and prostate cancer (Vermeeren et al., 2009).

5.1.4 Prostate cancer

FDA approved the use of Prostascint (In-111 capromab-pendetide), a monoclonal antibody-based imaging agent for detecting prostate cancer in 1996 but it was soon realized that the low tumour/background ratio and the lack of anatomical information necessitates hybrid imaging (Terence et al., 2005). With the limited sensitivity of contrast enhanced CT in prostate cancer, the contribution lies mainly in the improvement of topographical orientation and mapping for planning of external radiation therapy.

5.1.5 Dosimetry

SPECT/CT might be useful for performing valid and clinically applicable dosimetry, for improving treatment planning, and for ensuring safe and effective radionuclide therapy (Boucek & Turner 2005, Thierens et al., 2005, Prideaux et al., 2007, Lavely et al., 2007).

5.2 Endocrinology

5.2.1 99m-Tc MIBI parathyroid adenoma

CT co-registration is a valuable tool for the precise delineation of parathyroid adenomas with little incremental benefit from attenuation correction (Ruf et al., 2007) though others have seen little incremental benefit with non-diagnostic CT (Gayed et al., 2005).

5.3 Cardiology

SPECT attenuation correction with external sources was introduced in the early 1990s but, possibly due to financial and logistic problems got mixed reviews ever since (Dondi et al, 2004). Ten years later attenuation correction with CT was introduced (Masood et al., 2005) and the Society of Nuclear Medicine awarded its 2006 image of the year award to a cardiac SPECT/CT study (2006 Image of the year: focus on cardiac SPECT/CT. J Nucl Med. 2006; 47:14N–15N). Three different approaches were developed. The first was a low dose low resolution CT protocol aimed entirely at attenuation correction of SPECT data (Fricke et al., 2005), the second performed additional calcium scoring (Chang et al., 2009) and the third combined myocardial perfusion SPECT with a 64-slice CT angiography (CTA), initially only available on two different devices with digital fusion of the attenuation corrected SPECT and CTA (Gaemperli et al., 2007). Though feasible in principle and possibly identifying an independent risk, the value of assessing coronary calcifications or coronary morphology as part of a nuclear study needs to be validated in large prospective studies and appreciated in the light of the increased radiation exposure. At present attenuation correction in myocardial SPECT is especially useful in overweight patients and in women, however some degree of misregistration is still seen in the majority of the patients (Fricke et al., 2004, Goetze & Wahl, 2007) and CT artefacts may be a problem. Recent developments aimed to reduce imaging times by using semiconductor detectors and a converging collimator to increase sensitivity and a 3D iterative reconstruction utilizing the CT-based attenuation map enabling SPECT acquisitions in typically 5 minutes (IQ•SPECT technology Siemens) (Corbet et al., 2010).

5.4 Neurology

Until now no systematic analysis is available to assess differences between individually measured and conventionally calculated attenuation correction. Quantitative receptor imaging of fp-cit SPECT could be a perfect candidate for proving this principle.

5.5 Bone scans

Presently, SPECT/CT has added value in improved localization and characterization of bone lesions, both increasing sensitivity and specificity of bone scintigraphy. This was mainly achieved by identifying benign bone conditions with increased bone turnover (Utsunomiya et al., 2006). Until the introduction of SPECT/CT this has been routinely performed by comparing bone scanning with conventional (planar) X-ray and until now no additional benefit over the visual fusion of bone SPECT with planar X-ray, CT, or MRI studies has been confirmed (Horger et al., 2007). Thus, the "one-stop-shop" SPECT/CT has the drawback of increased radiation exposure. Low dose SPECT/CT may be a feasible compromise but may miss osteolytic lesions (Horger et al., 2004). "SPECT-guided CT" may be a better solution to the problem if it can be achieved logistically and is supported by the hybrid system (Roemer et al., 2006). Playing the devils advocate one may also assume that some of the lesions described as indeterminate in those scans could have been correctly identified by classical image features like pattern recognition (Puig et al., 1998) as it has been the clinical practice in times before hybrid imaging has hit the market.

5.6 Infections

Ga-67 scintigraphy, In-111 and Tc-99m labelled white blood cell scintigraphy is used to visualize infection. Physiological uptake and excretion and the lack of topographical information may hamper scan interpretation. SPECT/CT has been useful in the differentiation between bone and soft tissue infection (Fillippi et al., 2009).

6. Unsolved challenges

6.1 Real integration in stead of two devices "glued" together

Some of the early systems required two consoles to operate the system, one for the CT and one for the PET or SPECT. Some early PET/CTs incorporated a patient bore size that started at 70 cm for the CT and narrowed to about 59 cm for the PET system. In contrast to the statements of all manufacturers most commercially available systems are in essence still two separate machines (Figure 3).

The software of commercially available systems although combined under an apparently homogeneous surface still shows it different origins. Until the development of new detector types for both signals, movement in the interval between SPECT and CT data collection will continue to pose a problem.

6.2 Imaging protocols

A simple combination of traditional imaging protocols might not be the optimal use of hybrid imaging. Procedure guidelines and protocols are available for PET/CT (Boellaard et al., 2010) and SPECT/CT (Delbeke et al., 2006, Buck et al., 2008) but little efforts have been published so far to downsize conventional CT protocols if combined with Nuclear Medicine. The possible trade off of this has not been investigated, yet. Discussions have already begun about the reimbursement of diagnostic imaging as it is not apparent to most that a previous

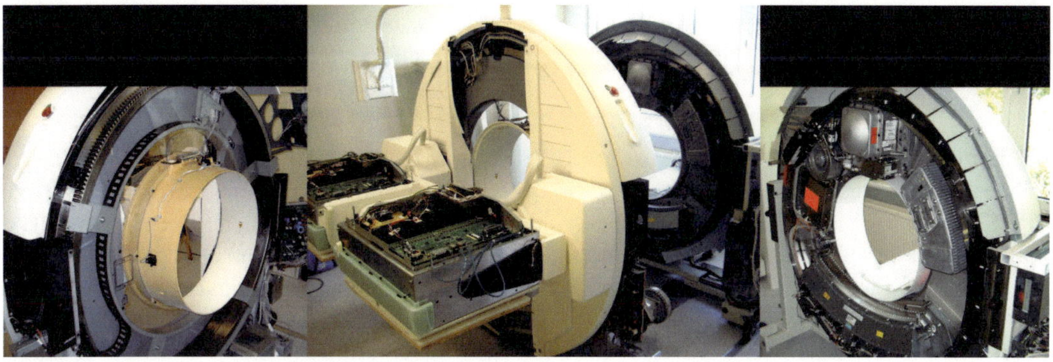

Fig. 3. Siemens Symbia T6: Left: Gantry of the dual head gamma camera, Center: both parts separated during service, Right: Gantry of the 6 slice MD CT

PET/CT study might not run other CT investigations obsolete. On the other hand, due to the higher number of CT investigations performed, many patients will already have undergone a diagnostic CT investigation before referral to their first Nuclear Medicine study and the duplicated CT further boosts the radiation burden. Current trends indicate that more and more centres use contrast enhancement and some regard the CT contrast agents and PET tracers as complementary (Antoch et al., 2004) but this may reflect common practice in radiology more than hard scientific evidence.

6.3 Education and training, data reporting

At present Nuclear Medicine and Radiology are different specialities in many countries with different training and licensing systems. Consequently the results of PET/CT and SPECT/CT require the competency and accreditation of individuals from both Nuclear Medicine and Radiology. Proposals for future training models have been put forward (White Paper, 2007) but first studies claim that only minimal additional training may be necessary to interpret both modalities (Narayanan et al., 2011). None of the commercially available RIS-NIS programmes is capable of simultaneous data reporting and validation by two different professionals. Standardization is mandatory as a recent survey (Cuocolo & Breatnach, 2010) revealed a wide heterogeneity in the current practice of multimodality imaging in Europe.

6.4 Diagnostic pathways

All current clinical recommendations are based on the sequential use of different imaging modalities. If hybrid imaging should be used to its full diagnostic utility, we will have to re-write conventional diagnostic paths as in many cases the optimized approach will start with hybrid imaging. However most of these pathways assume that the referrer has considerably narrowed the spectrum of possible differential diagnoses for a given problem, otherwise many conventional imaging steps will be necessary to narrow the problem to such an extent that a tailored approach is possible.

6.5 Forensic liabilities

The new hybrid devices produce a lot of additional information, not necessarily expected by the referrer. Data are accumulating that unexpected findings in PET/CT and SPECT/CT

(Goetze & Wahl 2007) as solitary pulmonary nodules, pneumonitis, and pleural effusion have clinical significance. The same problem has occurred in coronary CT protocols (Onuma et al., 2006, Schietinger et al., 2008).

6.6 Improved PET/CT correction, quantitative imaging

Whereas PET imaging was at least semi quantitative right from the start, quantitative SPECT has - in spite of early efforts (Rosenthal et al., 1995) - never reached prime time. The contribution of scatter, collimator response, depth dependent resolution and partial volume effect for accurate quantification have been determined for some investigations (Buvat et al., 2000), but only few data are available for the additional utility of CT for advanced data processing (Shcherbinin et al., 2008). On the other hand, contrast media and CT artefacts may severely hamper quantification of PET or SPECT (Sureshbabu & Mawlawi, 2005).

6.7 Costs

It is often overlooked that the increased costs for hybrid imaging are not only due to equipment costs but also to room preparation and energy supply. In those institutions where only Nuclear Medicine or Radiology has been practiced in the past, structural radiation protection for the other modality has to be installed. CT has a higher energy demand than conventional gamma cameras and produces more heat, thus energy supply and air conditioning have to be adapted. Usually hybrid systems require larger space than conventional systems. Both, radiation protection and space requirements stress the statics of some buildings.

7. Acknowledgement

The project was in part supported by the "Medical Research Society Vienna D.C."

8. References

Abraham, T. & Schöder, H. (2011). Thyroid cancer--indications and opportunities for positron emission tomography/computed tomography imaging. *Semin Nucl Med,* 41(2):121-38. 0001-2998

Almuhaideb, A., Papathanasiou, N., Bomanji, J. (2011). 18F-FDG PET/CT imaging in oncology. *Ann Saudi Med,* 31(1):3-13. 0975-4466

Ambrose, J. & Hounsfield, G. (1973). Computerized transverse axial tomography. *Br J Radiol,* 46(542):148-9. 0007-1285

Antoch, G., Kanja, J., Bauer, S., et al. (2004). Comparison of PET, CT, and dual-modality PET/CT imaging for monitoring of imatinib (STI571) therapy in patients with gastrointestinal stromal tumors. *J Nucl Med,* 45:357–365. 0161-5505

Basu, S., Urhan, M., Rosenbaum, J., Alavi, A. (2011). PET and PET/CT in the Management of Thyroid Cancer. *Meth Mol Biol,* 727:205-24. 1064-3745.

Bauhs, JA., Vrieze, TJ., Primak, AN., Bruesewitz, MR., McCollough, CH. (2008). CT dosimetry: comparison of measurement techniques and devices. *Radiographics,* 28(1):245-53. 0271-5333

BEIR VII (2006) Committee to Assess the Health Risks from Exposure to Low Levels of Ionizing Radiation, National Research Council. Health Risks From Exposure to Low Levels of Ionizing Radiation. Washington, DC: *National Academies Press.*

Beyer, T., Czernin, J., Freudenberg, LS. (2011). Variations in clinical PET/CT operations: results of an international survey of active PET/CT users. *J Nucl Med,* 52(2):303-10. 0161-5505

Beyer, T., Townsend, DW., Brun, T., et al. (2000). A combined PET/CT scanner for clinical oncology. *J Nuc Med,* 41:1369-1379. 0161-5 505

Boellaard, R., O'Doherty, MJ., Weber, WA., et al. (2010), FDG PET and PET/CT: EANM procedure guidelines for tumour PET imaging: version 1.0. *Eur J Nucl Med Mol Imag,* 37(1):181-200. 1619-7070

Boucek, JA. & Turner, JH. (2005), Validation of prospective whole-body bone marrow dosimetry by SPECT/CT multimodality imaging in 131I-anti-CD20 rituximab radioimmunotherapy of non-Hodgkin's lymphoma. *Eur J Nucl Med Mol Imag,* 32:458–469. 1619-7070

Bruzzi, JF., Munden, RF., Truong, MT., et al. (2007), PET/CT of esophageal cancer: its role in clinical management. *Radiographics,* 27(6):1635-52. 0271-5333

Buck, AK., Nekolla, S., Ziegler, S., et al. (2008). SPECT/CT. *J Nucl Med,* 49(8):1305-19. 0161-5505

Burnham, C. & Brownell, G., (1972). A multi-crystal positron camera. *IEEE Trans Nucl Sci,* 19:201-205, 0018-9499

Buvat, I., Soret, M., Hapdey, S., et al. (2000). Respective importance of scatter, collimator response, and partial volume effect corrections for accurate quantification 123I dopamine receptor imaging. *IEEE Nucl Sci Symp Rec,* 13:15–13/19

Büther, F., Stegger, L., Dawood, M., et al. (2007). Effective methods to correct contrast agent-induced errors in PET quantification in cardiac PET/CT. *J Nucl Med,* 48(7):1060-8. 0161-5505

Chang, SM. et al. (2009). The coronary artery calcium score and stress myocardial perfusion imaging provide independent and complementary prediction of cardiac risk. *J Am Coll Cardiol,* 54(20), 1872-82. 0735-1097

Chowdhury, FU. & Scarsbrook, AF. (2008). The role of hybrid SPECT-CT in oncology: current and emerging clinical applications. *Clin Radiol,* 63(3):241-51. 0009-9260

Chowdhury, FU., Shah, N., Scarsbrook, AF., Bradley, KM. (2010). 18F FDG PET/CT imaging of colorectal cancer: a pictorial review. *Postgrad Med J,* 86(1013):174-82. 0032-5473

Coleman, RE., Delbeke, D., Guiberteau, MJ., et al. (2005). Joint Working Group of the American College of Radiology; Society of Nuclear Medicine; Society of Computed Body Tomography and Magnetic Resonance. Concurrent PET/CT with an integrated imaging system: intersociety dialogue from the Joint Working Group of the American College of Radiology, the Society of Nuclear Medicine, and the Society of Computed Body Tomography and Magnetic Resonance. *J Am Coll Radiol,* 2(7):568-84. 1546-1440

Cooper, KL., Harnan, S., Meng, Y., et al. (2011). Positron emission tomography (PET) for assessment of axillary lymph node status in early breast cancer: A systematic review and meta-analysis. *Eur J Surg Oncol,* 37(3):187-98. 0748-7983

Corbett, J. et al. (2010) Clinical Validation of Attenuation Corrected Cardiac Imaging with IQ-SPECT SPECT/CT. Abstract from the 2010 Society of Nuclear Medicine Meeting

Cronin, CG., Swords, R., Truong, MT., et al. (2010). Clinical utility of PET/CT in lymphoma. *AJR*, 194(1):W91-W103. 1067-8654.

Cuocolo, A. & Breatnach, E., (2010). Multimodality imaging in Europe: a survey by the European Association of Nuclear Medicine (EANM) and the European Society of Radiology (ESR). *Eur J Nucl Med Mol Imag*, 37(1):163-7. 1619-7070

Czernin, J., Benza, MR., Allen-Auerbacha, MS., (2010). PET/CT imaging: The incremental value of assessing the glucose metabolic phenotype and the structure of cancers in a single examination. *Europ J Radiol*, 73 (3) 470-480. 0720-048X

Delbeke, D., Coleman, RE., Guiberteau, MJ., et al., (2006). Society of Nuclear Medicine (SNM). Procedure Guideline for SPECT/CT Imaging 1.0. *J Nucl Med*, 47(7):1227-34. 0161-5505

Delbeke, D. & Israel, O. (eds.), *Hybrid PET/CT and SPECT/CT Imaging*. Springer Science+Business Media 2010. Chapter I.1 History and Principles of Hybrid Imaging by JA Patton p. 28. ISSN 9780387928203.

Delbeke, D., Schöder, H., Martin, WH., Wahl, RL., (2009). Hybrid imaging (SPECT/CT and PET/CT): improving therapeutic decisions. *Semin Nucl Med*, 39(5):308-40. 0001-2998

Di Carli, MF., Dorbala, S., Meserve, J., et al., (2007), Clinical myocardial perfusion PET/CT. *J Nucl Med*, 48(5):783-93. 0161-5505

Dondi, M., Fagioli, G., Salgarello, M., Zoboli, S., et al., (2004). Myocardial SPECT: what do we gain from attenuation correction (and when)? *Q J Nucl Med Mol Imag*, 48:181–187. 1824-4785

Engles, JM., Quarless, SA., Mambo, E., et al. (2006), Stunning and its effect on 3H-FDG uptake and key gene expression in breast cancer cells undergoing chemotherapy. *J Nucl Med*, 47(4):603-8. 0161-5505

Eschmanna SM., Friedel, G., Paulsenc, F., et al., (2007). Repeat 18F-FDG PET for monitoring neoadjuvant chemotherapy in patients with stage III non-small cell. *Lung cancer*, 55 (2):165-171. 0169-5002

Even-Sapir, E., Keidar, Z., Sachs, J., et al. (2001). The New Technology of Combined Transmission and Emission Tomography in Evaluation of Endocrine Neoplasms. *J Nucl Med*, 42(7): 998-1004. 0161-5505

Even-Sapir, E., Lerman, H., Lievshitz, G., et al. (2003). Lymphoscintigraphy for sentinel node mapping using a hybrid SPECT/CT system. *J Nucl Med*, 44: 1413–1420. 0161-5505

Facey, K., Bradbury, I., Laking, G., Payne, E.. (2007). Overview of the clinical effectiveness of positron emission tomography imaging in selected cancers. *Health Technol Assess*, 11(44):iii-iv, xi-26. 1366-5278

Farid, K., Sibon, I., Fernandez, P., et al. (2009). Tc-99m HMPAO-SPECT with CT attenuation correction improves detection of epileptogenic areas. *Clin Nucl Med*, 34:290Y291. 0363-9762

Fillipi, L., Uccioli, L., Giurato, L., Schillaci, O., (2009). Diabetic Foot Infection: Usefulness of SPECT/CT for 99mTc-HMPAO-Labeled Leukocyte Imaging. *JNM*, 50(7), 1042-1046. 0161-5505

Filippi, V., Malamitsi, J., Vlachou, F., et al. (2011). The impact of FDG-PET/CT on the management of breast cancer patients with elevated tumor markers and negative or equivocal conventional imaging modalities. *Nucl Med Comm*, 32(2):85-90. 0143-3636

Fletcher, JW., Djulbegovic, B., Soares, HP., et al. (2008). Recommendations on the use of 18F-FDG PET in oncology. *J Nucl Med*, 49(3):480-508. 0161-5505

Franzius, C., Hermann, K., Weckesser, M., et al., (2006). Whole-body PET/CT with 11Cmeta-hydroxyephedrine in tumors of the sympathetic nervous system: feasibility study and comparison with 123I-MIBG SPECT/CT. *J Nucl Med*, 47:1635–1642. 0161-5505

Freudenberg, LS., Antoch, G., Schütt, P., et al. (2004). FDGPET/CT in re-staging of patients with lymphoma. *Eur J Nucl Med Mol Imag*, 31:325–329. 1619-7070

Fricke, H., Fricke, E., Weise, R., et al., (2004). A Method to Remove Artifacts in Attenuation-Corrected Myocardial Perfusion SPECT Introduced by Misalignment Between Emission Scan and CT-Derived Attenuation Maps. *J Nucl Med*, 45(10), 1619–1625. 0161-5505

Fricke, E., Fricke, H, Weise R, et al. (2005). Attenuation Correction of Myocardial SPECT Perfusion Images with Low-Dose CT: Evaluation of the Method by Comparison with Perfusion PET. *J Nucl Med*, 46(5), 736–744. 0161-5505

Fulham, MJ., Carter, J., Baldey, A., et al., (2009). The impact of PET-CT in suspected recurrent ovarian cancer: A prospective multi-centre study as part of the Australian PET Data Collection Project. *Gynecol Oncol*, 112(3):462-8. 0090-8258

Gabriel, M., Hausler, F., Bale, R., et al., (2005). Image fusion analysis of 99mTc-HYNICTyr(3)-octreotide SPECT and diagnostic CT using an immobilisation device with external markers in patients with endocrine tumours. *Eur J Nucl Med Mol Imag*, 32:1440–1451. 1619-7070

Gaemperli, O., Schepis, T., Valenta, I., et al., (2007). Cardiac Image Fusion from Stand-Alone SPECT and CT: Clinical Experience. *J Nucl Med*, 48:696–703. 0161-5505

Gallowitsch, HJ., Kraschl, P., Igerc, I., et al., (2007). Sentinel node SPECT-CT in breast cancer: can we expect any additional and clinically relevant information? *Nucl Med*, 46:252–256. 0029-5566

Gambhir, SS., Hoh, CK., Phelps, ME., et al., (1996). Decision tree sensitivity analysis for cost-effectiveness of FDG-PET in the staging and management of non-small-cell lung carcinoma. *J Nucl Med*, 37(9):1428-36. 0161-5505

Gámez, C., Rosell, R., Fernández, A., et al., (2006). PET/CT fusion scan in lung cancer: current recommendations and innovations. *J Thorac Oncol*, 1(1):74-7. 1556-0864

Gayed, IW., Kim, EE., Broussard, WF., et al., (2005). The value of 99mTc-sestamibi SPECT/CT over conventional SPECT in the evaluation of parathyroid adenomas or hyperplasia. *J Nucl Med*, 46:248–252. 0161-5505

Gearhart, SL., Frassica, D., Rosen, R., et al. (2006). Improved staging with pretreatment positron emission tomography/computed tomography in low rectal cancer. *Ann Surg Oncol*, 13: 397-404. 1068-9265

Goetze, S., Brown, TL., Lavely, WC., et al., (2007). Attenuation correction in myocardial perfusion SPECT/CT: effects of misregistration and value of reregistration. *J Nucl Med*, 48:1090–1095. 0161-5505

Goetze, S. & Wahl, RL. (2007). Prevalence of misregistration between SPECT and CT for attenuation-corrected myocardial perfusion SPECT. *J Nuc Cardiol*, 14, 200-206. 1071-3581

Groheux, D., Giacchetti, S., Espié, M., et al., (2011). Early monitoring of response to neoadjuvant chemotherapy in breast cancer with (18)F-FDG PET/CT: defining a clinical aim. *Eur J Nucl Med Mol Imag*, 38(3):419-25. 1619-7070

Hasegawa, BH., Lang, TF., Brown, EL., et al., (1993). Object specific attenuation correction of SPECT with correlated dual-energy x-ray CT. *IEEE Trans Nucl Sci*, NS-40:1242–1252. 0018-9499

Heller, GV., Calnon, D., Dorbala, S,. (2009). Recent advances in cardiac PET and PET/CT myocardial perfusion imaging. *J Nucl Cardiol*, 16(6):962-9. 1071-3581

Hillel, PG., van Beek, EJ., Taylor, C., et al., (2006). The clinical impact of a combined gamma camera/CT imaging system on somatostatin receptor imaging of neuroendocrine tumours. *Clin Radiol*, 61:579–587. 0009-9260

Hoffmann, EJ., Phelps, ME., Mullani, NA., et al., (1976). Design and performance characteristics of a whole-body positron transaxial tomograph. *J Nucl Med*, 17(6):493-502. 0161-5505

Horger, M., Eschmann, SM., Pfannenberg, C., et al., (2004). Evaluation of Combined Transmission and Emission Tomography for Classification of Skeletal Lesions. *Am J Roentgenol*, 183, 655-661. 0361-803X

Horger, M. & Bares, R. (2006). The role of single-photon emission computed tomography/computed tomography in benign and malignant bone disease. *Semin Nucl Med*, 36(4):286-94. 0001-2998

Horger, M., Eschmann, SM., Pfannenberg, C., et al., (2007). Added value of SPECT/CT in patients suspected of having bone infection: preliminary results. *Arch Orthop Trauma Surg*, 127(3):211-21. 0936-8051

Hutchings, M. & Barrington, SF. (2009). PET/CT for therapy response assessment in lymphoma. *J Nucl Med*, 50 Suppl 1:21S-30S. 0161-5505

Hyde, NC., Prvulovich, E., Newman, L., et al., (2003). A new approach to pre-treatment assessment of the N0 neck in oral squamous cell carcinoma: the role of sentinel node biopsy and positron emission tomography. *Oral Oncol*, 39(4):350-60. 1368-8375

ICRP publication 105 (2007). Radiation protection in medicine. *Ann ICRP*; 37(6):1-63. 0146-6453

Jeong, HS., Baek, CH., Son, YI., et al., (2007). Use of integrated 18F-FDG PET/CT to improve the accuracy of initial cervical nodal evaluation in patients with head and neck squamous cell carcinoma. *Head Neck*, 29(3):203-10. 1043-3074

Kantorva, I., Lipska, L., Belohlavek, O., et al., (2003). PET preoperative staging of colorectal cancer comparison with conventional staging and its impact on treatment decision making. *J Nucl Med*, 44: 1784-8. 0161-5505

Kessler, ML. (2006). Image registration and data fusion in radiation therapy, *Br J Rad*, 79: 99–108, 0007-1285

Kim, TJ., Kim, HY., Lee, KW., Kim, MS. (2009). Multimodality assessment of esophageal cancer: preoperative staging and monitoring of response to therapy. *Radiographics*, 29(2):403-21. 0271-5333

Kinahan, PE., Hasegawa, BH., Beyer T. (2003). X-Ray-Based Attenuation Correction for Positron Emission Tomography/Computed Tomography Scanners. *Sem Nucl Med*, 33: 166-179. 0001-2998

Klabbers, BM., Lammertsma, AA., Slotman, BJ. (2003). The value of positron emission tomography for monitoring response to radiotherapy in head and neck cancer. *Mol Imaging Biol*, 5(4):257-70. 1536-1632

Kohlfürst, S., Igerc, I., Lobnig, M., et al., (2009). Posttherapeutic 131I SPECT-CT offers high diagnostic accuracy when the findings on conventional planar imaging are inconclusive and allows a tailored patient treatment regimen. *Eur JNuc Med Mol Imag*, 36(6), 886-893. 1619-7070

Kramer, EL. & Noz, ME. (1991). CT/SPECT fusion for analysis of radiolabled antibodies: applications in gastrointestinal and lung cancinoma. *Int J Rad Appl InstrumB*, 18:27-42. 0883-2897

Krishnasetty, V., Bonab, AA., Fischman, AJ., et al., (2008). Comparison of standard-dose vs low-dose attenuation correction CT on image quality and positron emission tomographic attenuation correction. *J Am Coll Radiol*, 5(4):579-84. 1546-1440

Krug, B., Crott, R., Roch, I., et al., (2010). Cost-effectiveness analysis of FDG PET-CT in the management of pulmonary metastases from malignant melanoma. *Acta Oncol*, 49(2):192-200. 0284-186X

Lang, TF., Hasegawa, BH., Liew, SC., et al., (1991). A prototype emission-transmission imaging system. *IEEE Nucl Sci Symp Conf Rec*, 3:1902-1906. 0018-9499

Leitha T. & Staudenherz A. (2003). Frequency of diagnostic dilemmas in 131I whole body scanning. *Nuc Med*, 42(2):55-62. 0029-5566

Langer A. (2010). A systematic review of PET and PET/CT in oncology: a way to personalize cancer treatment in a cost-effective manner? *BMC Health Serv Res*, 10:283. 1472-6963

Lavely, WC., Goetze, S., Friedman, KP., et al., (2007). Comparison of SPECT/CT, SPECT, and planar imaging with single- and dual-phase 99mTc-sestamibi parathyroid scintigraphy. *J Nucl Med*, 48:1084–1089. 0161-5505

Lejeune, C., Bismuth, MJ., Conroy, T., et al., (2005). Use of a decision analysis model to assess the cost-effectiveness of 18F-FDG PET in the management of metachronous liver metastases of colorectal cancer. *J Nucl Med*, 46(12):2020-2028. 0161-5505

MacManus, M., Nestle, U., Rosenzweig, KE., et al., (2009). Use of PET and PET/CT for radiation therapy planning: IAEA expert report 2006-2007. *Radiother Oncol*, 91(1):85-94. 0167-8140

Mahmarian, JJ. (2007). Hybrid SPECT-CT: integration of CT coronary artery calcium scoring and angiography with myocardial perfusion. *Curr Cardiol Rep*, 9(2):129-35. 1523-3782

Mankoff DE. (2007). A Definition of Molecular Imaging. *JNM*; 48:18 -21N. 0161-5505

Masood, Y., Liu, YH., Depuey, G., et al. (2005). Clinical validation of SPECT attenuation correction using x-ray computed tomography-derived attenuation maps: multicenter clinical trial with angiographic correlation. *J Nucl Cardiol*, 12:676–686. 1071-3581. 1071-3581

Moore, KL., Palaniswaamy, G., White, B., et al., (2010). Fast, low-dose patient localization on TomoTherapy via topogram registration. *Med Phys*, 37(8):4068-77. 0094-2405

Munden, RF., Macapinlac, HA., Erasmus, JJ.. (2006). Esophageal cancer: the role of integrated CT-PET in initial staging and response assessment after preoperative therapy. *J Thorac Imag*, (2):137-45. 0883-5993

Nakamoto, Y., Senda, M., Okada, T., et al., (2008). Software-based fusion of PET and CT images for suspected recurrent lung cancer. *Mol Imaging Biol*, 10(3):147-53. 1536-1632

Narayanan D., Mdsen KS, Kalinyak JE., Berg WA. (2011). Interpretation of Positron Emission Mammography and MRI by Experienced Breast Imaging Radiologists: Performance and Observer Reproducibility, *AJR*, 196:971-981. 1067-8654

Neuwirth, J., Hefner, A., Ernst G., Staudenherz A. (2010). Does decreasing of setting parameters of the CT at PET/CT devices minimize patient-dose without noteworthy degradation of attenuation correction? S02-07 *Third European IRPA Congress*, Helsinki, F Publisher: NSFS - Nordic Society for Radiation Protection

O'Daniel, JC., Stevens, DM., Cody, DD. (2005). Reducing radiation exposure from survey CT scans. *AJR*, 185(2):509-15. 1067-8654

Onuma, Y., Tanabe, K., Nakazawa, G., et al. (2006). Noncardiac findings in cardiac imaging with multidetector computed tomography. *J Am Coll Cardiol*, 48: 402–406. 0735-1097

Pan, T., Mawlawi, O., Nehmeh, SA., et al., (2005). Attenuation correction of PET images with respirators-averaged CT images in PET/CT. *J Nuc Med*, 46:1481-1487. 0161-5505

Patton JA. & Turkington TG. (2008). SPECT/CT Physical Principles and Attenuation Correction. *J Nuc Med Tech*, 36 (1): 1-10. 0091-4916

Paulino, AC., Thorstad, WL., Fox T. (2003). Role of fusion in radiotherapy treatment planning. *Semin Nucl Med*, 33(3):238-43. 0001-2998

Pennant, M., Takwoingi, Y., Pennant, L., et al., (2010). A systematic review of positron emission tomography (PET) and positron emission tomography/computed tomography (PET/CT) for the diagnosis of breast cancer recurrence. *Health Technol Assess*, 14(50):1-103. 1366-5278

Perigauda, C., Bridjic, B., Roussela, JC., et al., (2009). Prospective preoperative mediastinal lymph node staging by integrated positron emission tomography–computerised tomography in patients with non-small-cell lung cancer. *Eur J Cardio Thorac Surg*, 36:731-736. 1010-7940

Pfannenberg, AC., Eschmann, SM., Horger, M., et al., (2003). Benefit of anatomical-functional image fusion in the diagnostic work-up of neuroendocrine neoplasms. *Europ J Nuc Med Mol Imag*, 30(6), 835-843. 1619-7070

Phelps, ME., Hoffman, EJ., Mullani, NA., Ter-Pogossian, MM., (1975). Application of annihilation coincidence detection to transaxial reconstruction tomography. *J Nucl Med*, 16(3):210-24. 0161-5505

Pichler, BJ., Wehrl, HF., Kolb, A., Judenhofer, MS. (2008). Positron emission tomography/magnetic resonance imaging: the next generation of multimodality imaging? *Semin Nucl Med*, 38(3):199-208. 0001-2998

Prideaux, AR., Song, H., Hobbs, RF., et al., (2007). Three-dimensional radiobiologic dosimetry: application of radiobiologic modeling to patient-specific 3-dimensional imaging-based internal dosimetry. *J Nucl Med*, 48:1008–1016. 0161-5505

Puig, S., Staudenherz, A., Steiner B, et al., (1998). Differential diagnosis of atypically located single or double hot spots in whole bone scanning. *J Nucl Med*, 39(7):1263-6. 0161-5505

Reinartz, P., Wieres, FJ., Schneider, W., et al., (2004). Side-by-side reading of PET and CT scans in oncology: which patients might profit from integrated PET/CT? *Eur J Nucl Med Mol Imag*, 31:1456–1461. 1619-7070

Römer, W., Nömayr, A., Uder, M., et al., (2006). SPECT-Guided CT for Evaluating Foci of Increased Bone Metabolism Classified as Indeterminate on SPECT in Cancer Patients. *J Nuc Med*, 47(7), 1102–1106. 0161-5505

Rosenthal, MS., Cullom, J., Hawkins, W., et al., (1995). Quantitative SPECT Imaging: A Review and Recommendations by the Focus Committee of the Society of Nuclear

Medicine Computer and Instrumentation Council. *J Nucl Med*, 36:1489-1513. 0161-5505

Ruf, J., Seehofer, D., Denecke, T., et al. (2007). Impact of image fusion and attenuation correction by SPECT-CT on the scintigraphic detection of parathyroid adenomas. *Nuc Med*, 46:15–21. 0029-5566

Schietinger, BJ., Bozlar, U., Hagspiel, KD., et al. (2008). The prevalence of extracardiac findings by multidetector computed tomography before atrial fibrillation ablation. *Am Heart J*, 155:254–259. 0002-8703

Schillaci, O. (2005). Hybrid SPECT/CT: a new era for SPECT imaging? *Eur J Nucl Med Mol Imag*, 32:521–524. 1619-7070

Schöder, H., Yeung, HW., Gonen, M., et al., (2004). Head and neck cancer: clinical usefulness and accuracy of PET/CT image fusion. *Radiology*, 231(1):65-72. 0033-8419

Schwaiger, M., Ziegler, SI., Nekolla, SG. (2010). PET/CT challenge for the non-invasive diagnosis of coronary artery disease. *Eur J Radiol*, 73(3):494-503. 0720-048X

Shcherbinin, S., Celler, A., Belhocine, T., et al., (2008). Accuracy of quantitative reconstructions in SPECT/CT imaging. *Phys Med Biol*, 53: 4595–4604. 0031-9155

Segaert, I., Mottaghy, F., Ceyssens, S., et al., (2010). Additional value of PET-CT in staging of clinical stage IIB and III breast cancer. *Breast J*, 16(6):617-24. 1075-122X

Sherif, A., Garske, U., de la Torre, M., Thorn, M. (2006). Hybrid SPECT-CT: an additional technique for sentinel node detection of patients with invasive bladder cancer. *Eur Urol*, 50:83–91.

Slomka PJ. (2004). Software Approach to Merging Molecular with Anatomic Information *J Nucl Med*, 45:36S–45S. 0161-5505

Stabin, M., Stubbs, JB., Toohey, RE. (1996). Radiation Dose Estimates for Radio-pharmaceuticals. Oak Ridge, TN: *Radiation Internal Dose Information Center, ORNL*

Stemberger, A., Leitha, T., Staudenherz, A. (2011). Diagnostic reference value. Critical evaluation of the term with the example of nuclear medicine studies in Austria. *NucMed*, Feb 21;50(2). [Epub ahead of print]

Strobel, K., Dummer, R., Husarik, DB., et al., (2007). High-risk melanoma: accuracy of FDG PET/CT with added CT morphologic information for detection of metastases. *Radiology*, 244(2):566-74. 0033-8419

Sureshbabu, W., Mawlawi, O., (2005). PET/CT Imaging Artifacts, *J Nuc Med Tech*, 33 (3): 156-161. 0091-4916

Tang, HR., Da Silva, AJ., Matthay, KK., et al., (2001). Neuroblastoma Imaging Using a Combined CT Scanner–Scintillation Camera and 131I-MIBG. *J Nucl Med*, 42(2), 237-247. 0161-5505

Terence, Z., Wong, TZ., Turkington, TG., et al., (2005). ProstaScint (Capromab Pendetide) Imaging Using Hybrid Gamma Camera–CT Technology. *AJR*, 184(2):676-80. 1067-8654

Ter-Pogossian, MM., Phelps, ME., Hoffman, EJ., Mullani, NA. (1975). A positron-emission transaxial tomograph for nuclear imaging (PET). *Radiology*, 114(1):89-98. 0033-8419

Thierens HM, Monsieurs MA, Bacher K. (2005). Patient dosimetry in radionuclide therapy: the whys and the wherefores. *Nucl Med Comm*, 26:593–599.

Townsend, DW., Beyer, T., Kinahan, PE., et al., (1998). The SMART scanner: A combined PET/CT tomography for clinical oncology. *IEEE Nucl Sci Symp Conf Rec*, 2:1170-1174, paper M5-1. 0018-9499

Utsunomiya, D., Shiraishi, S., Imuta, M., et al., (2006). Added value of SPECT/CT fusion in assessing suspected bone metastasis: comparison with scintigraphy alone and nonfused scintigraphy and CT. *Radiology*, 238(1):264-71. 0033-8419

Veena, R., Iyer, VR., Lee, SI. (2010). MRI, CT, and PET/CT for Ovarian Cancer Detection and Adnexal Lesion Characterization. *AJR*, 194:311–321. 1067-8654

Vermeeren, L., Valdés Olmos, RA., Meinhardt, W., et al., (2009). Value of SPECT/CT for dectection and anatomic localization of sentinal lymph nodes before laparascopic sentinel node lymphadenectomy in prostate cardinoma. *J Nuc Med*, 50(6), 865-870. 0161-5505

von Schulthess, GK. & Pelc, NJ. (2002). Integrated-modality imaging: the best of both worlds. *Acad Radiol*, 9:1241–4. 1076-6332

Wagner, A., Kermer, C., Zettinig, G., et al., (2007). Validity of sentinel lymph node (SLN) detection following adjuvant radiochemotherapy (RCT) in head and neck squamous cell carcinoma (HNSCC). *Technol Cancer Res Treat*, 6(6):655-60. 1533-0346

Wahl, RL., Jacene, H., Kasamon, Y., Lodge, MA. (2009). From RECIST to PERCIST: Evolving Considerations for PET response criteria in solid tumors. *J Nucl Med*, 50 Suppl 1:122S-50S. 0161-5505

Walker, AJ., Spier, BJ., Perlman, SB., et al., (2011). Integrated PET/CT fusion imaging and endoscopic ultrasound in the pre-operative staging and evaluation of esophageal cancer. *Mol Imag Biol*, 13(1):166-71. 1536-1632

White Paper: http://www.spmn.org/documentos/2007_FINAL_White_Paper_Cuocolo_Adam_23_05_07.pdf

Wiering, B., Vogel, WV., Ruers, TJ., Oyen WJ. (2008). Controversies in the management of colorectal liver metastases: role of PET and PET/CT. *Dig Surg*, 25(6):413-20. 0253-4886

Weber, WA. & Figlin, R. (2007). Monitoring Cancer Treatment with PET/CT: Does it make a difference. *J Nucl Med*, 48:36S-44S. 0161-5505

Weber, WA., Ott, K., Becker, K., et al., (2001). Prediction of response to preoperative chemotherapy in adenocarcinomas of the esophagogastric junction by metabolic imaging. *J Clin Oncol*, 19(12):3058-65. 0732-183X

Yamamoto, Y., Nishiyama, Y., Monden, T., et al., (2003). Clinical usefulness of fusion of 131I SPECT and CT images in patients with differentiated thyroid carcinoma. *J Nucl Med*, 44:1905–1910. 0161-5505

Yang, DH., Min, JJ., Song, HC., et al., (2011). Prognostic significance of interim (18)F-FDG PET/CT after three or four cycles of R-CHOP chemotherapy in the treatment of diffuse large B-cell lymphoma. *Eur J Cancer*, Feb 17. [Epub ahead of print]

Yen, RF., Yen, MF., Hong, RL., et al., (2009). The Cost-utility Analysis of 18-Fluoro-2-Deoxyglucose Positron Emission Tomography in the Diagnosis of Recurrent Nasopharyngeal Carcinoma. *Acad Radiol*, 16(1):54-60. 1076-6332

Zhang, WJ., Zheng, R., Wu, LY., et al., (2006). Clinical application of sentinel lymph node detection to early stage cervical cancer [in Chinese]. *Chin J Canc/Ai Zheng*, 25:224–228. 1000-467X

18

The Role of Contrast Enhanced Computed Tomography in Integrated Positron Emission Tomography Computed Tomography Study

Abdul Jalil Nordin[1], Noraini Abdul Rahim[2],
Fathinul Fikri Ahmad Saad[1] and Ahmad Zaid Fattah Azman[1]
[1]Diagnostic Nuclear Imaging Centre , Universiti Putra Malaysia, Serdang
[2]Radiology Department, Serdang Hospital, Serdang
Malaysia

1. Introduction

Integrated Positron Emission Tomography Computed Tomography (PET/CT) is becoming an important tool for clinical investigation with increase clinical utilization. Technology evolution has brought tremendous improvement in lesion detection by integrating morphological and functional informations in a single study. Improved technical specification for CT and PET camera is translated into shorter time spent in image acquisition and reconstruction with improved PET temporal resolution. Both systems complement each other in improving diagnostic capabilities by enabling accurate lesion localization unlike stand alone PET or CT system .

A combined PET/CT system involves the use of a full-ring detector PET scanner with a multi-detector helical CT scanner in combination, allowing the PET scan to be acquired sequentially after the CT scan. The images are then fused to give a precise localization of PET-positive lesions. When integrated PET/CT system was initially introduced, CT scan was performed using low dose exposure without intravenous contrast administration.

This new integrated technology imaging diagnostic system improved lesion detectability, localization, and characterization in up to 30% of 204 cases as demonstrated by Rachel and her colleague (1). The greatest impact was in abdominal and pelvic diagnostic interpretations than any other sites.

To optimize the diagnostic capability of both systems during an integrated PET/CT study, variations to the basic CT practice has been employed.(2). In addition to useful diagnostic informations obtained, the advantage of advance CT protocol can be observed in cases where lesions are non PET-avid, and alternative diagnostic imaging study is needed. Thus, higher diagnostic CT quality performed during integrated PET/CT study will avoid the hassle for a separate diagnostic CT appointment.

This chapter will highlight the advantages of contrasted CT over low dose CT in a contemporaneous integrated FDG PET/CT study. The capability of both modalities would be optimized if such technique is employed . The technical aspects of multi detector CT and PET and the specifications are discussed elsewhere.

2. PET technique – Basic and advance

2.1 Basic PET technique

PET is a nuclear imaging technique which detects abnormal tissues with the help of molecular imaging probe like flurodeoxyglucose (FDG), dopa, fluoroethylcholine (FLT) and fluoroethylthymidine (FET). These probes can be tagged with radioisotopes like 18-Fluorine (^{18}F) and carbon (^{11}C ,^{12}C). These unstable isotopes while emitting beta plus (β^+) rays will enable the PET camera to localize the highest decaying activity in the body. The process can be captured and image. However, due to poor resolution of PET camera, a standalone PET system yields poor lesion localization. To improve the resolution, transmission from Germanium-68 isotope was utilized for attenuation correction but the technique is time consuming. All new PET systems are now improved by incorporation with a CT system. The CT parameters are used for attenuation correction of PET images. The new integrated system is capable in delivering higher quality images with improved resolution (Figure 1) . The time spent for each examination is shorter in comparison to using the conventional old PET system.

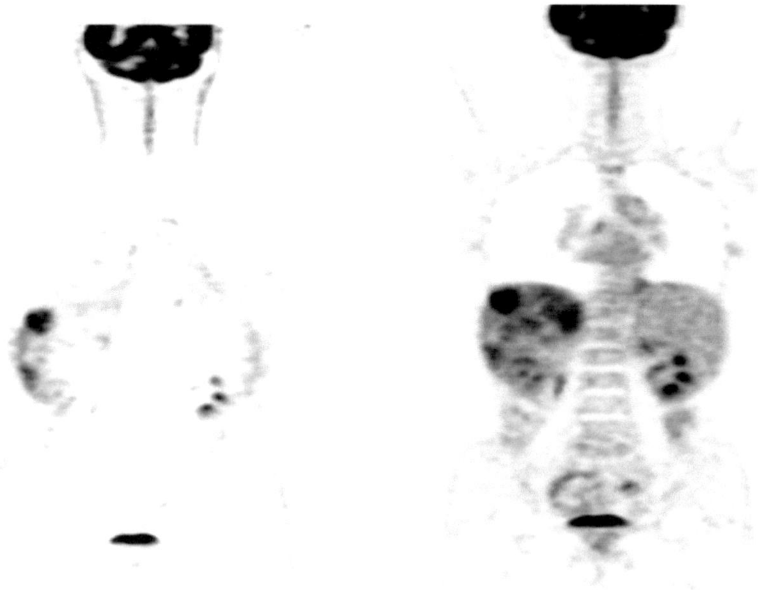

(a) (b)

Fig. 1. Coronal view of PET image in grey scale demonstrating non attenuation corrected image (a) and attenuation corrected image (b) using CT parameters.

The widely recommended protocol for a PET study is intravenous injection of 8-12mci of ^{18}F-FDG isotope after ensuring that the patient is fasting by obtaining fasting blood sugar. Prior to intravenous administration of isotope, the height and weight of the patient will also be recorded. These essential parameters are important for accurate calculation of standardized uptake value (SUV), a recognized method in semiquantifying the FDG uptake in avid lesions. PET/CT image acquisition will start after 45 minutes post injection rest to ensure good FDG uptake and distribution in the body. Image acquisition will start with a

scanogram for planning the study followed by low dose CT from eyes to the thigh with exception in cases of melanoma and childrens. Images acquired in 2D or 3D mode with 2-3 minutes per bed position ending with 5-7 bed positions will depend on the dose of isotope injected and size of the patient. Tall patients may require more time to complete the eyes and thigh protocol as compared to shorter individuals.
This recommended basic PET imaging technique is practiced with minor variation from one institution to another depending on camera specification and work load.

2.2 Advance PET technique

Advance whole body FDG PET study includes delayed or dual- time point imaging techniques.
In delayed PET image acquisition technique, imaging is delayed after 90 minutes following an earlier acquisition at 45 minutes (3).Russ et al observed a significant increase in standard uptake value (SUV) of liver lesions between early and delayed acquisition ($p< 0.001$) in 30 patients without significant reduction in liver background activity between the two studies allowing better lesion detection by visual inspection. Delayed phase PET protocol also revealed new lesions in 17% of the patients thus improved lesion detectability in primary and metastatic liver disease. Thus, the technique may be deemed beneficial in oncology work-up to obtain detail information on extension of lesions .
Another advance PET technique is the dual-time point imaging. The technique has been utilized to differentiate inflammatory from malignant lesions (4,5,6). Lesion of inflammatory in origin demonstrate peak FDG uptake at approximately 30 minutes post FDG injection. As opposed to aggressive malignant lesions which peak is seen much later depending on histopathological variation and degree of aggressiveness.

3. Contrast Enhanced Computed Tomography (CECT)

Computed tomography is a diagnostic radiological imaging modality commonly employed to assist physicians in the clinical management. CT is a useful tool in cancer staging, localizing infection and inflammatory lesions and evaluation of treatment response. In clinical practice, a stand- alone CT system is often the first choice of cross sectional imaging modality to be employed in making a diagnosis. This is attributed to its accessibility, fast, relatively cheap and its capability in demonstrating morphological abnormalities. In addition, CT procedures are somehow standardized and reproducible.
Technological development focusing on CT helical systems resulted in increased gantry speed rotation, increasing number of detector rows, and increased tube outputs to maintain adequate signal-to-noise ratio (SNR) leading to improved image resolution. New development involving PET systems are now incorporated into multidetector CT with full diagnostic capability.
In this section, we highlight the benefit of using contrast enhanced CT during integrated FDG PET/CT study.
Although low dose CT has been an acceptable norm in PET/CT practice, contrast enhanced CT integrated with PET can be considered as the protocol of choice in recent days especially if the technique will benefit the patient's clinical management .
Advance CT protocol is useful in demonstrating pathology accurately. This can be achieved through dynamic and sequential image acquisition protocols to be incorporated into multiplanar PET images. The technique is capable in characterizing tumour physiology with improved

visual delineation of tumour margins (7). Inflammatory lesions and infection can also be highlighted and shall gain advantage from this technique. The new multidetector CT scanners can achieve a high temporal resolution in monitoring contrast agent first-pass effects(8).
Lesion characterization on CT are through morphological changes , homogeneity, size, outline, vascularity and adjacent structure involvement. Lesion characterization through enhancement properties depends on whether they are hyper or hypovascular in nature as different types of lesions enhance differently during each phase of image acquisition.

	Very Low Dose CT	Intermediate dose CT	Diagnostic CT
MAs	Less 35	40-80mAs	>80mAs
Description	No oral, rectal, intravenous contrast	Oral and rectal contrast may be administered	Oral, rectal , intravenous contrast administrered

Table 1. Recommended CT doses during whole body FDG PET/CT study

There is increasing evidence in the literature to support the incremental benefit of FDG-PET/ CT in tumour staging and monitoring treatment response. The latest generation of PET/CT machines incorporates multi-detector CT allowing diagnostic quality CT images to be obtained. As such, CT images acquired during integrated PET/CT examination can be used to avoid separate CT examination for staging or treatment response assessment. Low-dose CT protocols allow attenuation-correction of PET images and accurate anatomical localization. However, image quality is compromised with poor resolution and inability to exclude an involvement of surrounding organs and vascular structures. Informations obtained at visual image interpretation are vital informations to support clinical decisions. It is also vital consideration to the non-specificity of fluorodeoxyglucose (FDG) to malignant lesions. Some malignancies demonstrate poor or non FDG-avidity. In these circumstances, an alternative imaging modality is needed. Integrated diagnostic contrast enhance-CT during PET/CT study potentially avoid another CT session which is inconvenient to the patient which lead to delay in diagnosis and treatment delivery. This can be avoided if a diagnostic CT is integrated concurrently with PET imaging in a single seating.
A diagnostic CT procedure incorporated in a PET/CT study may comprise either a single phase or a multiphase contrast enhanced CT. Image acquisition during a single phase study starts 60-80s following bolus intravenous contrast administration at a rate of 2-3 mls/second while multiphase CT comprise of arterial, venous and delayed phase CT where images are acquired at different time frame.
During study of patient with suspicious intracranial pathology, physiological high intracerebral FDG uptake will mask the visibility of lesions. Contrasted CT image acquisition during the study can potentially identify intracranial structural abnormalities (figure 2).
Non invasive CT angiography of cerebral circulation can be a useful technique for demonstrating vascular involvement . This technique can be incorporated into a PET/CT study mapping the course of nearby vessels. The information is useful in excluding specific vascular involvement and choosing the correct vessel for intra arterial embolization procedures.
In head and neck malignancy involving the neck nodes, contrasted CT during FDG PET/CT study can provide useful information prior to CT guided histo-pathological sampling procedure in establishing the clinical diagnosis.

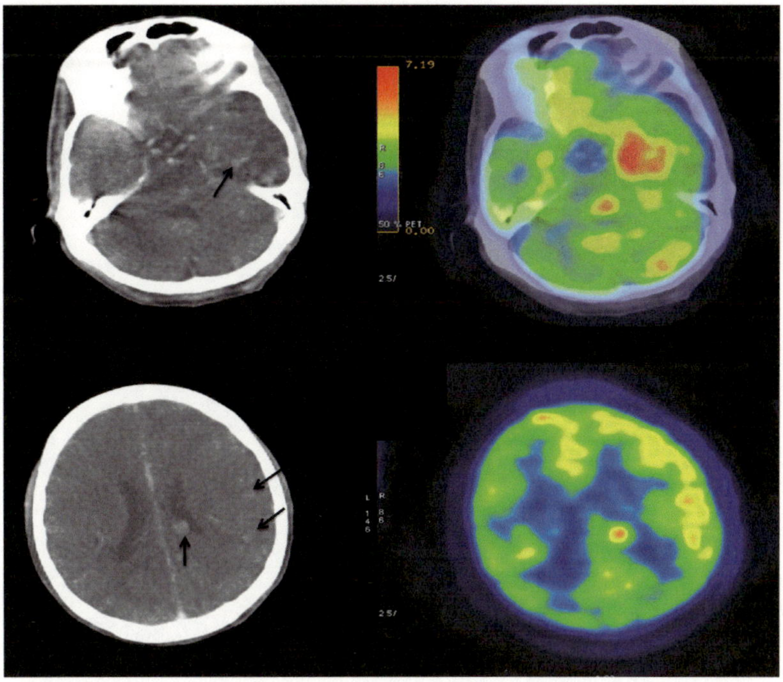

Fig. 2. Single phase contrast enhanced PET CT in a 28-year old man demonstrating subtle enhancing intracerebral (black arrows) tuberculosis abcess in the brain.

In thoracic malignancy , particularly carcinoma of the lungs involving mediastinal nodes, contrast enhanced PET/CT study can be a useful technique in affirming T-staging by excluding local invasion, guiding invasive interventional tissue sampling procedure by avoiding vital structures and characterizing tumour resectability (figure 3).

A single phase PET/contrast enhance CT can also be carried out in patients with mediastinal malignancy including carcinoma of esophagus (figure 4).

A 4- phase CT technique involves CT image acquisition at different time phases including a plain non contrasted study prior to contrast administration , arterial phase (30 seconds delay imaging) , venous phase (70-90 seconds delay imaging) and delayed phase (5-10 minutes delay imaging). Technical softwares are usually available in prescribing the protocol depending on the type and specification of the equipment. These include smartprep, care-bolus or bolus tracking.

CT is a valuable tool in assessing liver pathology. Informations acquired is very useful in planning clinical management especially in cases of hepatocellular carcinoma and metastasis. A 4- phase CT liver and a single phase CT can be used in the former and latter conditions respectively.

FDG avidity of hepatocellular carcinoma in PET imaging varies. Most of the time they demonstrate low avidity except in aggressive tumour sub-types which usually demonstrate higher uptake and activity. Similar to metastatic lesions where tumours with tendency to develop cystic liver metastasis will demonstrate low FDG avidity than the more aggressive solid liver lesions. In the event of non FDG-avid or unidentified malignant liver lesions during a PET/CT study, an alternative imaging modality is sought for to help solving the clinical diagnosis (figure 5).

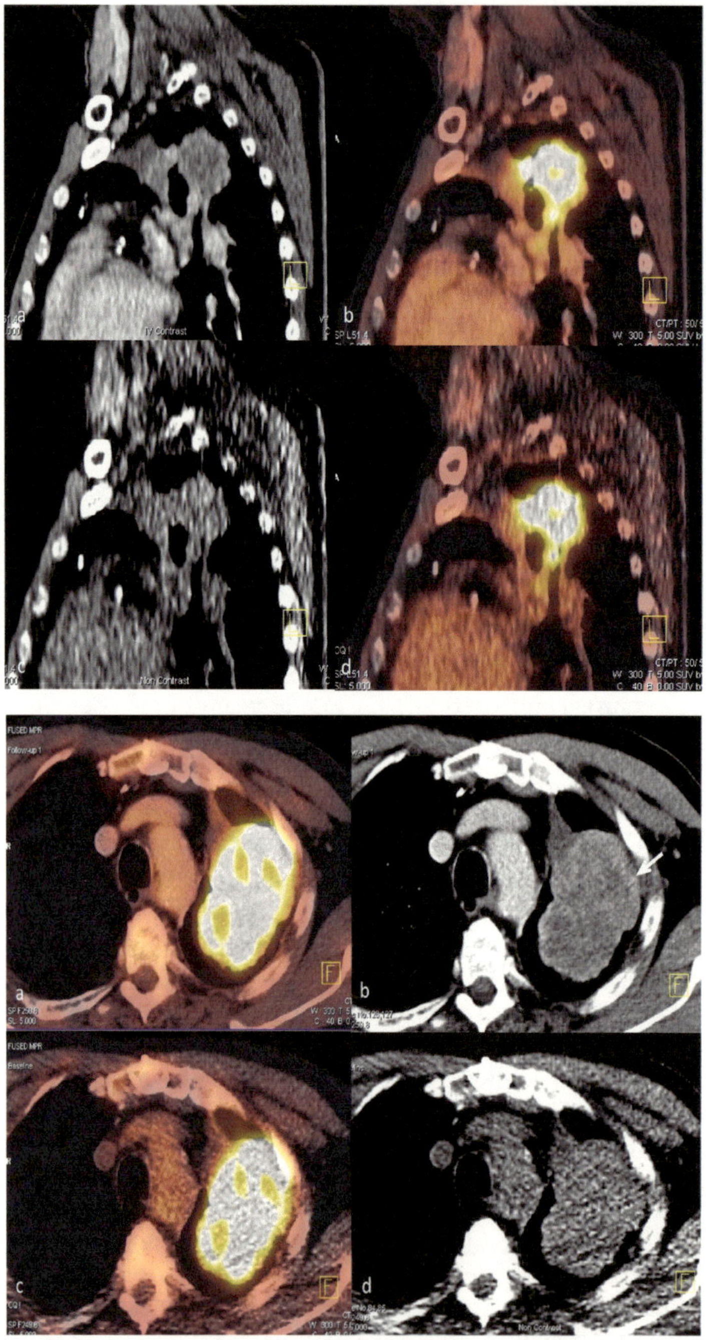

Fig. 3. FDG PET/CT study of a 56 year old man with carcinoma of the left lung. FDG PET study in sagittal (top) and axial (bottom). Top row (a and b) demonstrate PET/CT study with intravenous contrast administration and bottom row (c and d) demonstrate FDG PET/CT with low dose non contrasted CT. Intravenous contrast sharply delineating tumour outline (white arrow axial CT image) excluding thoracic wall invasion and vascular involvement.

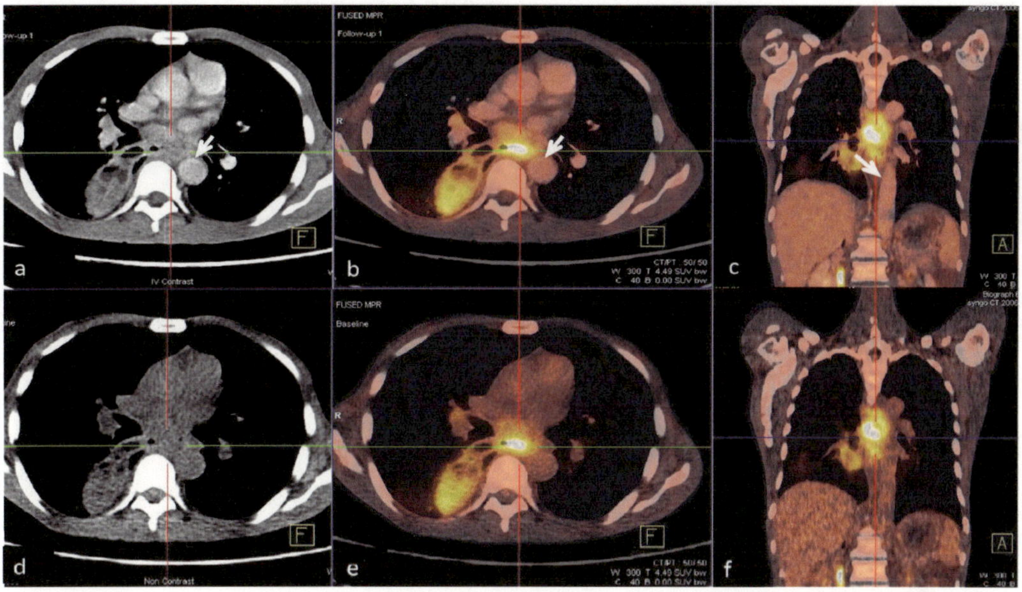

Fig. 4. Whole body FDG PET/CT study showing contrast enhanced CT (a,b,c) and non contrast enhanced CT(d,e,f) in a patient diagnosed with carcinoma of esophagus. In axial and coronal planes (c,f) . Poor definition of descending aortic wall in non enhanced CT was solved after giving intravenous contrast administration (white arrow). Contrast enhanced CT helped in determining tumour resectability and treatment planning in this patient

^{18}F-FDG-PET in combination with low dose CT in the evaluation of hepatocellular carcinoma has low sensitivity (55%) in comparison to multiphase contrast enhanced CT (90%). Since the role of PET in detecting primary carcinoma is limited, contrasted multiphase CT during PET/CT study can be a very useful protocol in detecting liver pathology (9).

The accuracy of low dose CT during qualitative assessment of the liver can be jeorpardized in cases where the CT value of the lesions fall within the range of normal liver parenchyma. In such situation, contrast enhanced CT can delineate these lesions through enhancing pattern of normal liver parenchyma against the lower attenuation value of the lesion itself rendering visibility of the lesions separable from the normal liver parenchyma (10,11,12, 13).

The successful use of contrast enhanced CT during PET/CT examination has been clearly demonstrated by Patrick VH and his colleagues. In his study, he reported the integration of a combined CT-perfusion in FDG PET study without the use of additional contrast media compared to a standard contrast enhance PET/CT study in patients with intra abdominal malignancy (14).

CT is more sensitive than FDG-PET in detecting colorectal metastases following neo-adjuvant therapy. According to Lubezky and his group (15), the sensitivity of CT in comparison to FDG PET is 65% versus 49% (n=27; p<0.0001). The lower sensitivity of FDG PET in detecting liver metastasis during this time are attributed by various factors including post-chemotherapeutic 'metabolic shutdown' phenomenon, small size lesions and non FDG avidity. Baseline FDG PET/CT studies prior to neo-adjuvant therapy in colorectal cancer patients are known to be mandatory, thus contrast enhanced CT during this time may deemed appropriate. From the study conducted by Lubezky, the technique is obviously beneficial in demonstrating non avid smaller liver lesions which may be limited by PET camera's spatial resolution.

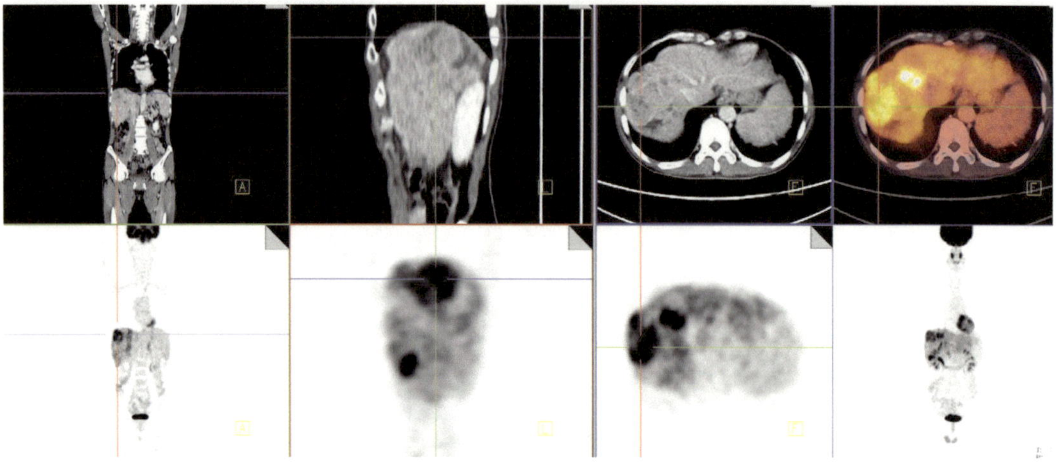

a. FDG PET/CT study using intravenous non ionic contrast enhanced CT

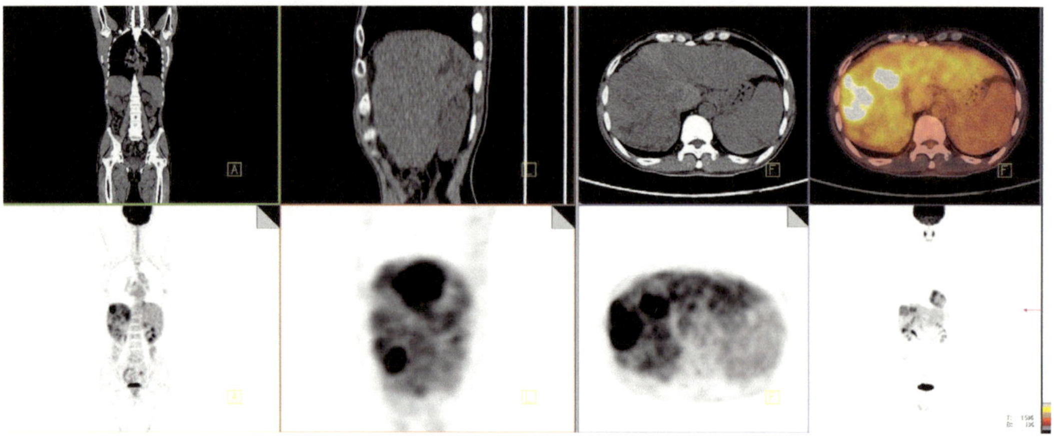

b. FDG PET/CT study with low dose CT

Fig. 5. Multiplanar images acquired for a 56 year old patient diagnosed with hepatocellular carcinoma in FDG PET/CT study using intravenous contrast (a), and using low dose CT (b). There are multifocal high metabolic activity lesions seen in segment VIII of the liver clearly demonstrate in the study as ill defined heterogenous contrast enhancement within the affected segment (a) as compared to low dose CT (b).

As an alternative to using positive contrast media during PET/CT study, negative contrast like gas can also be used. In the assessment of intraabdominal malignancy arising from the bowels, cross-sectional imaging study of the bowels using CT is capable in demonstrating the entire intraluminal, wall thickness and extraluminal involvement (16,17).

Non invasive virtual CT colonoscopy (VCTC) using thin-slice cross-sectional imaging techniques with multiplanar 3D reconstruction is another procedure capable in evaluating the entire large bowel. The technique has positive impact in screening patients with intermediate risk for malignant colonic polyps (18,19). Integrating VCTC with FDG PET will perfect the diagnostic value of both modalities. This technique may be useful especially in the evaluation of focal increase bowel activity commonly addressed as physiological bowel uptake (20,21). The sensitivity and specificity of VCTC in detecting polyps ranging between 48-85% and 91-97% depending on polyp size (Mulhall et al) while the sensitivity of FDG PET to detect pre-malignant adenomatous polyps also correlated with grading of polyp dysplasia (20) and generally non pre-malignant hyperplastic polyps do not tend to be FDG avid. The intensity of FDG uptake is also incapable to discriminate malignant, pre-malignant and benign lesions (23,24). Thus incidental focal colonic uptake on PET deserves further confirmatory investigations to exclude a malignant pathology. CT can play an important role in localizing these lesions.

The advantage of combining VCTC into FDG PET study has been proven by Veit-Haibach and his colleagues where the tehnique improved the accuracy of staging in 47 patients with colorectal carcinoma (25).

Integrated PET/ low dose CT has limited role in local staging of rectal and colonic cancers except in the assessment of metastatic disease and potential recurrence (26,27) . The value of diagnostic CT with intravenous contrast can be optimized during integrated imaging PET/CT in rectal and colonic cancers especially in complicated cases of gross invasion of adjacent organs (T4). Contrast enhancement of the surrounding organs of the lesion can assess local invasion. Since CT is routinely employed as a primary tool in the detection of metastatic disease in rectal carcinoma, combining FDG PET and CECT will provide 'one stop shop ' for the patient (28)

The feasible role of combined FDG PET/VCTC may also be applicable in combined FDG PET/CT enterography (CTE) which involves enteroclysis using low-density oral contrast agents , intravenous contrast and thin slice CT image acquisition. The technique can be useful in small bowel infections, neoplasms, adhesions, polyps, vascular malformations and inflammatory bowel diseases. (29) The protocol can potentially provide better clues on the cause of pitfalls in FDG PETCT imaging of the bowels which are currently addressed as physiological activity in most cases .

The role of FDG PET / CT cholangiography using biliary excreted contrast agent should be further evaluated (30)

High resolution advanced MDCT technique has become the mainstay of pancreatic tumor imaging. Multiphase CT allow accurate detection, staging and assessment of tumor resectability (31,32). In general, the differentiation of malignant and inflammatory lesions on FDG PET images are crucial. Multiphase CT angiography has the potential to increase the diagnostic value of FDG PET/CT study in pancreatic carcinoma especially in determining tumour resectability by excluding vascular invasion. Contrast enhanced PET/CT is also a recommended imaging procedure in carcinoid and non-carcinoid neuroendocrine tumours (33).

In any clinical situation, decision should adhere to ALARA principle. Perhaps, in view of clinical benefits to patients, contrast enhanced FDG PET/CT protocol should be recommended as a first line tool in imaging of selected malignant diseases.

4. Implications

4.1 Radiation dose

Recent advances in CT equipment has enable high resolution imaging of smaller anatomical structures which has made imaging more feasible for small to medium size vessels but resulting in higher radiation dose delivered to the patients.

Increasing concern over radiation dose have been addressed by vendors through technical improvement of X-ray tubes (34). Other strategies to reduce dose include the awareness of referring doctors especially the capability of 'one stop shop' of PET CT facilities. These attempts to reduce patients' radiation dose according to the 'As Low As Reasonably Achievable' (ALARA) principle(35). The opportunity to reduce dose exposure should be seize during whole body PET/CT study by optimizing the diagnostic role of contrasted CT. Each PET/CT study would lead to radiation exposure ranging from 14 to 32 mSv in adults depending on CT parameters. The PET component typically contributes 8–9 mSv to the overall radiation dose based on a standard 10mCi dose of tracer. Importantly, avoiding duplication of studies also reduces overall radiation exposure.

4.2 Standardized uptake value

Standardized uptake value (SUV) is the most commonly used method for assessing tumor glucose metabolism in clinical studies (36) where it can be measured with relative ease.
The basic concept underlying the SUV is that the activity concentration after injection is correlated with FDG phosphorylation rates where it is approximately proportionate to the activity concentration in the tissue and inversely correlated to the ratio of the injected dose to the body weight (37).The rate of FDG phosphorylation is a measure to tumor glucose utilization which can be influenced by multiple factors including patient size, blood glucose level, extravascular injection and others (38).
In addition to FDG PET/CT study before the start of treatment, semiquantitative analysis of FDG uptake is also needed in assessing early tumour response during the course of treatment (39,40). This can help differentiate between responders and non responders. The controversial effect of contrasted PET/CT study on SUV readings is highlighted in the following section.

4.3 Effects of contrasted PET/CT on semiquantitative uptake value (SUV)

Following the work of Kinahan and his colleagues (39), improved function of PET/CT scanner by CT-attenuation correction eliminated the need for orbiting transmission sources. The quality of joint PET/CT procedure can be improved further by performing contrast enhance study. Thus a separate diagnostic CT scan can be avoided.
Studies from several groups (41,42,43,44) including Berthelsen (45) demonstrated the feasibility of intravenous contrast administration in PET/CT scanning without changing the clinical diagnostic interpretation. These studies demonstrated the effects of intravenous CT contrast in malignancy.
We observed the effect of contrast CT in PET/CT study in 19 patients investigated for infections. In our study, whole body PET/CT scan were conducted using a standard protocol. Two sets of datas where low dose CT and diagnostic contrasted CT were obtained. Both parameters were utilized for attenuation correction of PET images. During image analysis, we compared the percentage difference of CT value in Hounsfield unit (HU) and Standardized Uptake Value (SUV) PET at 4 different anatomical sites including the right lobe of liver, spleen, right heart chamber and urinary bladder. We tabulated our findings and performed statistical analysis.

Result

The percentage differences of HU and SUV were calculated in all 4 different sites for all patients and tabulated in table 2-6.

No	Computed Tomography (CT)						Positron Emission Tomography (PET)					
	NECT mean	NECT Max	CECT mean	CECT Max	HUmean % Δ	HUmax % Δ	NECT mean	NECT Max	CECT mean	CECT Max	SUVmean % Δ	SUVmax % Δ
1	52	110	89.5	127	-72.1	-15.5	2.6	3.7	3	4.2	-15.4	-13.5
2	56	136	85.4	138	-52.5	-1.5	2.8	3.6	2.9	3.8	-3.6	-5.6
3	60.8	110	107.3	164	-76.5	-49.1	2.3	3	2.4	3.1	-4.3	-3.3
4	57.4	123	100.7	165	-75.4	-34.1	2.4	2.9	2.2	2.8	8.3	3.4
5	50.8	93	92.4	186	-81.9	-100.0	3.1	3.6	2.8	3.2	9.7	11.1
6	54.2	124	95.3	136	-75.8	-9.7	1.8	2	1.7	2.2	5.6	-10.0
7	58.8	83	41.5	61	29.4	26.5	1.6	2.1	1.7	2	-6.2	4.8
8	33.5	114	84.3	127	-151.6	-11.4	2.6	3.5	2.4	3.3	7.7	5.7
9	62.1	87	98.9	128	-59.3	-47.1	2.2	2.5	1.9	2.4	13.6	4.0
10	63	108	124.4	193	-97.5	-78.7	2.2	2.8	2.3	2.7	-4.5	3.6
11	48	73	86.6	120	-80.4	-64.4	2.5	2.9	2.1	2.9	16.0	0.0
12	58.8	91	45.3	77	23.0	15.4	2.4	3.1	2.3	3.1	4.2	0.0
13	44.7	74	84.6	122	-89.3	-64.9	2.2	3	2.3	2.6	-4.5	13.3
14	105.9	798	104.1	137	1.7	82.8	1.7	2.2	1.8	2.1	-5.9	4.5
15	66	89	89	68.3	-34.8	23.3	0.9	1.3	1.1	1.3	-22.2	0.0
16	47.9	76	105.5	128	-120.3	-68.4	0.9	1.2	1.2	1.5	-33.3	-25.0
17	44	306	134	107.1	-204.5	65.0	1.1	1.3	1.1	1.4	0.0	-7.7
18	61.4	104	92.5	128	-50.7	-23.1	2.1	3.4	2.1	2.4	0.0	29.4
19	53.7	123	84	141	-56.4	-14.6	1.6	2.4	1.6	2.6	0.0	-8.3
				mean	-69.7	-19.4				mean	-1.8	0.3
				sd	55.1	48.1				sd	12.1	11.4

Table 2. The percentage differences in HU and SUVmax and SUVmean obtained from the right lobe of the liver.

No	Computed Tomogaphy (CT)						Positron Emission Tomography (PET)					
	NECT mean	NECT max	CECT mean	CECT max	HUmean % Δ	HUmax % Δ	NECT mean	NECT max	CECT mean	CECT max	SUVmean % Δ	SUVmax % Δ
1	47	92	118.2	183	-151.5	-98.9	1.5	1.8	2.1	5.9	-40.0	-227.8
2	43	112	121.4	164	-182.3	-46.4	2.1	2.8	2.2	2.7	-4.8	3.6
3	47	81	154.6	188	-228.9	-132.1	1.5	2.1	1.7	2	-13.3	4.8
4	47.2	86	130.5	159	-176.5	-84.9	1.9	2.3	2	2.4	-5.3	-4.3
5	25.8	57	153	175	-493.0	-207.0	2	2.3	1.6	1.9	20.0	17.4
6	39.8	70	156.3	177	-292.7	-152.9	1.4	1.5	1.3	1.5	7.1	0.0
7	78.9	126	42.9	56	45.6	55.6	1.5	1.6	1.5	1.7	0.0	-6.2
8	90	190	142	214	-57.8	-12.6	2.4	3.1	2.3	2.9	4.2	6.5
9	38.4	54	148	177	-285.4	-227.8	1.9	2.5	1.7	2.1	10.5	16.0
10	45.9	72	145.8	175	-217.6	-143.1	2	2.3	1.8	2.1	10.0	8.7
11	24.6	44	118.7	187	-382.5	-325.0	1.7	2	1.6	2	5.9	0.0
12	30.5	60	87.2	123	-185.9	-105.0	1.5	1.9	1.9	1.5	-26.7	21.1
13	39.5	63	133.1	165	-237.0	-161.9	2.6	3.5	2.5	3.2	3.8	8.6
14	129.8	155	132.4	159	-2.0	-2.6	1.3	1.6	1.4	1.7	-7.7	-6.2
15	68	84	85.1	108	-25.1	-28.6	1	2.5	0.8	1	20.0	60.0
16	59.9	78	172.8	197	-188.5	-152.6	0.6	0.9	1.1	1.4	-83.3	-55.6
17	25.4	40	71.2	193	-180.3	-382.5	0.7	1.1	1.9	10.8	-171.4	-881.8
18	69.4	131	95	132	-36.9	-0.8	1.3	1.8	1.4	1.8	-7.7	0.0
19	61.8	102	99.3	123	-60.7	-20.6	1.9	2.4	2.6	2.9	-36.8	-20.8
				mean	-175.7	-117.3				mean	-16.6	-55.6
				sd	134.7	113.2				sd	44.9	208.1

Table 3. The percentage differences in HU and SUVmax and SUVmean obtained from the right heart chamber

No	Computed Tomography (CT)						Positron Emission Tomography (PET)					
	NECT mean	NECT Max	CECT mean	CECT Max	HUmean % Δ	HUmax % Δ	NECT mean	NECT Max	CECT mean	CECT Max	SUVmean % Δ	SUVmax % Δ
1	42.3	75	93.3	130	-120.6	-73.3	2.2	2.7	2.7	3.7	-22.7	-37.0
2	46.4	107	86.4	128	-86.2	-19.6	2.4	2.7	2.5	3.2	-4.2	-18.5
3	48.2	83	102.1	128	-111.8	-54.2	2.3	3.1	2.1	2.7	8.7	12.9
4	44.5	75	87.2	116	-96.0	-54.7	2.4	2.7	2.1	2.9	12.5	-7.4
5	47.8	98	99	126	-107.1	-28.6	2.6	3.1	2.6	2.9	0.0	6.5
6	56.1	110	99.9	122	-78.1	-10.9	1.8	2.2	1.7	2	5.6	9.1
7	61.8	79	45.1	61	27.0	22.8	1	1.3	1.2	1.4	-20.0	-7.7
8	38.7	79	88.3	124	-128.2	-57.0	2.6	3	2.8	3.4	-7.7	-13.3
9	45.8	71	96.3	119	-110.3	-67.6	1.8	2.3	1.8	2.1	0.0	8.7
10	50	86	118.4	161	-136.8	-87.2	2.4	2.7	2.4	2.7	0.0	0.0
11	44.3	71	90.3	129	-103.8	-81.7	2	2.3	1.9	2.6	5.0	-13.0
12	68.1	99	47.9	73	29.7	26.3	1.7	2.2	1.7	2	0.0	9.1
13	52.6	74	97.4	125	-85.2	-68.9	1.9	2.6	1.8	2.4	5.3	7.7
14	92.9	114	95.2	130	-2.5	-14.0	1.5	1.7	1.5	1.8	0.0	-5.9
15	66.7	91	67.1	83	-0.6	8.8	1.2	2.1	1.1	1.4	8.3	33.3
16	51.7	70	106.6	123	-106.2	-75.7	1.5	1.9	1.6	1.9	-6.7	0.0
17	47.2	633	102	123	-116.1	80.6	1.4	2.8	1.5	1.6	-7.1	42.9
18	61.8	110	77.8	125	-25.9	-13.6	2.1	3.2	1.7	2.5	19.0	21.9
19	50	107	72.9	129	-45.8	-20.6	1.4	1.8	1.4	2.3	0.0	-27.8
				mean	-73.9	-31.0				mean	-0.2	1.1
				sd	53.7	44.4				sd	10.1	19.6

Table 4. The percentage differences in HU and SUVmax and SUVmean obtained from the spleen.

No	Computed Tomography (CT)						Positron Emission Tomography (PET)					
	NECT mean	NECT Max	CECT mean	CECT Max	HUmean % Δ	HUmax % Δ	NECT mean	NECT Max	CECT mean	CECT Max	SUVmean % Δ	SUVmax % Δ
1	-1.2	45	16.9	47	1508.3	-4.4	7.9	9.7	7.7	9.8	2.5	-1.0
2	1.8	105	0.8	40	55.6	61.9	6.3	8.1	6.8	8	-7.9	1.2
3	-4	42	6.3	33	257.5	21.4	5.8	6.6	5.9	6.7	-1.7	-1.5
4	-4.7	37	2.3	37	148.9	0.0	4.4	5.2	4.4	5.2	0.0	0.0
5	8.8	51	6.5	26	26.1	49.0	12.6	13.4	12.7	13.4	-0.8	0.0
6	-1	62	-7.5	21	-650.0	66.1	4.2	4.7	4.1	4.6	2.4	2.1
7	-1.3	25	1.8	20	238.5	20.0	3.5	3.8	3.5	3.8	0.0	0.0
8	-4.3	26	-5.7	56	-32.6	-115.4	5.2	6.2	5.3	6	-1.9	3.2
9	-1.4	19	5.4	23	485.7	-21.1	5.5	6.9	5.7	7	-3.6	-1.4
10	4.2	38	-2.2	15	152.4	60.5	5.2	6	4.6	5.3	11.5	11.7
11	-4.6	21	0.5	28	110.9	-33.3	7.3	7.8	7.6	8.9	-4.1	-14.1
12	11.8	43	5.6	32	52.5	25.6	11.3	12.8	11.9	13.1	-5.3	-2.3
13	-2.3	26	32.7	67	1521.7	-157.7	2.8	3.8	2.6	3.1	7.1	18.4
14	41.2	82	38.4	70	6.8	14.6	3.1	3.5	2.9	3.1	6.5	11.4
15	0.5	48	81.3	113	-16160.0	-135.4	1.9	2.6	1.8	2.5	5.3	3.8
16	-2.8	18	34.1	55	1317.9	-205.6	2.1	2.6	2	2.4	4.8	7.7
17	-1.8	16	28.7	58	1694.4	-262.5	2.2	2.5	2.2	3.4	0.0	-36.0
18	8.1	63	8.9	66	-9.9	-4.8	2.1	2.7	2.1	2.7	0.0	0.0
19	64.6	199	14.8	103	77.1	48.2	6.6	8.6	5.7	7.4	13.6	14.0
				mean	-484.1	-30.1				mean	1.5	0.9
				sd	3849.6	97.3				sd	5.6	11.5

Table 5. The percentage differences in HU and SUVmax and SUVmean obtained from the bladder

The average mean and the maximum percentage differences were calculated and tabulated as following:

Site	Computed Tomography		Positron Emission Tomography	
	% Δ HUmean	% Δ HUmax	% Δ SUVmean	% Δ SUVmax
Liver	71.6	19.5	2.1	0.9
Spleen	78.4	32.7	1.4	-1.6
Heart	190.7	129.9	2.3	10.4
Bladder	545	36.2	-0.9	-0.2

Table 6. The average mean and maximum percentage differences in all sites.

Statistical analysis

Nineteen patients were subjected to Non-Contrast Enhanced CT (NECT), Contrast Enhanced CT (CECT), Non-Contrast Enhanced PET (NEPET) and Contrast Enhanced PET (CEPET). For analyses purpose, the clinically-relevant and quantifiable HU-Mean and SUV-Max were treated as unit values of observations for CT (NECT & CECT) and PET (NEPET & CEPET) respectively. Observations between Non-Contrast Enhanced and Contrast Enhanced were not treated as independent of each other because the changes in unit values of Contrast Enhance depended on the initial unit values (Non-Contrast Enhanced) of each patient. Thus, values of CT HU-Max (i.e. NECT and CECT) were treated as paired data. Values of PET SUV-Max (i.e. NEPET and CEPET) were also treated as paired data. All HU-Mean and SUV-Max values were originally continuous data but subsequently ranked as most did not conform to Gaussian distribution. Observations of NECT were compared against CECT and observations of NEPET were compared against CEPET. Medians and Interquartile Ranges (IQR) were used as summary measures for HU-Means, SUV-Maxes and percentage of change in HU-Means and SUV-Maxes. Non-parametric (Wilcoxon Signed Ranks) test were used. Alpha (α) was set at 0.05 thus statistical significance was achieved where p-value was less than 0.05. Summary results are shown in Table 7. Graphic comparison between Non-Contrast Enhanced and Contrast Enhanced observations were also shown in figure 6-9.

Interpretation

At 3 different sites (Liver, Heart & Spleen), we are able to show that the HU-Mean of Non-Contrast Enhanced CT (NECT) differ than that of Contrast Enhanced CT (CECT). This difference is statistically significant, $p<0.05$ (Table 7). In other words, administrations of contrast in CT will yield higher HU-Mean values than plain CT (without contrast). In the liver, the median increase in HU-Mean is 75.4% (+/38.6%). Results of observations in the heart and spleen also showed similar trend. Only in the bladder the values of HU-Mean did not differ statistically (p=0.147).

SITE	IMAGING TEST (Values Used)	HU-Mean/SUV-Max	% Change in HU-Mean/SUV-Max	*p*-value
		Median(IQR)	Median(IQR)	
LIVER	NECT (HU-Mean), n=19	56 (13.4)	75.4 (38.6)	**<0.001***
	CECT (Hu-Mean), n=19	92.4 (19.5)		
	NEPET (SUV-Max), n=19	2.9 (1.3)	0 (12.5)	0.814
	CEPET (SUV-Max), n=19	2.6 (1.0)		
HEART	NECT (HU-Mean), n=19	47 (29.6)	182.3 (179.2)	**<0.001***
	CECT (HU-Mean), n=19	130 (53.0)		
	NEPET (SUV-Max), n=19	2.1 (0.9)	0 (14.9)	0.876
	CEPET (SUV-Max), n=19	2 (2.2)		
SPLEEN	NECT (HU-Mean), n=19	50 (16)	96.0 (86.0)	**0.001***
	CECT (HU-Mean), n=19	93.3 (22.1)		
	NEPET (SUV-Max), n=19	2.6 (0.7)	0 (80.0)	0.721
	CEPET (SUV-Max), n=19	2.4 (1.0)		
BLADDER	NECT (HU-Mean), n=19	-1.2 (10.9)	-110.9 (12854.4)	0.147
	CECT (HU-Mean), n=19	6.3 (27.9)		
	NEPET (SUV-Max), n=19	6 (4.6)	0 (9.1)	0.440
	CEPET (SUV-Max), n=19	5.3 (4.9)		

*statistically significant difference, $p<0.05$ (Wilcoxon Signed Ranks Test)

Table 7. Comparing Non-Contrast Enhanced CT versus Contrast Enhanced CT and Non-Contrast Enhanced PET versus Contrast Enhanced PET at 4 sites in 19 subjects

On the other hand, contrast administrations apparently did not affect the results of PET as evidenced by its SUV-Max values. Non-contrasted PET (NEPET) and Contrasted PET (CEPET) yield similar values of SUV-Max (median % change in SUV-Max=0). They were not statistically different in the liver (p=0.814), heart (p=0.876), spleen (p=0.721) and bladder (p=0.44). Comparing the effects of contrasts on CT and PET can be easily seen by eyeballing. Thus we were able to show that contrast may change the result of CT (by increasing its HU-Mean) but not PET (SUV-Max). How this can affect diagnosis or clinical decision is a question that must be explored further.

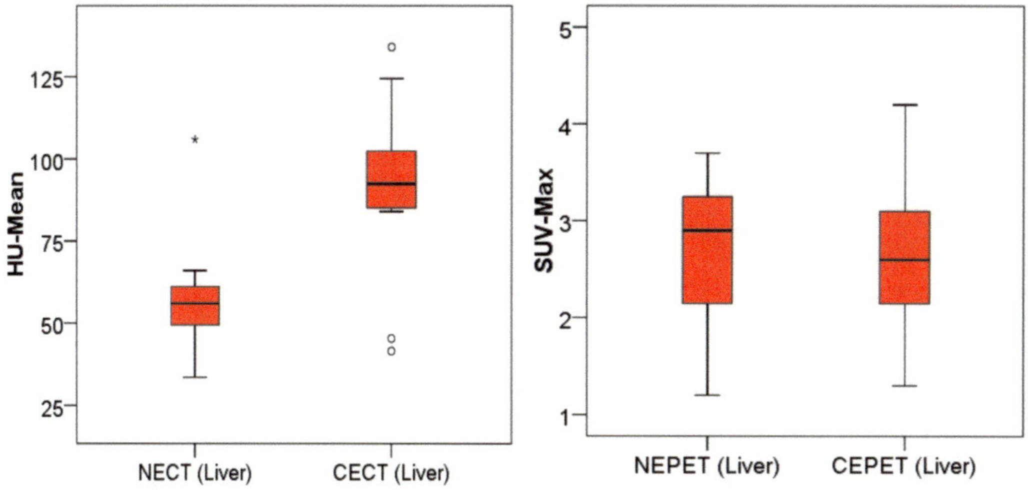

Fig. 6. Side-by-side box & whisker plots of HU-Mean/SUV Max distributions comparing Non-Contrast Enhanced (left within) and Contrast Enhanced (right within) in CT (left) and PET (right) of the Liver.

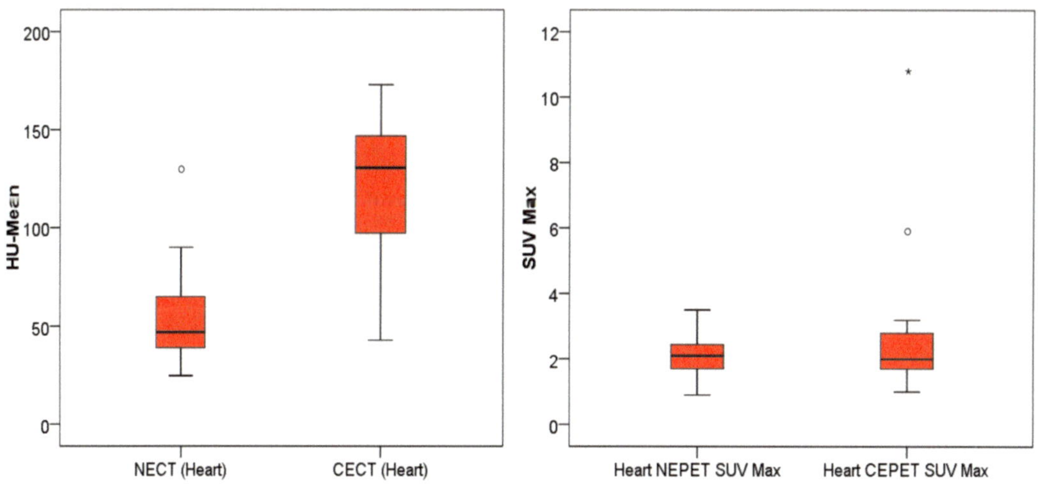

Fig. 7. Side-by-side box & whisker plots of HU-Mean/SUV Max distributions comparing Non-Contrast Enhanced (left within) and Contrast Enhanced (right within) in CT (left) and PET (right) of the Heart.

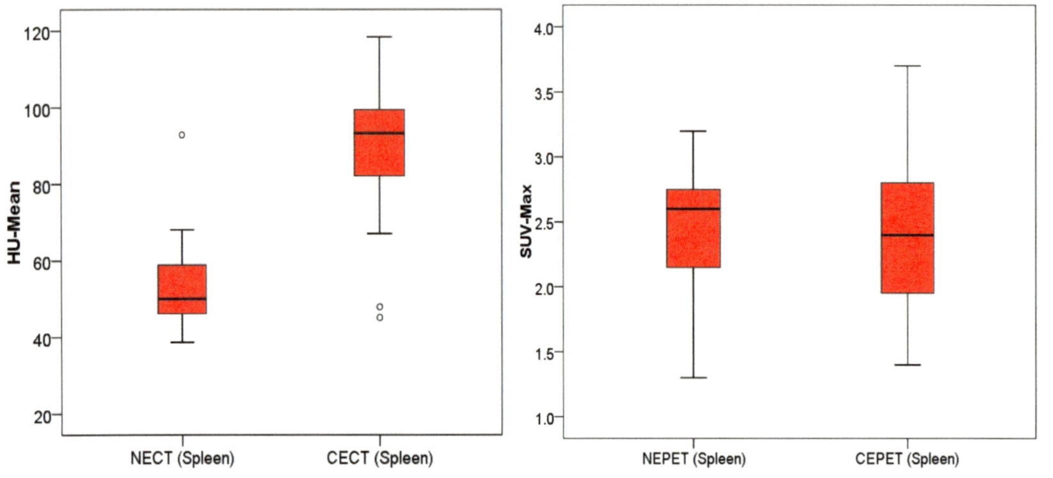

Fig. 8. Side-by-side box & whisker plots of HU-Mean/SUV Max distributions comparing Non-Contrast Enhanced (left within) and Contrast Enhanced (right within) in CT (left) and PET (right) of the Spleen.

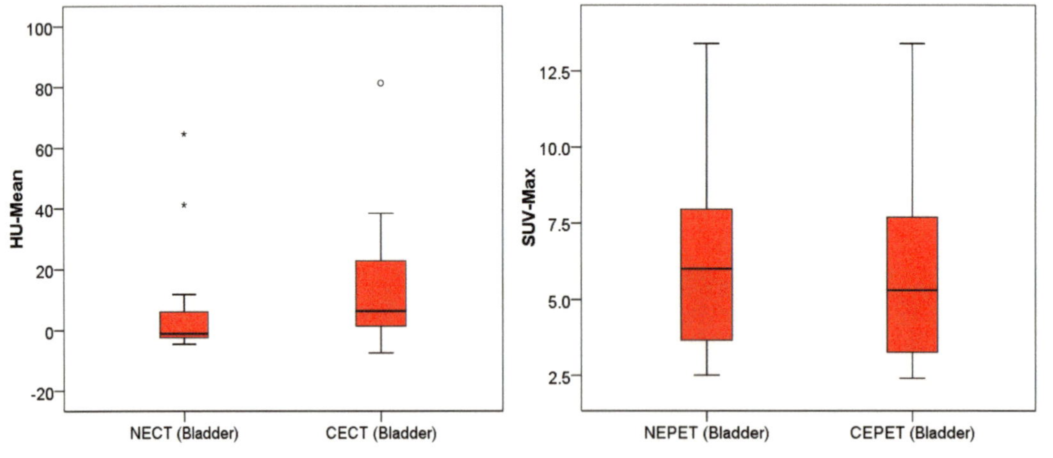

Fig. 9. Side-by-side box & whisker plots of HU-Mean/SUV Max distributions comparing Non-Contrast Enhanced (left within) and Contrast Enhanced (right within) in CT (left) and PET (right) of the Bladder.

5. Conclusions

In conclusion, contrast enhanced PET/CT study provide detail anatomical imaging descriptions obviating the need for a separate CT study and improve lesion characterization including surrounding organs and vascular involvement. Detail CT informations can be optimized and utilized in patient clinical management. Thus the protocol can be recommended as a first line tool in the investigation of oncology patients.

6. References

[1] Rachel Bar-Shalom, Nikolai Yefremov,Ludmila Guralnik, Diana Gaitini, Alex Frenkel, Abraham Kuten, Hernan Altman, Zohar Keidar, Ora Israel. (2003) Clinical Performance of PET/CT in Evaluation of Cancer: Additional Value for Diagnostic Imaging and Patient Management. The Journal of Nuclear Medicine 44(8) 2003

[2] Terence Z. Wong, Erik K. Paulson, Rendon C. Nelson, Edward F. Patz, Jr., R. Edward Coleman (2007) Practical Approach to Diagnostic CT Combined with PET . AJR,188,622–629

[3] Russ A Kuker, Geraldine Mesoloras, Seza A Gulec. Optimization of FDG-PET/CT imaging protocol for evaluation of patients with primary and metastatic liver disease. Semin Surg Oncol, 4, 17.

[4] Ichiya Y, Kuwabara Y, Sasaki M, *et al (1996)* FDG PET in infectious lesions: the detection and assessment of lesion activity. *Ann Nucl Med*.10,185- 191.

[5] Wang Y, Chiu E, Rosenberg J, Gambhir S (2007). Standardized Uptake Value Atlas: Characterization of Physiological 2-Deoxy-2-[18F]fluoro-d -glucose Uptake in Normal Tissues. Mol Imaging Biol, 9, 83-90.

[6] Nakamoto Y, Higashi T, Sakahara H, *et al (2000)*. Delayed 18F-fluoro-2-deoxy-D-glucose positron emission tomography scan for differentiation between malignant and benign lesions in the pancreas. *Cancer*, 89, 2547-2554.

[7] Bisdas S, Baghi M, Smolarz A et al (2007). Quantitative measurements of perfusion and permeability of oropharyngeal and oral cavity cancer, recurrent disease, and associated lymph nodes using first-pass contrast- enhanced computed tomography studies. Invest Radiol, 42,172–17

[8] Sotirios Bisdas , Leon Medov , Mehran Baghi , George N. Konstantinou, Jens Wagenblast, Choon Hua Thng, Thomas J. Vogl, Tong San Koh (2008) A comparison of tumour perfusion assessed by deconvolution-based analysis of dynamic contrast-enhanced CT and MR imaging in patients with squamous cell carcinoma of the upper aerodigestive tract . Eur Radiol,18, 843–85

[9] Khan MA, Coms CS, Brunt EM, et al (2000). Positron emission tomography scanning in the evaluation of hepatocellular carcinoma. J Hepatol, 32, 792-7

[10] Choti MA, Sitzmann JV, Tiburi MF, Sumetchotimetha W, Rangsin R, Schulick RD, Lillemoe KD, Yeo CJ, Cameron JL. (2002) Trends in long-term survival following liver resection for hepatic colorectal metastases. Ann Surg, 235, 759–66.

[11] Elias D, Sideris L, Pocard M, Ouellet JF, Boige V, Lasser P, Pignon JP, Ducreux M (2004). Results of R0 resection for colorectal liver metastases associated with extrahepatic disease. Ann Surg Oncol. 11, 274–80.

[12] Tanaka S, Noguchi N, Ochiai T, Kudo A, Nakamura N, Ito K, Kawamura T, Teramoto K, Arii S. (2007).Outcomes and recurrence of initially resectable HCC meeting Milan criteria: Rationale for partial hepatectomy as first strategy J Am Coll Surg, 204,1–6

[13] Hanazaki K, Kajikawa S, Shimozawa N, Shimada K, Hiraguri M, Koide N, Adachi W, Amano J. (2001). Hepatic resection for large hepatocellular carcinoma. Am J Surg. 2001;181:347–53.

[14] Patrick Veit-Haibach, Valerie Treyer, Klaus Strobel, Jan D. Soyka, Lars Husmann, Niklaus G. Schaefer, Alois Tschopp, Thomas F. Hany (2010) Feasibility of integrated CT-liver perfusion in routine FDG-PET/CT Abdom Imaging (2010) 35:528–536

[15] Nir Lubezky, Ur Metser, Ravit Geva, Richard Nakache, Einat Shmueli, Joseph M. Klausner, Einat Even-Sapir, Arie Figer, Menahem Ben-Haim (2007) J Gastrointest Surg,11,472–478.

[16] Paulsen SR, Huprich JE, Hara AK (2007). CT enterography: Noninvasive evaluation of Crohn's disease and obscure gastrointestinal bleed. Radiol Clin North Am, 45, 303-15.

[17] Fidler J. (2007) MR imaging of the small bowel. Radiol Clin North Am, 45, 317-31.

[18] Kinner S, Lauenstein TC (2007). MR colonography. Radiol Clin North Am 45, 377-87.

[19] Landeras LA, Aslam R, Yee J. (2007) Virtual colonoscopy: Technique and accuracy. Radiol Clin North Am,45,333.

[20] Mulhall BP, Veerappan GR, Jackson JL. (2005) Meta analysis: Computed tomographic colonography. Ann Intern Med ,142, 635-50.

[21] Johnson CD, Chen MH, Toledano AY, Heiken JP, Dachman A, Kuo MD, et al. (2008) Accuracy of CT colonography for detection of large adenomas and cancers. N Engl J Med, 359, 1207-17

[22] YasudaS, Fujii H, NakaharaT, et al. (2001) 18F-FDGPET detection of colonicadenomas. J Nucl Med, 42, 989–92.

[23] Van Kouwen MCA, Nagengast FM, Jansen JBMJ, Oyen WJG, Drenth JPH. (2005)2-(18F)-fluoro-2-deoxy-d-glucose positron emission tomography detects clinical relevant adenomas of the colon: a prospective study. J Clin Oncol 23, 3713–7.

[24] Israel O, Yefremov N, Bar-ShalomR, et al.(2005) PET/CT detection of unexpected gastrointestinal foci of 18F-FDG uptake: incidence, localization patterns, and clinical significance. J Nucl Med, 46, 758–62

[25] Veit-Haibach P, Kuehle CA, Beyer T, et al. (2006) Diagnostic accuracy of colorectal cancer staging with whole-body PET/CT colonography. JAMA, 296, 2590–600.

[26] Low G, Tho LM, Leen E, Wiebe E, Kakumanu S, McDonald AC, et al. (2008). The role of imaging in the pre-operative staging and post-operative follow-up of rectal cancer. Surgeon, 6, 222-31

[27] Shin SS, Jeong YY, Min JJ, Kim HR, Chung TW, Kang HK (2008). Preoperative staging of colorectal cancer: CT vs integrated FDG PET/CT. Abdom Imaging, 33, 270-7.

[28] Gollub MJ, Schwartz LH, Akhurst T. (2007). Update on colorectal cancer imaging. Radiol Clin North Am, 45, 85-118.

[29] Dave-Verma H, Moore S, Singh A, Martins N, Zawacki (2008). J. Computed tomographic enterography and enteroclysis: Pearls and pitfalls. Curr Probl Diagn Radiol , 37, 279-87.

[30] Hashimoto M, Itoh K, Takeda K, Shibata T, Okada T, Okuno Y, et al. (2008). Evaluation of biliary abnormalities with 64-channel multidetector CT. Radiographics, 28,119-34.

[31] Kwon RS, Brugge WR.(2005). New advances in pancreatic imaging. Curr Opin Gastroenterol,2005,21,561-7.

[32] Kwon RS, Scheiman JM. (2006). New advances in pancreatic imaging. Curr Opin Gastroenterol, 22, 512-9.

[33] Robert Dudczak, Tatjana Traub-Weidinger (2010). PET and PET/CT in endocrine tumours. European Journal of Radiology, 73, 481–493

[34] McCollough C.H, Bruesewitz M.R, Kofler J.M. Jr. (2006). CT Dose Reduction and Dose Management Tools: Overview of Available Options. Radiographics, 3, 26.

[35] Valentin, J. (2007) ICRP Publication 103: The 2007 Recommendations of the International Commission on Radiological Protection. Elsevier.

[36] Thie J. (2004). Understanding the standardized uptake value, its methods, and implications for usage. J Nucl Med, 45, 1431–1434.

[37] Martin Allen-Auerbach, Wolfgang A.Weber (2009). Measuring Response with FDG-PET: Methodological Aspects . The Oncologist, 14, 369 –377.

[38] MacManus MP, Hicks RJ, Matthews JP et al. (2003). Positron emission tomography is superior to computed tomography scanning for response-assessment after radical radiotherapy or chemoradiotherapy in patients with non-small- cell lung cancer. J Clin Oncol, 21, 1285–1292.

[39] Hawkins DS, Schuetze SM, Butrynski JE et al. (2005). [18F]-Fluorodeoxyglucose positron emission tomography predicts outcome for Ewing sarcoma family of tumors. J Clin Oncol, 23, 8828 – 8834.

[40] P. E. Kinahan, D. W. Townsend, T. Beyer, and D. Sashin, Kinahan PE,Townsend DW, Beyer T, Sashin D. (1998). Attenuation correction for a combined 3D PET/CT scanner Med Phys,25,2046 –2053.

[41] Dizendorf E, Hany TF, Buck A, von Schulthess GK, and Burger C. (2003). Cause and magnitude of the error induced by oral CT contrast agent in CT-based attenuation correction of PET emission studies. J Nucl Med, 44, 732-738.

[42] Dizendorf EV, Treyer V, Von Schulthess GK,Hany TF. (2002). Application of oral contrast media in coregistered positron emission tomography CT. AJR Am J Roentgenol, 179, 477-481

[43] Antoch G, Kuehl H, Kanja J, Lauenstein TC, Schneemann H, Hauth E, et al. (2004) Dual-modality PET/CT scanning with negative oral contrast agent to avoid artifacts: introduction and evaluation. Radiology,230, 879-885.

[44] Antoch G, Saoudi N, Kuehl H, Dahmen G, Mueller SP, Beyer T, et al. (2004). Accuracy of whole-body dual-modality fluorine-18-2-fluoro-2-deoxy-D-glucose positron emission tomography and computed tomography (FDG-PET/CT) for tumor staging in solid tumors: comparison with CT and PET. J Clin Oncol, 22, 4357-4368.

[45] Berthelsen AK, Holm S, Loft A, Klausen TL, Andersen F, Hoigaard L (2005) PET/CT with intravenous contrast can be used for PET attenuation correction in cancer patients. Eur J Nucl Med Mol Imaging. 10, 32:1167-75.

19

Cumulative Radiation Effective Dose

Nelofur Hayat, Eshrak Hassanein and Mohamed Shoukry
Saad Specialist Hospital
Saudi Arabia

1. Introduction

The CT scanners on the market offer a multitude of procedure protocols that enable many clinical questions to be answered quickly. CT scanners can be used to image all parts of the body, some common uses in our hospital include; acute inflammatory bowel diseases; acute appendicitis, trauma including head, spine and skeletal trauma, renal diseases including congenital, inflammatory and neoplastic, temporal bone diseases, neck swelling, diagnosing and staging cancer (using PETCT when appropriate) and planning radiotherapy treatment (using PETCT when appropriate).

Whatever the reason for a procedure a radiation dose is associated with the exam and this can range from a relatively small to a relatively large amount depending on the clinical requirements of the diagnostic test.

Since x-rays have the potential to damage cells in the body and there is no "safe" dose of radiation, the body's exposure to radiation should be kept to a minimum, a challenging task for CT imaging.

The radiation effective dose is a calculated quantity that is intended to give an estimate of the relative biological detriment resulting from a radiation exposure and is measured in units called Sieverts (Sv).

As the x-ray tube rotates around the patient it takes hundreds of x-ray pictures of a thin section of the body. In one rotation the "thin section" is determined by the number of detector rows and their collimation. Many rotations around the patient result in large body volumes being imaged. The images obtained from each section can be reconstructed to any slice width down to the width of the collimation of a single detector.

Technological advances in CT scanners have seen increases in the number of slices and detector rows leading to wider coverage of the patient anatomy per rotation of the x-ray tube around the patient. Helical scanners have led to even greater coverage of the patient anatomy in faster examinations.

However, CT procedures are inherently high radiation effective dose procedures, although the actual scanning takes from a few seconds to a few minutes, depending on the examination and type of scanner, it's easy to lose track of the actual radiation exposure to the patient.

The images obtained from CT provide much more diagnostic information than conventional radiographs or fluoroscopy but the radiation effective doses are much higher than for other x-ray exams.

Contrast agents enable multiple phases to be evaluated during procedures, the difference between pre and post contrast images can give the radiologist valuable information; a single procedure may therefore result in a multiple of scans over the same body region.
In itself, the radiation effective dose from a CT procedure may not differ greatly from one machine to another, nor will it be too large but used again and again on the same individual and multiple scans within those procedures will increase the cumulative effective dose to the patient and therefore increase the risk of chance effects, which have no threshold dose, called stochastic effects such as cancer induction. If left unmonitored, these risks will remain unknown.
The physician who requests a CT procedure for a patient must ensure that the benefits provided by the information obtained outweigh the risks associated with the radiation effective dose and that if the information required can be obtained by an alternative modality that does not involve ionising radiation such as MRI or ultrasound it should be used. In order to do this the physician needs to know the estimated effective dose of the procedure and must also be aware of other modalities that perform the required tests.
Moreover, since radiation dose is cumulative it is not enough for the physician to consider a radiation dose for a procedure in isolation for a patient as it may not be the only dose that the patient has received and it may not be the only dose that the patient is likely to receive in the future. A clear indication of radiation exposure history of the patient is needed at the point of request for a CT procedure, and the possibility of further CT procedures based on current practice for the diagnosis or follow up should be considered. Used responsibly, CT procedures should not cause unnecessary additional radiation risks to the individual.
The benefits in CT imaging are not in question here, however, rapid growth in the use of CT and PETCT in organizations where radiation safety programs focused on dose reduction are not in place, setup or maintained should be a cause for concern for unaware patients and physicians.
The cumulative dose received by the patient can be alarmingly high and it is likely that it will increase in the future as the utilization of CT further increases. A consequence of this may be a significant increased incidence of radiation related cancer in the future.
The International Commission on Radiation Protection, (ICRP, 1991) specifies that the nominal risk coefficient for induction of fatal cancer is 5% per Sv and total detriment, induction of all cancers and genetic effects is 7.3% per Sv when risk factors are averaged over the whole population. For doses over 100mSv there is little doubt over the potential for increased cancer risks (Wall et al, 2006).
This cumulative study of radiation effective dose reveals the current practice patterns and areas of improvement in a tertiary private hospital in Saudi Arabia. It has required good electronic records to piece together exposure history of its patients. Only CT and the CT part of PETCT have been included in the data so the results of the cumulative doses are conservative and do not include contributions from nuclear medicine studies, general radiographic, dental, fluoroscopic or interventional fluoroscopic procedures.

2. Materials and methods

The Siemens Definition 64 slice CT scanner is the main CT scanner used in the Radiology Department. The scanner provides a large number of preset protocols, the most commonly used of the Head, Chest/Thorax and Abdomen/Pelvis protocols along with the European Reference Levels for CT (Bongartz et al. 2004) are shown in Table 1. The European reference levels are not intended to be applied to individual exposures of individual patients but are aimed as guidance for standard procedures for groups of standard sized patients and are intended to assist in the optimization of protection by helping to avoid unnecessarily high doses to the patient.

Name	kV	mAs	mA	Rotation Time s	(Acquisition) Detectors x collimation n x mm	Pitch	CTDIvol mGy	Scanned Length cm	Dose Length Product (DLP) mGycm	Effect-ive Dose (E) mSv
Head 1	120	450	248	1	(19.2mm) 64 x 0.6	0.55	60.65	13	790	2.2
Head 2	120	450	248	1	(28.8mm) 24 x 1.2	0.55	55.69	12	670	1.9
European Reference Levels for Adult CT - Head							60	17.5	1050	-
Chest /Thorax 1	120	110	264	0.5	(19.2mm) 64 x 0.6	1.2	7.93	30	240	5.3
Chest /Thorax 2	120	170	408	0.5	(28.8mm) 24 x 1.2	1.2	11.24	27	305	6.7
European Reference Levels for Adult CT - Chest							30	21.7	650	-
Abdomen/ Pelvis1	120	210	378	0.5	(19.2mm) 64 x 0.6	0.9	15.14	27	410	8.9
Abdomen/ Pelvis 2	120	190	342	0.5	(28.8mm) 24 x 1.2	0.9	12.56	48	605	11
European Reference Levels for Adult CT - Abdomen							35	22.3	780	-

Table 1. Scanning protocols and effective dose (E) of typical Adult protocols for the Siemens Definition 64 slice CT Scanner and European guidance reference levels for Adult CT.

The scan parameters kV, mAs, mA, rotation time, acquisition, detectors and collimation and pitch used for an individual scan result in the associated volume computed tomography dose index (CTDIvol) and an associated dose length product (DLP) of the scan as shown in table 1.

The CTDIvol is a quantity that tells the operator how much radiation dose will be absorbed in a single rotation according to the specific setup. It is a measure of the average dose delivered to the scan volume and its numeric value depends only on the spatial distribution of individual rotations and is unrelated to the total scan length determined by the total number of successive rotations.

For helical scanners, the spatial distribution of individual rotations is dependent on the pitch; this is the ratio of the table movement per tube rotation to the beam width (number of detectors x collimated slice). Pitch conveys the degree of overlap of the radiation beam, a value of 1 indicates contiguous slices, less than 1 indicates overlap (hence a larger CTDIvol) and greater than 1 indicates a gap between slices (hence a lower CTDIvol). The pitch can be determined from the mAs, mA and rotation time of the scan and is equal to the product of the mA and rotation time divided by the effective mAs.

The dose length product, DLP, is a product of the CTDIvol dose and the scanned length, it is independent of what is actually being scanned; the reported DLP is the same whether a newborn or adult is being exposed if the scan length and other scan parameters are the same.

The scanned length shown in table 1. for the European reference level has been calculated from the DLP and CTDIvol; the scanned length in cm is equal to the DLP (mGy.cm) divided by the CTDIvol (mGy).

The adult protocols shown in table 1 represent a single scan of the indicated body region, the effective dose derived from the scanning parameters has been calculated using the ImPACT CT patient dosimetry calculator (version 1.0.2 12/11/2009) and associated NRPB-SR250 Normalised Organ Doses for X-ray Computed Tomography Calculated using Monte Carlo Techniques software (Jones & Shrimpton, 1993).
Variations in the protocols shown in table 1 are also used which can result in different doses, the benefit of the CTDIvol on the display is in allowing the operator to compare the radiation doses from different imaging protocols.
Children are particularly sensitive to radiation and have an increased susceptibility due to their developing bodies and smaller size; the risk of cancer induction is greater in children due to their longer potential life span. (Mettler et al., 2000 & Brody et al., 2007 & Stecker et al., 2009).
To estimate pediatric effective doses, results from the ImPACT CT patient dosimetry software can be multiplied by the age appropriate factors shown in table 2. The values shown in table 2 give a range of normalized effective doses at each age, relative to the adult dose (Khursheed et al. 2002). The minimum values were used in this study as representative for the Siemens Definition scanner.

	Newborn 0y	1 y	5 y	10 y	15 y	Adult
Head and Neck	2.3 - 2.6	2.2	1.6 - 1.7	1.2 - 1.3	1.1	1.0
Chest	1.4 - 2.2	1.3 - 1.9	1.2 - 1.6	1.1 - 1.4	1.0 - 1.1	1.0
Abdomen and Pelvis	1.4 - 2.4	1.3 - 2.0	1.2 - 1.6	1.2 - 1.5	1.0 - 1.1	1.0

Table 2. Typical normalized effective doses to pediatric patients relative to adults (ImPACT CT Patient Dosimetry software)

Techniques used in pediatric CT imaging may not necessarily be tailored to children's smaller bodies and adult protocols are used, resulting in radiation effective doses much greater than necessary. To illustrate the consequence of not adjusting parameters to pediatric sizes table 3 shows the effective doses estimated for the head protocols shown in table 1 if used unadjusted.

Name	kV	mAs	mA	Rotation Time s	(Acquisition) Detectors x collimation n x mm	Pitch	CTDIvol mGy	Scanned Length cm	Dose Length Product (DLP) mGycm	Effect-ive Dose (E) mSv
Head 1 Adult	120	450	248	1	(19.2mm) 64 x 0.6	0.55	60.65	13	790	2.2
Head 1 10 yr-old	120	450	248	1	(19.2mm) 64 x 0.6	0.55	60.65	13	790	3.5
Head 1 5 yr-old	120	450	248	1	(19.2mm) 64 x 0.6	0.55	60.65	13	790	4.8
Head 1 Newborn	120	450	248	1	(19.2mm) 64 x 0.6	0.55	60.65	13	790	5.1

Table 3. Estimate of effective dose for adult head protocols unadjusted for pediatric patients

Using techniques appropriate for pediatric CT imaging will result in much lower effective doses (Fujii et al., 2007) without detriment to the image quality required for the diagnostic image. Simply adjusting the protocol for kV, mAs and mA can significantly reduce the effective dose to the pediatric patient. A useful reference for assessing local optimization techniques in pediatric CT are found in the proposed diagnostic reference levels for pediatric patients for the head and chest (ICRP, 2007 and Shrimpton et al, 2005), as shown in table 4.

Examination	CTDIw (mGy)	CTDIvol (mGy)	Scanned Length (cm)	Dose Length Product, DLP (mGy.cm)
Head 0-1 yr old	23	12	17	204
Head 5 yr old	20	13	17.5	228
Head 10 yr old	26	17	21.6	368
Chest 0-1 yr old	28	28	9.6	270
Chest 5 yr old	43	43	10.8	465
Chest 10 yr old	52	51	12.1	619

Table 4. Proposed Diagnostic Reference levels for pediatrics

The weighted computed tomography dose index, CTDIw is a measure of the average dose delivered to the scan volume in polymethylmethacrylate, PMMA cylinders of 16cm diameter, representing adult head, pediatric head and pediatric body and 32cm diameter, representing adult body. CTDIw is used to account for the variation in the CTDI across the field of view which is higher at the surface of a body relative to the centre, CTDIw is equal to 1/3 CTDIcentre + 2/3 CTDIperiphery.

In pediatric patients, due to their smaller size, the difference between the dose at the surface and at the centre is not as large as it is in adults.

The CTDIvol is equal to the CTDIw divided by the pitch. Both quantities are equivalent if the pitch has a value of 1 and CTDIvol is less than CTDIw if the pitch has a value greater than 1. Both quantities indicate the average dose within the scan volume for a particular protocol but the displayed CTDIw does not account for the pitch.

Multiple scans involving contrast and phases such as arterial, venous and delayed are also used in many protocols, typically doubling, tripling and quadrupling the effective dose of the procedure. So although the effective dose for a single scan is low, care must be taken to ensure that the numbers of scans in a procedure are known and the consequence on the effective dose is understood.

This study was designed to provide a snapshot of the CT imaging procedures being undertaken on pediatric patients in the Radiology Department. Stage 1 involved data collection from the Hospital Radiology Information System (RIS). Cohort selection was an all inclusive group of pediatric patients (newborn to 18 years old) undergoing CT procedures in October 2010. Figure 1 shows a breakdown of the frequency of daily procedures performed on 53 patients, male pediatrics n=31, female pediatrics n=22.

A total of 55 procedures on the 53 patients were performed in the one month period of October 2010. Details about the procedures were recorded in an excel spreadsheet. To assess the number of cumulative CT procedures performed on the patients and the interval period between procedures, data collection expanded to include all previous CT procedures and all post October 2010 procedures performed up to March 2011 in the identified patients. Figure 2 shows the number of procedures and scans involved in those procedures on the patients.

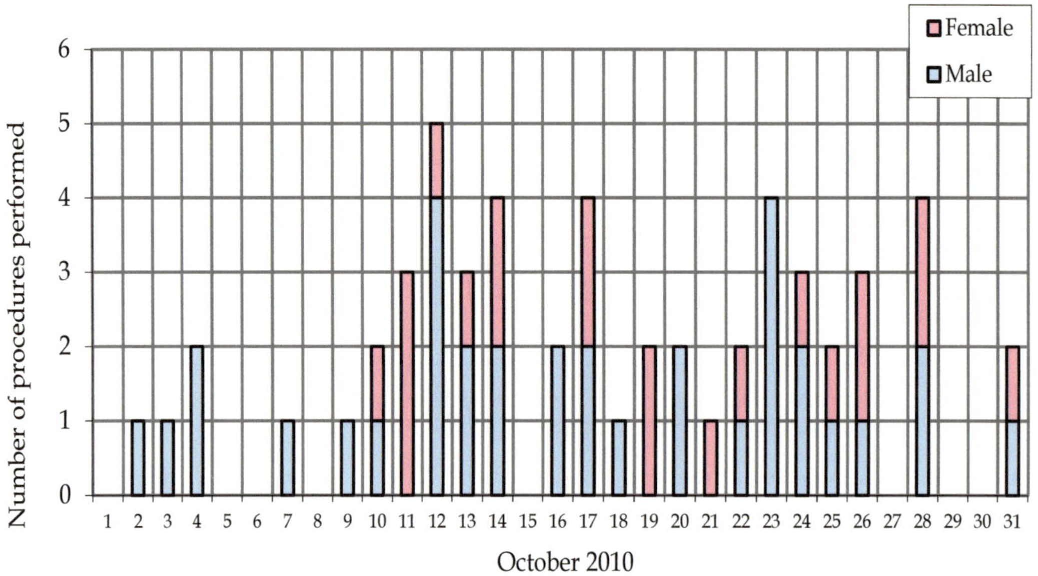

Fig. 1. Number of Procedures performed in October 2010.

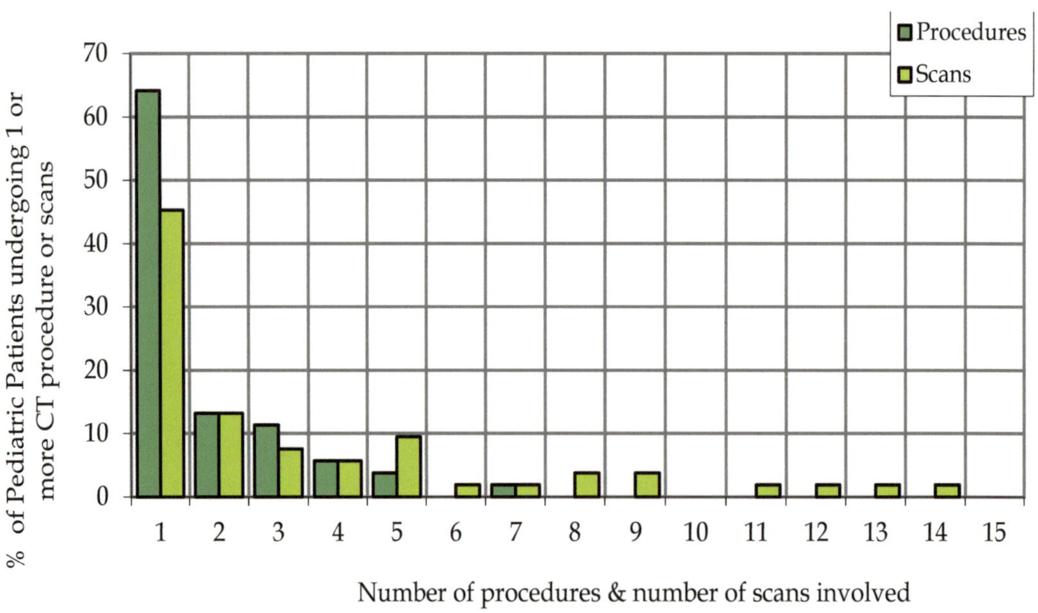

Fig. 2. Number of procedures & scans performed on pediatric patients.

A total of 95 procedures involving 184 scans were performed on the 53 pediatric patients ranging a 7 year period from October 2004 to March 2011.
For pediatric patients undergoing CT procedures consisting of one or more scans, 64% (n=34) underwent a single procedure, 24.5% (n=13) underwent 2-3 procedures and the remaining 11.5% (n=6) underwent between 4-7 procedures. Multiple procedures were performed on 36% (n=19) of the pediatric patients, for these patients the mean number of procedures was 3.2 ± 1.9 procedures/ patient.
Whilst only 45% (n=24) underwent a single scan, 21% (n=11) underwent 2-3 scans and the remaining 34% (n=18) underwent between 4-14 scans. Multiple scans were performed on 55% (n=29) of the pediatric patients, for these patients the mean number of scans per patient was 5.5 ± 4.2 scans/ patient.
Only 32.6% (n=24) procedures involved 1 scan per procedure, for the remaining 67.4% (n=64) procedures the mean number of scans per procedure was 3.5 ± 2.8 scans/ procedure
For patients undergoing multiple procedures, 69% (n=29) of the multiple procedures were performed within 6 months of a previous procedure. The interval period between multiple procedures is shown in figure 3.

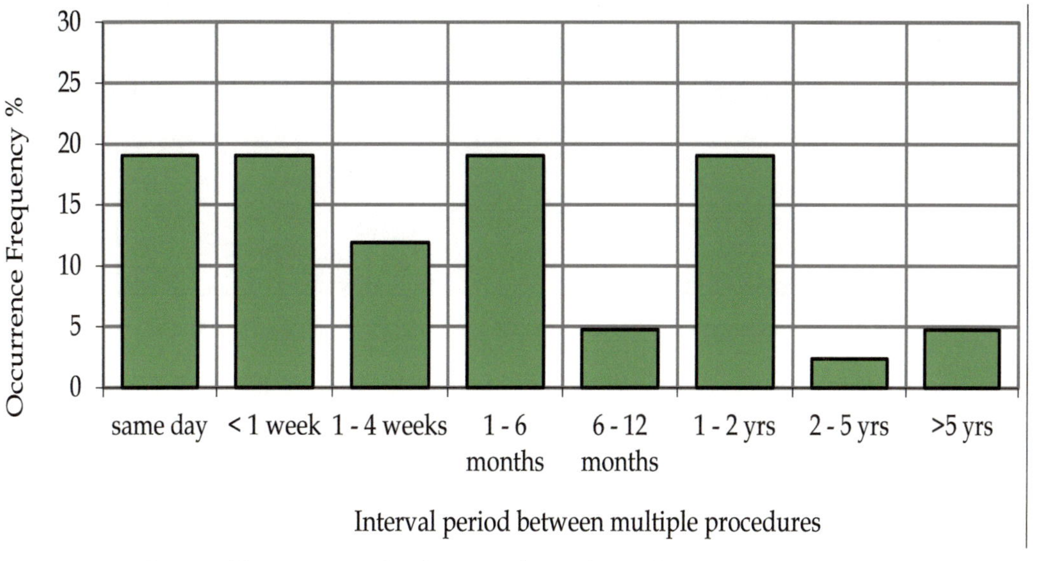

Fig. 3. Interval period between multiple procedures for pediatric patients.

In order to assess the effective dose of the scan, specific technical information of the parameters and techniques used in the actual scans was collected from the patient protocol and DICOM information from images obtained by the procedure.
The patient protocol is generated at the end of the exam for a patient and summarizes each exposure, giving the number of scans and phases along with technical parameters of the procedure. It is department policy to archive the patient protocol with the CT images as it provides much of the information required for assessing the effective dose of the procedure.
Data contained in the patient protocol is shown in figure 4 which was generated by the Definition 64-slice CT scanner during the performance of a routine abdomen scan with contrast on a 17 year old male patient. All the data required to calculate effective doses of the procedures was collected.

The volume computed tomography dose index (CTDIvol) for the individual scan at the parameters used and the associated dose length product (DLP) of the scan are shown in the patient protocol as well as the total DLP and total mAs of the procedure.
The total DLP for the whole procedure is the sum of the individual DLP's for each scan. The DLP as a dose metric has limited value but is a useful indicator of relative technique.

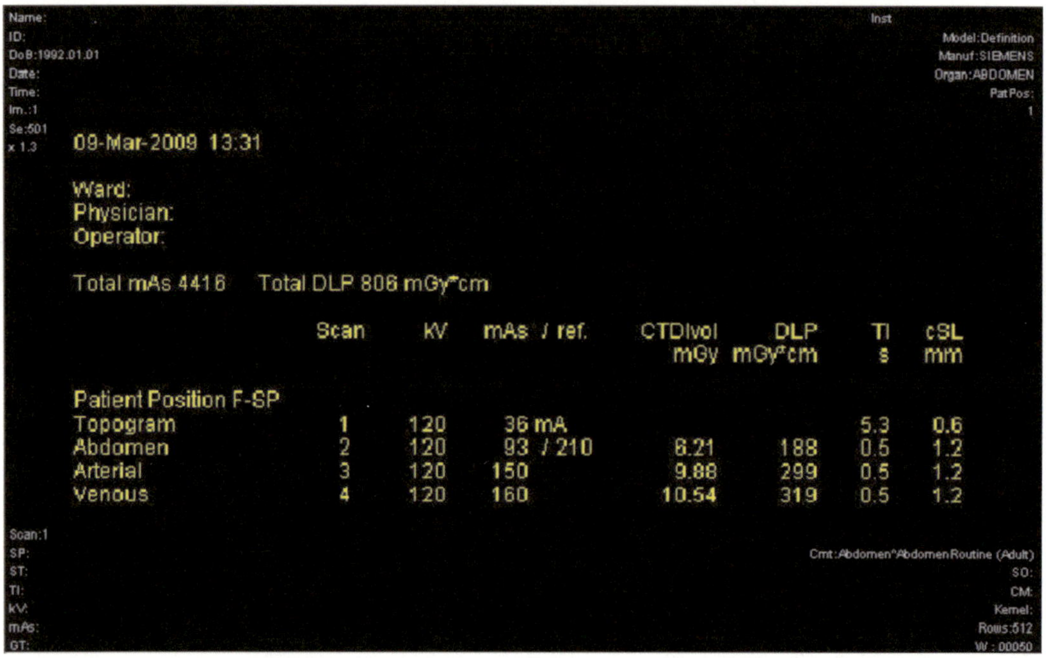
Name:
ID:
DoB:1992.01.01
Date:
Time:
Im.:1
Se:501
x 1.3

Inst
Model:Definition
Manuf:SIEMENS
Organ:ABDOMEN
PatPos:
1

09-Mar-2009 13:31

Ward:
Physician:
Operator:

Total mAs 4416 Total DLP 806 mGy*cm

	Scan	KV	mAs / ref.	CTDIvol mGy	DLP mGy*cm	TI s	cSL mm
Patient Position F-SP							
Topogram	1	120	36 mA			5.3	0.6
Abdomen	2	120	93 / 210	6.21	188	0.5	1.2
Arterial	3	120	150	9.88	299	0.5	1.2
Venous	4	120	160	10.54	319	0.5	1.2

Scan:1
SP:
ST:
TI:
kV:
mAs:
GT:

Cmt:Abdomen^AbdomenRoutine (Adult)
SO:
CM:
Kernel:
Rows:512
W : 00050

Fig. 4. Patient protocol generated by the Siemens Definition 64 slice CT scanner

Some relevant information not provided in the patient protocol is the body region actually covered, often an abdomen scan covers both abdomen and pelvis, the scanned volume was therefore determined from the first and last image of each scan.
The pitch is also not provided in the patient protocol but can be determined from the mAs, mA and rotation time of the scan and is equal to the product of the mA and rotation time divided by the effective mAs.
Depending on the level of information available two methods for assessment of effective dose were applied in this study.
Method 1 was used where all the information was available in the data and the patient protocol had been archived, for the earlier procedures before archiving of the patient protocol was adopted the patient protocol had not been stored, for these procedures the reference effective dose for the typical procedure was used.
Method 1 uses values of kV, mAs, mA, rotation time, collimation, pitch and scanned body region from the patient protocol and CT images on the MiPACS MedView/CS (version MiPACS MedView 1.6.0_SP1 and the 1.7.0 update on 11/12/2010) along with measurements of CT dose index in air, CTDIair and weighted, CTDIw, made using a 10cm ionisation chamber during quality assurance tests on the CT scanner.
CTDIair is the average dose in air in the central region of a scan volume specific for the type of scanner and scanning parameters used.

All required fields were input into the ImPACT patient dosimetry software (version 1.0.2 12/11/2009) to calculate the effective dose of the scan. The effective dose of each scan in a procedure was summed to provide the effective dose of the procedure.
Method 2 was used if the CT scanner used for the procedure was not the Definition. This method for estimating effective dose involved calculating the product of the DLP and a conversion factor. Table 5 shows the conversion factors used in this study (k, mSv.mGy-1.cm-1) (ICRP, 2007 & Bongartz, et al. 2004, Shrimpton et al. 2006). The table gives the normalized effective dose per dose length product for adults (standard physique) and pediatric patients of various ages for various body regions. Although full range of pediatric sizes is not represented by the data, the method offers an approximation of the effective dose and has value due to its ease of use, providing a useful indicator of dose levels.

k mSv.mGy-1.cm-1	0-year-old	1-year-old	5-year-old	10-year-old	Adult
Head and Neck	0.013	0.0085	0.0057	0.0042	0.0031
Head	0.011	0.0067	0.004	0.0032	0.0021
Neck	0.017	0.012	0.011	0.0079	0.0059
Chest	0.039	0.026	0.018	0.013	0.014
Abdomen and Pelvis	0.049	0.030	0.020	0.015	0.015
Trunk	0.044	0.028	0.019	0.014	0.015

Table 5. Normalized effective dose per dose length product for adults (standard physique) and pediatric patients of various ages for various body regions.

For the routine abdomen protocol shown in figure 4 the two methods gave the following effective doses;

Method 1:

Information from routine quality assurance of the CT scanner and data collected yielded the information and result of the effective dose for the procedure shown in table 6. The dosimetry phantom range was estimated from the coverage of the organs as seen in the images. In this case the same coverage for all three phases was observed. However because the tube current (mA) used for each phase was varied, a different effective dose resulted, the non contrast abdomen scan resulted in the lowest effective dose due to the use of CAREdose. CAREdose is a feature of the Siemens scanners that provides current (mA) modulation over the scanned region according to body size. The effect on the effective dose is significant and can be achieved without loss of image quality for small and average sized patients. CAREdose is recommended for use with all pediatric scans.

Scan	Start Loca-tion	End Loca-tion	Phantom Range	mA	Effective mAs	pitch	kV	Rotation time s	Slice collima-tion mm	Effective dose (mSv)	
Abdomen	390.5	650.5	27 - 47	168	93	0.9	120	0.5	1.2	2.8	12.1
Arterial	390.5	650.5	27 - 47	270	150	0.9	120	0.5	1.2	4.5	
Venous	390.5	650.5	27 - 47	288	160	0.9	120	0.5	1.2	4.8	

Table 6. Method 1 Data obtained from images (MiPACS MedView) and DICOM information input into the ImPACT CT dosimetry calculator yielding results for effective dose

Method 2:

Using the formula DLP mGy.cm x k mSv.mGy-1.cm-1 and values of DLP from the patient protocol and values of k from table 5 the results shown in table 7 were obtained;

Scan	DLP mGy.cm	k mSv.mGy-1.cm-1	Effective dose (mSv)	
Abdomen	188	0.015	2.8	12.1
Arterial	299	0.015	4.5	
Venous	319	0.015	4.8	

Table 7. Method 2 calculation of effective dose

Although in this case the two methods gave the same result, in general it was found that using conversion factors resulted in effective dose estimates that ranged 40% lower to 60% higher than those calculated using method 1.

3. Pediatric results

53 pediatric patients were identified as undergoing a CT procedure in October 2010; the age range of the patients in October 2010 and at their first procedure is shown in figure 5. The mean age in October 2010 was 8.6 ± 6.2 years. 58.5% (n=31) of the pediatric patients were male with a mean age of 8.2 ± 5.8 years and 41.5% (n=22) were female with a mean age of 9.3 ± 6.7 years.

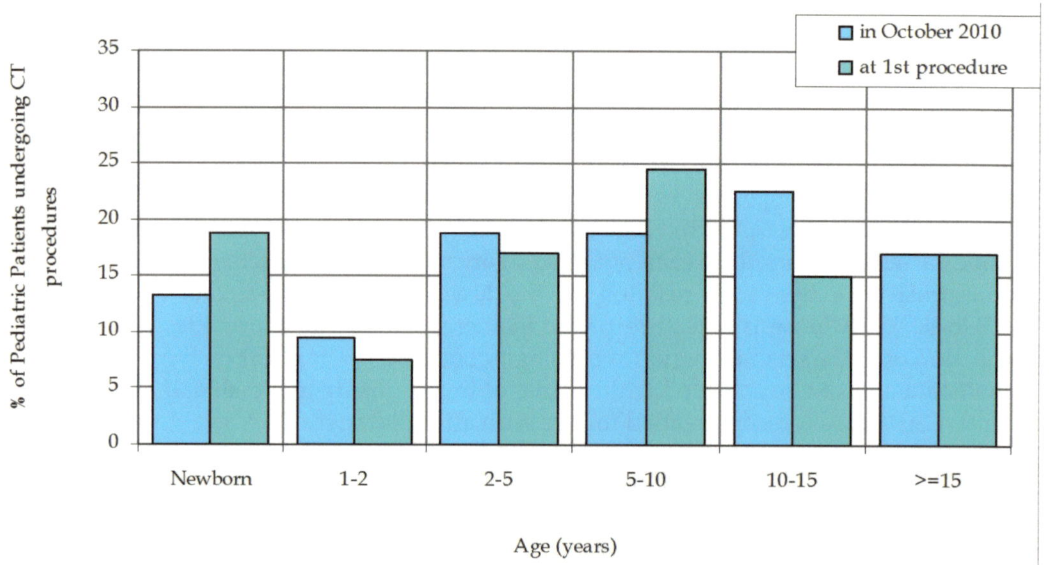

Fig. 5. Age Distribution of Pediatric Patients in October 2010 and at 1st procedure.

A total of 95 procedures were performed on these pediatric patients, 61% (58 procedures) on the male patients and 39% (37 procedures) on the female patients.
A total of 184 scans resulted from these procedures, 60% (110 scans) were performed on the male patients and 40% (74 scans) were performed on the female patients.

A breakdown of the scans performed according to gender and body region exposed is shown in figure 6.

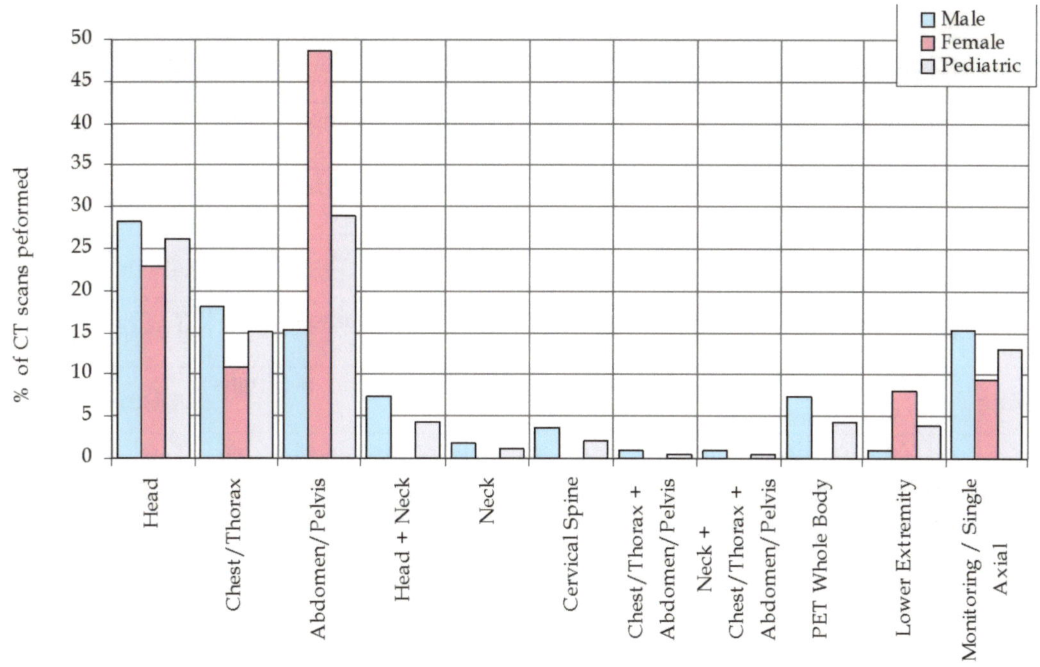

Fig. 6. Pediatric patients undergoing scans according to body region and gender

The most commonly exposed body regions and scans undertaken by the patients are shown in table 8.

Body Region	Parameter	Male	Female	All pediatrics
Head	Scans	28% (n=31 scans)	23% (n=17 scans)	26% (n=48 scans)
	Patients involved	64.5% (n=20)	54.5% (n=12)	60% (n=32)
Chest/Thorax	Scans	18% (n=20 scans)	11% (n=8 scans)	15% (n=28 scans)
	Patients involved	19% (n=6)	14% (n=3)	29% (n=9)
Abdomen/Pelvis	Scans	16% (n=17 scans)	49% (n=36 scans)	29% (n=53 scans)
	Patients involved	25% (n=8)	41% (n=9)	32% (n=17)

Table 8. Exposed body regions and scans undertaken by pediatric patients

For female pediatrics, abdomen/pelvis scans were the most performed, involving 41% (n=9) of the female patients. For male pediatrics, head scans were the most performed, involving 28% (n=31) of the male patients.

The patients could be grouped according to their number of procedures, scans and body regions exposed. Table 9 shows the group specification and the number of patients involved.

Group	Specification	Patients Involved
Group 1	Single Procedure involving a Single Scan on a Single Body Region	45.3% (n=24)
Group 2	Multiple Procedures involving a Single Scan/procedure on a Single Body Region	3.8% (n=2)
Group 3	Multiple Procedures involving a Single Scan/procedure on Multiple Body Regions	9.4% (n=5)
Group 4	Single Procedure involving Multiple Scans on a Single Body Region	18.9% (n=10)
Group 5	Multiple Procedures involving Multiple Scans on a Single Body Region	9.4% (n=5)
Group 6	Multiple Procedures involving Multiple Scans on Multiple Body Regions	13.2% (n=7)

Table 9. Patient exposure groups

To use the number of procedures or the number of scans as a cumulative radiation dose indicator would imply that Group 1 patients have the lowest cumulative effective doses and group 6 patients have the highest. However, the body region affects this.

For the purpose of this study cumulative effective dose levels for individuals have been specified according to the values shown in table 10.

Cumulative effective dose Level	Very Low	Low	Moderate	High	Very High
Effective dose range mSv	< 5	> 5 - 10	> 10 - 20	> 20 - 50	> 50 - 100

Table 10. Cumulative effective dose level categories

Figure 7 shows the cumulative effective dose to pediatric patients according to age and gender.

The distribution of cumulative effective dose varies considerably across all age groups, with a tendency of increasing for the over 10 year olds. Since the cumulative effective dose is dependent on the type of procedures carried out, the older age groups are more likely to have multiple phases and are likely being imaged as small adults, with protocols not being adjusted for size and weight unless the scanner specifies the appropriate child protocol. Childhood diseases and their detection and diagnosis using CT in pediatrics needs careful consideration to ensure that cumulative effective doses are minimized.

Figure 8 shows the cumulative effective doses received by pediatric patients according to the dose levels assigned.

The majority of pediatric patients, 64% (n=34) receive very low to moderate levels of cumulative dose. However, 28% (n=15) received high levels and 7.5% (n=4) received very high levels.

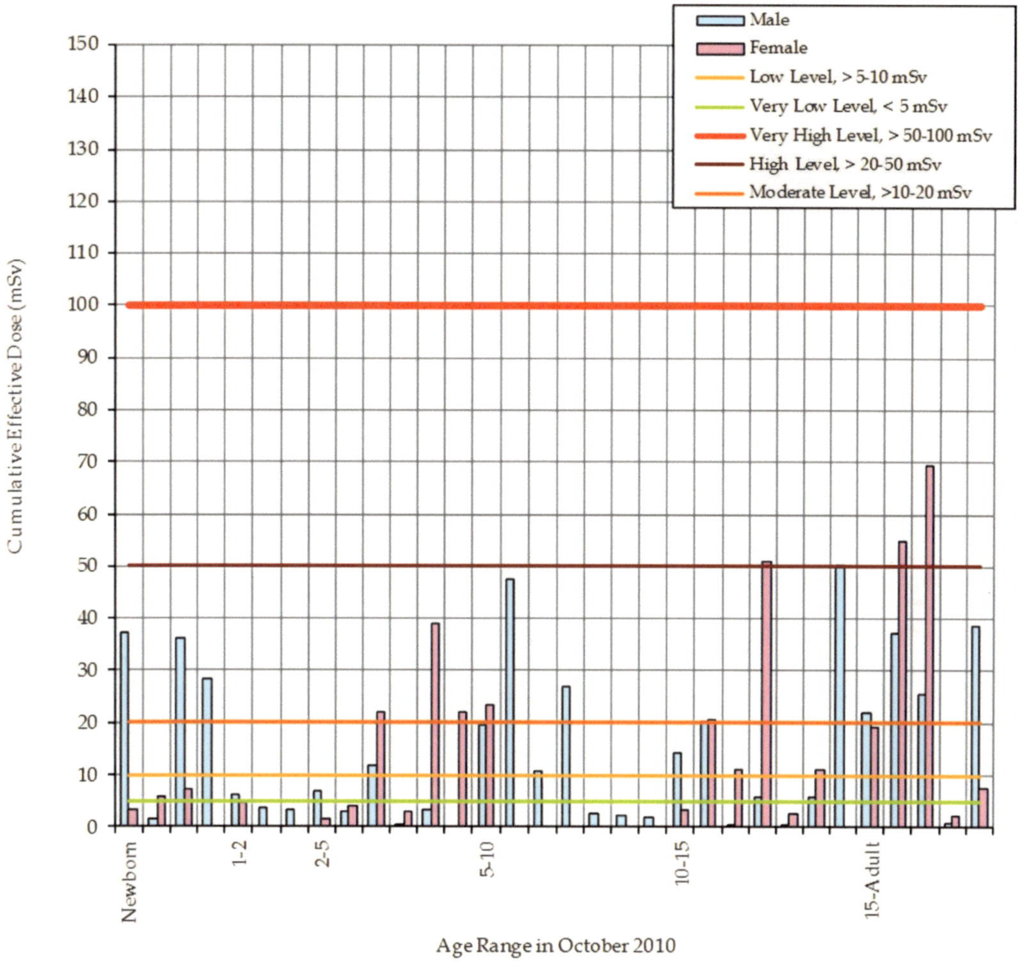

Fig. 7. Cumulative effective dose of pediatric patients according to age and gender

4. Discussion

Increased use of CT from new protocols and advances in technology means higher radiation dose in the patient population. Knowing the doses for CT protocols delivered through actual clinical studies in any radiology department is an important step towards developing reasonable strategies to optimize CT protocols and minimize unnecessary exposure. Understanding the physician's referral process and quantitative data about the numbers and types of procedures a patient has undergone is a useful aid to assessing the cumulative dose received by the patient.

Recent studies (Fazel et al., 2009 & Berrington et al., 2009) revealed higher-than-expected radiation dose in clinical CT studies and increased lifetime potential cancer risks as a result. The Northern California Childhood Leukemia Study in October 2010 has shown an increased risk of leukemia in pediatric patients that have had 3 or more radiology exams.

This study was intended to reveal the level of exposure and establish the scale of cumulative dose received by the pediatric patient population in a Private Tertiary Hospital in Saudi

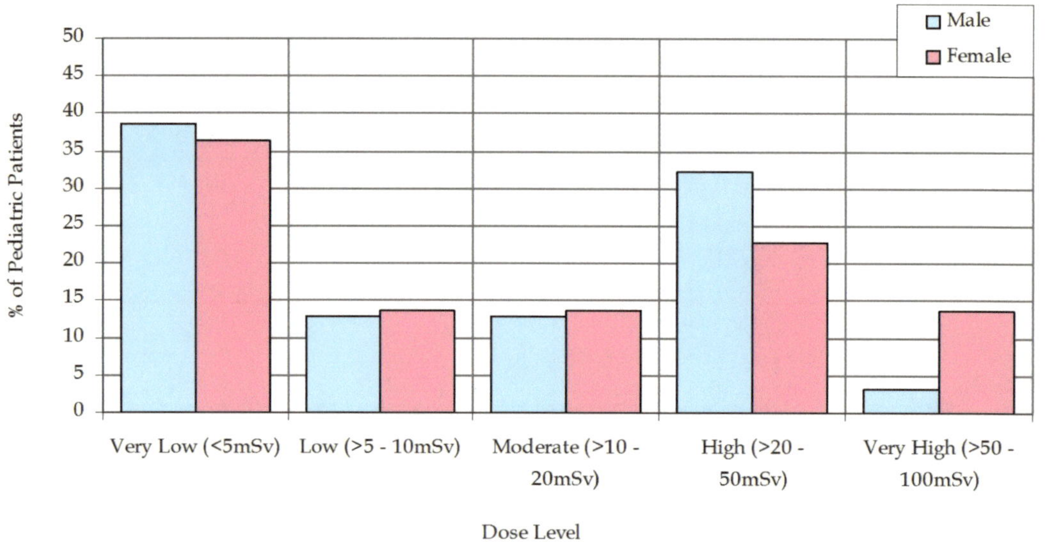

Fig. 8. Frequency of cumulative Effective Dose of pediatric patients according to dose level

Arabia. Calculating the radiation dose in clinical CT studies helped to establish reference dose levels for standard routine exams. In order to ensure justification of the exposure, benefit to the patient and to minimize risk to the individual, findings of the study have helped to develop protocols to address any inappropriate CT use and also started a process for monitoring cumulative dose to patients.

Considering the significant proportion of patients (55%, n=29, of our patient) undergoing multiple CT scans, often of the same body region, the cumulative effective dose easily reaches moderate to high levels and a small proportion, (7.5%, n=4, of our patients) reach very high levels of cumulative effective dose from CT alone.

As an indicator of the level of exposure and associated risk patients have accumulated from CT imaging procedures, simply knowing the number of procedures is not adequate, the type of procedure, body region exposed and number of scans in each procedure should also be known. From the number of scans a patient has undertaken, the body region and technique should also be known.

Using the dose length product as a dose metric is limited unless body region is also known. The effective dose calculated for a scan technique is the only indicator at present that provides the information necessary to estimate the associated biological damage and risk from cumulative procedures.

In order to provide accurate estimates, complete details of the procedure are necessary. However effective dose was not intended to provide individual doses but to provide a reference for the level of radiation dose to a standard sized adult phantom exposed under specific conditions. To measure the true dose to a patient would require direct measurement at the time of scanning.

Children are particularly sensitive to radiation from imaging scans and cumulative radiation dose to their developing bodies could well have adverse effects over time

In this study we have looked at the main clinical applications of CT in symptomatic pediatric patients and focused on the increasing number of CT scans being obtained and the associated radiation effective doses. To find that over one third of the pediatric patients have reached high to very high levels of effective dose from just CT imaging is of great concern.

The 7.5% (n=4) of pediatric patients who have reached very high levels of cumulative effective dose were reviewed for justification and benefit and to assess if any recommendations regarding future CT imaging can be determined.

Investigation of and justification of the 4 patients receiving very high levels of cumulative effective dose are now presented.

The first case was a 14.9 year old female who underwent a single procedure, dual source Coronary CTA child protocol, involving 3 helical scans, 1 pre monitoring axial scan and 4 IV bolus monitoring axial scans. Her resulting cumulative effective dose was estimated to be 51 mSv.

This patient had previous cardiac surgery and congenital anomaly of the aorta (right sided aortic arch and descending aorta), she had CT thorax (3 phases), an un-enhanced phase needed to trigger the contrast during maximum arterial opacification in the next arterial phase. The Venous phase was also done (resulting in approximately 18mSv, but could have been avoided).

The second case was a 17year old female who underwent a single urogram procedure involving 5 helical scans, (un-enhanced, arterial, venous and two delayed). Her resulting cumulative effective dose was estimated to be 55 mSv.

This patient's radiation exposure history also revealed 3 dynamic functional scintigraphy renograms using Tc-99m. The CT was performed to know the cause of bilateral pelviureteric junction partial obstruction, and the renogram preoperative to assess split renal function, intraoperative fluoroscopic guidance and postoperative renogram to asses split renal function. Proper and complete preoperative assessment necessitated the 5 phases in this patient.

The third case was a 12.8 year old male who underwent 2 procedures, the first procedure Carotid DSACT in May 2009 involved 3 helical scans plus 1 pre-monitoring axial scan and 3 IV bolus monitoring axial scans. The second procedure in October 2010 involved 4 helical scans (un-enhanced, arterial, venous and delayed). His resulting cumulative effective dose was estimated to be 51mSv.

This patient with neurofibromatosis diagnosed first by MRI of the neck and the brain had CTA of the neck for preoperative assessment of cervical carotid arteries and internal jugular veins. His follow-up examination was requested by the radiologist to be MRI but the patient had a CT of the head and neck to avoid the long MRI procedure and cost.

The final case was a 17.6 year old female who underwent 3 procedures, the first procedure, CT head in May 2009 involved 1 helical scan, the second procedure, CT Urogram in September 2009 involved 5 helical scans and the third procedure, CT pelvis involved 3 helical scans. Her resulting cumulative effective dose was estimated to be 69mSv.

This patient presented to the ER with severe headache, CT of the brain was done which showed abnormalities, further assessment was done by MRI. She had cerebral sinus thrombosis so, as diagnostic work-up CT of the abdomen and pelvis was done to exclude malignancy, it showed ovarian mass which was operated upon, her follow-up CT examination revealed, contralateral ovarian mass, all her follow-up examinations are now MRI and US.

Recommendations; reduce the scan range, reduce the number of phases, avoid un-enhanced and venous phases if possible and promote an awareness to the physician, radiologist and technologist about which procedures require high dose protocols. Record the estimated effective dose of the procedures in the patient's health records to avoid or minimize future CT imaging and follow up using Ultrasound and MRI.

Before this study was undertaken these figures were untracked and unmonitored. These results have helped to look at ways to implement guidelines for utilizing CT whilst balancing the risks of CT imaging with the clinical benefits.

Pediatric radiologists are best able to appreciate the challenges of imaging a child's small anatomy, faster breathing and heartbeat and the challenges of minimizing radiation dose to these patients. The challenge starts with the proper order of test, minimizing the area exposed, proper use of child settings, weight dependent to avoid over exposure, the use of special protocols for children and a full understanding of the childhood disorder.

The Image Gently campaign is an effort to ensure that medical protocols for imaging children keep pace with technological advances. It focuses on reducing CT dose for individual protocols and procedures, but a bigger concern is raised here about the use of CT diagnostic imaging and the consequence in cumulative effective dose to pediatric patients. Efforts to reduce the radiation effective dose to children if and when they need a CT scan must always be made. Any measure taken and every effort made for each individual child has a collective effect on the whole population.

Some of the steps that can be taken to reduce cumulative effective dose to children include applying measures to reduce, or child-size, the amount of radiation used for imaging children. Scanning only when necessary, ensuring that the risk benefit ratio is in favor of the exam ensuring that all previous and possible future exams are considered.

Only scanning the indicated region and only scanning once. Reducing the scan length and multiphase imaging can significantly reduce effective dose. Due to their smaller body size, organs are much closer and likely to receive greater levels of scattered radiation, reducing the scan region can help to reduce the amount of scattered radiation reaching critical organs not required in the image. Multiphase imaging significantly increases the effective dose of a procedure, it should rarely be used in children and each phase should be justified.

The Image Gently campaign also urges providers who perform imaging exams on children to work with medical physicists in order to monitor pediatric CT techniques, and to involve the radiology technologists to optimize scanning. The Image Gently website (www.imagegently.org) provides information describing how to achieve these goals. Achieving CT dose optimization and utilization is a team effort that will ensure that the radiation safety of the patient is considered and balanced with the clinical needs of the patient. A system of monitoring needs to be established in order to track dose, procedures and associated risks for individuals.

5. Conclusions

The likely effective doses received have been estimated with an acceptable level of accuracy for the purposes of risk assessment. The effective doses estimated support the conclusion that the level of exposure is high from CT and monitoring CT procedures performed on individuals certainly needs to be established. At the very minimum an easy to obtain dose metric such as the dose length product from a procedure should be considered for record in the patient file. Ideally effective dose, calculated for the individual undergoing the procedure to better estimate the risk estimates could be determined for that individual. These conclusions reflect the difference in the magnitude and circumstances of an individual's exposure.

Publication of the dose assessment, either the total dose length product or the effective dose of the procedure on the final CT report will benefit the physician and radiologist in providing quantitative information to the extent of doses received by the individual to enable appropriate risk benefit and justification of future procedures involving ionising radiation to the individual.

However without prior knowledge of the extent of an individual patient's exposure to ionizing radiation, or the number of previous CT procedures performed, as was the current situation, the number of patients exceeding a high level of radiation effective dose can be much higher than expected.

This study shows that unless precautions are taken to control the use of CT, pediatric patients have the potential to receive doses in excess of 50mSv very easily and very quickly during a hospital stay.

Although doses to patients undergoing CT procedures will be of low radiological significance in the majority of circumstances, the potential for the numbers of these procedures to increase for an individual is there which can mean that for a small proportion of patient's very high cumulative radiation doses can be reached, increasing their personal stochastic risks to a significant level.

Children are at a greater risk of receiving higher doses over their lifetime. With a proportion already exceeding 50mSv by the age of 18, what lies ahead.........

6. Recommendations

Physicians need to be aware of estimates of the effective doses of procedures requested; this can be achieved by providing reference levels for commonly performed procedures and training programs.

Alternative modalities either not involving ionizing radiation such as MRI and Ultrasound or procedures involving less ionizing radiation such as certain nuclear medicine or general radiology procedures should be considered by physicians and radiologists.

Patient radiation exposure history needs to be included in the patient file and be reviewable by the physician and radiologist to help in the management of further imaging.

Patients undergoing CT should have the patient protocol of the procedure archived along with the images. The dose length product and scanned range should be included in the final CT report by the radiologist.

Precautions in over utilization of CT need to be established.

Optimized, appropriately used procedures performed with full justification and consideration of the risk benefit for the individual patients' circumstances prior to a procedure being performed do not pose concern, but it should be borne in mind that a CT procedure is always associated with a radiation effective dose to the patient which can increase their risk of a future cancer or other genetic or hereditary detriment and every effort should be made to reduce that risk. The control of CT exposure and associated issues should be under an organization management policy of dose reduction, particularly in consideration to pediatric CT imaging.

7. References

Berrington, A., González, D., Mahesh, M., et al., (2009). Projected Cancer Risks From Computed Tomographic Scans Performed in the United States in 2007. Archives of Internal Medicine Vol. 169 (22) (2009), 2071-2077.

Bongartz, G., Golding, S.J., Jurik, A.G. et al., (2004). European Guidelines for Multislice Computed Tomography. European Commission. URL:www.msct.eu/CT_Quality_Criteria.

Brody, A.S., Frush, D.P., Huda, W., et al. (2007). Radiation Risk to Children from Computed Tomography. Pediatrics Vol. 120 No. 3 (Sep 2007), 677-682.

Fazel, R., Krumholz, H.M., Wang, Y., et al., (2009). Exposure to Low-Dose Ionizing Radiation from Medical Imaging Procedures. The New England Journal of Medicine Vol. 361 No. 9 (Aug 2009),849-857.

Fujii, K., Aoyama, S. & Kawaura, C., (2007). Comparative evaluation of organ and effective doses for pediatric patients with those for adults in chest and abdominal CT examinations. The British Journal of Radiology, 80 (2007), 657-667.

ICRP (1991). 1990 Recommendations of the International Commission on Radiological Protection. ICRP Publication 60. Oxford: Pergamon Press, 1990.

ICRP (2007). Managing Patient Dose in Multi-Detector Computed Tomography (MDCT). ICRP Publication 102. Volume 37 No. 1 2007. Elsevier.

ImPACT: Imaging Performance Assessment of CT Scanners, ImPACT CT Patient Dosimetry Calculator. (2009), version 1.0.2 12/11/2009. URL:www.impactscan.org

Jones, D.J. & Shrimpton, P.C., (1993). Survey of CT Practice in the UK Part 3: Normalised Organ Doses Calculated using Monte Carlo Techniques. NRPB-R250 and associated Software NRPB-SR250. National Radiological Protection Board, Oxon.

Khursheed, A., Hillier, M.C., Shrimpton, P.C. et al. (2002). Influence of patient age on normalized effective doses calculated for CT examinations. The British Journal of Radiology; 75 (2002), 819-830.

Mettler, F.A., Wiest, P.W., Locken, J.A., et al., (2000). Radiation Risks to Children from Computed Tomography. Journal of Radiological Protection; 20 (2000), 353-359.

Shrimpton, P.C., Hillier, M.C., Lewis, M.A., et al., (2005). Doses from Computed Tomography (CT) Examinations in the UK – 2003 Review. NRPB-W67. National Radiological Protection Board, Oxon.

Stecker, M.S., Balter S., Towbin, R., et al., (2009). Guidelines for patient radiation dose management. Journal of Vascular and Interventional Radiology, 20 (2009), s263-s273.

Wall, B.F., Kedall. G.M., Edwards, A.A. et al., (2006),What are the risks from medical X-rays and other low dose radiation? The British Journal of Radiology, 79 (2006), 285-294.

20

Dose Reduction on Computed Tomography Angiography Using Adaptive Control Techniques

Zhijun Cai[1], Er-Wei Bai[1] and Ge Wang[2]
[1]*University of Iowa*
[2]*Virginia Polytechnic Institute & State University*
USA

1. Introduction

With the advent of multi-slice computed tomography (CT) scanner and the sophisticated CT reconstruction algorithm, CT Angiography (CTA) is increasingly used to evaluate patient with vascular diseases (Fleischmann et al., 2006; Chow & Rubin, 2002; Rubin at al., 2001). It has many advantages over the conventional catheter angiograms: 1) non-invasiveness, 2) short acquisition time, 3) multiple viewing methods, and 4) low cost. However, the radiation exposure of CT scan has become of a wide concern due to its induction to genetic, cancerous and other diseases (Brenner et al., 2001; de Gonzalez & Darby et al., 2004). According to (Mettler et al., 2000), CT scan delivers 2/3 of the total radiation dose every year in US, and this number is climbing. On June 19th, 2007, the New York Times reported that "the per-capita dose of ionizing radiation from clinical imaging exams in the U.S. increased almost 600% from 1980 to 2006". Brenner (Brenner et al., 2001) reported that diagnostic X-rays, indicating that radiation from medical and dental scans, cause about 700 cases of cancer per year in Britain and more than 5,600 cases in US. To that end, every effort to reduce the radiation dose is appreciated and the well-known ALARA (As Low As Reasonably Achievable) principle is widely accepted in the medical community.
There are many studies have been reported on dose reduction for CT scan. Wintersperger and his colleagues (Wintersperger et al., 2000) used lower kilo voltage and claimed the resultant image had similar sensitivity and accuracy. In Fraioli's studies (Fraioli et al., 2006), lower tube currents were used and the resultant image quality was claimed to be good enough for diagnosis. Generally, dose reduction is contrary to the image quality. In other words, reducing the radiation dose will sacrifice the image quality. However, with the advanced CT reconstruction algorithm (Yan et al., 2008; Zeng et al., 2007; Liu et al., 2009; Yin et al., 2009) and post-processing techniques (Salmon et al., 2009; Benitez et al., 2009; Zeng et al., 2008; Zhang et al., 2008), the resultant images could be held to certain diagnosis level while the radiation dose is reduced lot. Recently, control technique is found very useful in CT. It can be applied to improve the CT image quality (Lu et al., 2008; H. Bai et al., 2008), and to reduce the radiation dose reduction, for example, Automatic Exposure Control (AEC) program, which modulates the tube current to maintain the same x-ray attenuation level according to the scan angle/position of the human body.

In this chapter, we present a radiation dose reduction approach using adaptive control techniques. It is specifically for CTA scan and is based on the adaptive bolus chasing techniques. The adaptive bolus chasing techniques are capable of tracking the contrast bolus peak during the CTA scan, and ensure every segment of the blood vessel to be scanned with the possible highest bolus density. To that end, it is very likely that segment of vasculature is scanned with a much higher Contrast to Noise Ratio (CNR), which is better than enough for diagnosing. With the ALARA principle, it is straightforward to modulate the tube current and/or vary the table increment to reduce the radiation dose while keeping the resultant CT images at the same diagnosis level.

2. Method

Adaptive bolus chasing techniques, the basis of the proposed dose reduction approach, will be introduced first. After that, we will show how to estimate the radiation exposure during a CTA scan followed by the introduction of the proposed scan scheme to reduce the radiation exposure.

2.1 Adaptive bolus chasing CTA

The proposed dose reduction approach is made possible by the adaptive bolus chasing CTA techniques, which will be briefly introduced in this subsection. More details can be found in (E.W. Bai et al., 2007).

In a CTA scan, the contrast bolus is used to enhance the vasculature so that it can be distinguished from the surrounding soft tissue, which has similar physical property of the vasculature (Tublin et al., 1999; Sheafor et al., 1998). During the CTA san, it is desirable to synchronize the contrast peak and CT imaging aperture, in such a way, the CNR is maximized and the vascular diseases on resultant CT images are better shown. However, the current scan method uses a pre-set constant speed to move the CT table, which is problematic due to the complicated bolus dynamics influenced by many factors such as, patient characteristics, injection patterns, and vascular diseases (Cademartiri et al., 2002). The contrast bolus rarely flows constantly along the blood vessels. Therefore, the current constant-speed method either needs a large amount of contrast volume or results in lower CNR vascular images due to the unmatched the longitudinal position of the bolus peak and CT imaging aperture.

The adaptive bolus chasing techniques are illustrated in Fig. 1. The patient is feeding into the CT gantry at the speed of the CT table. The real-time CT images are reconstructed and meanwhile the intravascular bolus density information is extracted and fed into the adaptive bolus chasing controller. The controller uses the past and current bolus density information and the knowledge of the bolus dynamics to predict the bolus peak time for the next position and sends the signal to the table driver to vary the CT table speed accordingly. Thus, the synchronization of the bolus peak and CT imaging aperture will be realized.

2.2 Radiation dose calculation in CT scan

Generally, the effective radiation dose is affected by the tube voltage, collimator width, tube current, scanning time, and scan volume (Kalender, 2005). The following procedure is used to estimate the effective radiation dose for a CT scan.

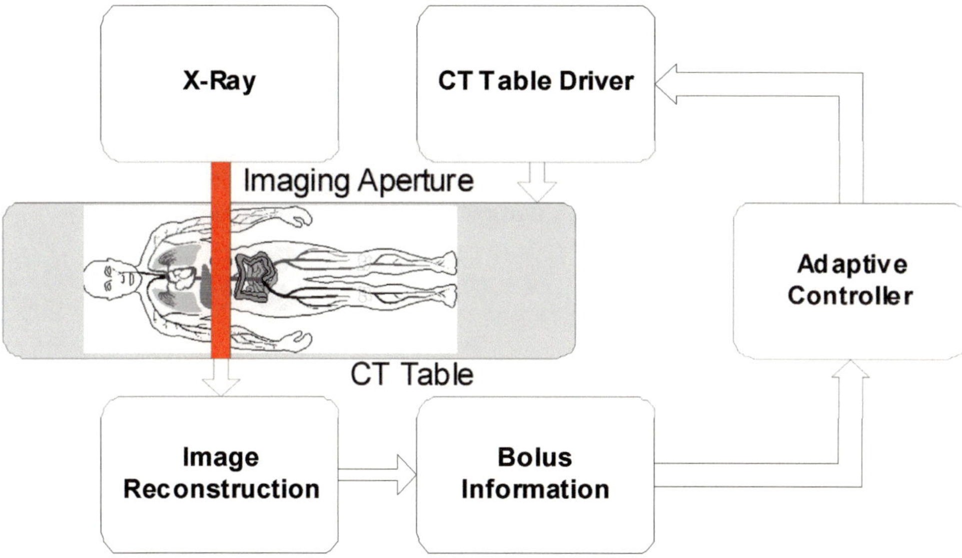

Fig. 1. Illustration of control scheme for adaptive bolus chasing CTA

1. Find the normalized weighted CT dose index (CTDI) at a specified voltage, which is given by

$$ {}_n\mathrm{CTDI}_w = \left(\frac{1}{3}\mathrm{CTDI}_{100,c} + \frac{2}{3}\mathrm{CTDI}_{100,p} \right) \tag{1} $$

where ${}_n\mathrm{CTDI}_w$ denotes the normalized CTDI at 100 mAs (product of tube current and gantry rotation time), and $\mathrm{CTDI}_{100,c}$ and $\mathrm{CTDI}_{100,p}$ represent the measurement of phantom center and the average measurement at four different locations around the periphery of the phantom, respectively. For instance, $\mathrm{CTDI}_{100,c}$ and $\mathrm{CTDI}_{100,p}$ are 4.6 and 9.7, respectively, for Siemens Volume Zoom CT scanner with 120kV.

2. Compute the CTDI_{vol}. Most CTA scans are spiral scan, and adaptive bolus chasing techniques are only applicable to spiral scan; therefore, we need to compute the CTDI_{vol} for spiral scan.

$$ \mathrm{CTDI}_{vol} = {}_n\mathrm{CTDI}_w \frac{W}{T} IT_r \tag{2} $$

where CTDI_{vol}, W, T, I and Tr denote CTDI volume, collimator width, tube current and gantry rotation time, respectively. W/T is called pitch in CT scan, and product of I and T_r is the effective tube current.

3. Calculate the dose length product (DLP), which is formulated as

$$ DLP = \mathrm{CTDI}_{vol} \times L \tag{3} $$

where L is the total scan length.

4. Convert the absorbed dose to effective radiation dose E

$$ E = E_{DLP} \times DLP \tag{4} $$

where E_{DLP} is the region-specific conversion factor, and it equals to 0.015 for abdomen and pelvis (Shrimpton, 2009).
The above calculation is based on the constant-pitch (speed), which is not the case for the adaptive bolus chasing CTA scan. In the adaptive bolus chasing CTA scan, the CT table speed varies according to the bolus movement in the patient's vasculature. To that end, we need to modify the formula accordingly. In step 2), CTDI_{vol} is computed at every step (gantry rotation time) under assumption that gantry rotation time is kept constant

$$\mathrm{CDTI}_{vol,i} = {}_{n}\mathrm{CDTI}_{w}\frac{W_i}{T_i}I_iT_r \tag{5}$$

Accordingly, the *DLP* is changed to

$$DLP = \sum_{i=1}^{N}\mathrm{CDTI}_{vol,i}T_i = \sum_{i=1}^{N}\underbrace{{}_{n}\mathrm{CDTI}_{w}T_r}_{C_D}W_iI_i \tag{6}$$

where T_i is the table increment at each step and N is total number of gantry rotation.

Remark

It seems that T_i is not related to *DLP* in Eq. (6); however, T_i affects the total number of gantry rotation. Higher average T_i results in smaller N. With all other parameters kept constant, total *DLP* is smaller.

2.3 Dose reduction approach using adaptive bolus chasing CTA techniques

Dose reduction can be achieved under the condition that the resultant CT images are good enough for diagnosis, which is subjective. Different physicians may have different diagnosis results for the same set of CT images. On the other hand, CT image quality is affected by many factors, such as, image noise, signal to noise ratio, antifacts and resolution. It is hard to find a standard that quantifies the image quality. Here, we focus on the CNR or Signal to Noise Ratio (SNR). Meanwhile, we restrict the spatial resolution (slice thickness) within some range.
The idea of the dose reduction approach is as follows. Since the proposed bolus chasing CTA techniques are capable of tracking the contrast bolus peak, and the scanned blood vessels are well enhanced, according to the literature, most of the segments have CT number greater than 250 HU. On the other hand, "the minimum adequate goal for contrast opcification of arterial system is 150 -200 HU" (Rubin & Rofsky, 2008). Therefore, we can modulate the tube current (and the collimator width) to achieve the desired CNR and reduce the radiation dose meanwhile.

2.3.1 Modulating the tube current

In this subsection, we propose a radiation dose reduction approach only through modulating the tube current to maintain the minimum CNR to certain level at each step. Varying the tube current and collimator width simultaneously will be presented in the next subsection.
Since we only modulate the tube current and the collimator width is kept constant, the image noise and CT number of blood vessel at step i is denoted by $\sigma_i = C_\sigma / \sqrt{I_i}$ and C_i, respectively, then the CNR at step i is $CNR_i = \sqrt{I_i}C_i / C_\sigma$ under assumption that the CT

number of the surrounding tissue is zero (or a constant value). In the adaptive bolus chasing techniques (E.W. Bai et al., 2007), we use a two-variate 2nd order polynomial to approximate the bolus density function,

$$B_i(z,t) = a_0(z_i,t_i) + a_1(z_i,t_i)t + a_2(z_i,t_i)z + a_3(z_i,t_i)t^2 + a_4(z_i,t_i)tz + a_5(z_i,t_i)z^2 \quad (7)$$

where t and z represent the time and distant starting at the current time and position, respectively. Substitute $t = T_r = \Delta t$ and replace z with T_i (table increment at the step i), then we have

$$CNR_i = C_c\sqrt{I_i}\left(\bar{a}_0 + \bar{a}_1 T_i + \bar{a}_2 T_i^2\right) \quad (8)$$

where $\bar{a}_0 = a_0(t_i,z_i) + a_1(t_i,z_i)\Delta t + a_3(t_i,z_i)\Delta t^2$, $\bar{a}_1 = a_2(t_i,z_i) + a_4(t_i,z_i)\Delta t$, and $\bar{a}_2 = a_5(t_i,z_i)$.

Now, we can formulate the problem as follows:

Minimize the radiation dose (DLP) normalized over the table increment at every step, $C_D I_i / T_i$, under condition that CNR is kept constant or above a designated value, that is $C_c\sqrt{I_i}\left(\bar{a}_0 + \bar{a}_1 T_i + \bar{a}_2 T_i^2\right) \geq CNR_0$, and the longitudinal resolution is not worsen very much, which is quantified by the slice thickness. The optimal solution will be given when $C_c\sqrt{I_i}\left(\bar{a}_0 + \bar{a}_1 T_i + \bar{a}_2 T_i^2\right) = CNR_0$.

Lagrange multiplier is used to solve this problem

$$J = C_D \frac{I_i}{T_i} + \lambda\left[C_c\sqrt{I_i}\left(\bar{a}_0 + \bar{a}_1 T_i + \bar{a}_2 T_i^2\right) - CNR_0\right] \quad (9)$$

The solution of the above problem is

$$T_i = \frac{-3\bar{a}_1 - \sqrt{9\bar{a}_1^2 - 20\bar{a}_0\bar{a}_2}}{10\bar{a}_2} \quad (10)$$

and the corresponding estimated bolus density at T_i is

$$\hat{B}_i = \bar{a}_0 + \bar{a}_1 T_i + \bar{a}_2 T_i^2 \quad (11)$$

Remark

Generally, the bolus density profile is bell-shaped (Cademartiri, 2002), to that end, $\bar{a}_2$ is negative, and $\bar{a}_1$ and $\bar{a}_0$ are positive. Without the dose reduction optimization, $T_0 = -\bar{a}_1 / (2\bar{a}_2)$ maximizes the bolus density at the next step. However, in the dose reduction approach, table increment

$$T_i = \frac{-3\bar{a}_1 - \sqrt{9\bar{a}_1^2 - 20\bar{a}_0\bar{a}_2}}{10\bar{a}_2} > \frac{-3\bar{a}_1}{5\bar{a}_2} > \frac{-\bar{a}_1}{2\bar{a}_2} > T_0$$

It is reasonable because table increment is expected to be maximized under the condition the next scan affords enough *CNR*.

Adaptive bolus chasing with dose optimization procedure through modulating tube current only

1. Identify the local bolus model, a two-variate 2nd order polynomial online as in Eq. (7). See details in (E.W. Bai et al., 2007)
2. Substitute the Δt in Eq. (7) to obtain $\overline{a}_0$, $\overline{a}_1$, and $\overline{a}_2$
3. Use Eq. (10) to compute T_i
4. Modulate tube current using $I_i = \left(B_0/\hat{B}_i\right)^2 I_0$
5. Translate the CT table for distance T_i in time Δt
6. Until the preset length is scanned.

Remark

This algorithm alone does not guarantee that the whole vasculature length be scanned. However, by setting the minimum moving distance at each step, it is no longer a problem. This is reasonable because scanning the vasculature forever contradicts minimizing the radiation dose.

2.3.2 Modulating the tube current and collimator width

Adaptive-chasing method varies the table increment T_i at each step, and changes the pitch p accordingly, since $p=T_i/W$, where W is the collimator width. Under condition that the collimator width is constant, the slice thickness, which depends on the collimator width and table increment (see (2)), also varies. This is not good to the image quality in the sense that the longitudinal spatial resolution is not uniform. To that end, we propose to modulate the tube current and collimator width simultaneously to reduce the radiation dose and maintain the slice thickness constant.

Assume uniform slice thickness, S_0, is expected for the whole scan. For a single slice CT and half-scan reconstruction method, the slice thickness is given by

$$S_0 = \sqrt{\frac{W^2}{12} + \frac{T^2}{24}} \tag{13}$$

see (Wang & Vannier, 1984).

To keep slice thickness constant, we need to vary the collimator width at each step

$$W_i = \sqrt{12S_0^2 - \frac{T_i^2}{2}} \tag{14}$$

Adaptive bolus chasing with dose optimization procedure through modulating tube current and collimator width

1. Identify the local bolus model, a two-variate 2nd order polynomial online as in Eq. (7)). See details in (E.W. Bai et al., 2007)
2. Substitute the Δt in Eq. (7) to have have $\overline{a}_0$, $\overline{a}_1$, and $\overline{a}_2$
3. Use Eq. (10) to obtain T_i
4. Use Eq. (14) to obtain W_i
5. Modulate tube current using $I_i = \left(B_0/\hat{B}_i\right)^2 I_0 W_0 / W_i$
6. Translate the CT table for distance T_i in time Δt
7. Until the preset length is scanned.

3. Results

We applied the proposed dose reduction approach on the referenced digital subtraction angiogram (DSA) data sets of four patients, among which, two had occlusive diseases; one had abdominal aneurysm and one was normal. To show the advantage of the proposed method, we compared the conventional constant-speed method on the same referenced data sets. The high frame DSA data sets were collected in University of Iowa Hospital and Clinic (UIHC). They recorded the bolus information in the abdominal-aorta to the femoral artery from the time of bolus injection to the end. We extracted the bolus information along the blood vessel from every frame and formed the bolus 3D profile (position-time-density), which would be used as the referenced bolus information. It is known that the CTA data sets do not have this ability due to its narrow FOV in the longitudinal direction short acquisition time.

The CTA scan is assumed to be performed on the Siemens SOMATON Volume Zoom four-row detector CT scanner, and spiral scan mode is used. The peak Kilo-Voltage is set to 120 kV for both adaptive-chasing and constant-speed method. As for constant-speed method, we set the effective tube-current and collimator width to be 240 mAs and 10 mm, respectively. The resultant CNR of the vasculature is expected to be greater than or equal to 200 HU over the noise level generated by the above voltage, current and collimator settings.

During the simulation, the constant speed is set as 30mm/sec for all four cases. For adaptive-chasing method, the collimator width is fixed at 10mm and the pitch varies between 0.5 and 2, which also limited the CT table speed. As for the case of varying collimator width, the scanned HU results will be same. The difference is on the reconstructed CT image, and it is not discussed in this Chapter. Both methods use auto-trigged technique to start the CT table, i.e., monitor the HU in the designated region of interest (ROI), and starts the CT table when the HU reaches the pre set threshold.

The effective radiation doses for four patients are estimated in the way aforementioned in Section 2.2. To show the performance of the adaptive-chasing method and the constant-speed method, we use the performance index (PI), which is defined as

$$PI = \frac{\sum_{k=1}^{N} \hat{B}\left(z_k, \hat{t}_k\right)}{\sum_{k=1}^{N} B\left(z_k, t_k\right)} \tag{15}$$

where $B\left(z_k, t_k\right)$ is the actual maximum density at position z_k, which happens at time t_k, and $\hat{B}\left(z_k, \hat{t}_k\right)$ is the observed density at position z_k, scanned at time $\hat{t}_k$. The higher the PI, the better the performance is. However, due to the limitation on the CT table velocity and acceleration, *PI* is less than 1.

Fig. 2 to Fig. 5 show the patient vascular diseases and corresponding simulated scan results (CT number of the vasculature) of the adaptive-chasing and constant-speed method results. In most of the time, the scanned CT number of adaptive-chasing method (dash-dot curve) is greater than that of the constant-speed method (dashed curve).

Table 1 shows the estimated effective dose and PI for adaptive-chasing and constant-speed method, respectively. We can see that adaptive-chasing method reduces the effective dose, on average, 39% of the constant-speed method, and PI increases about 17%.

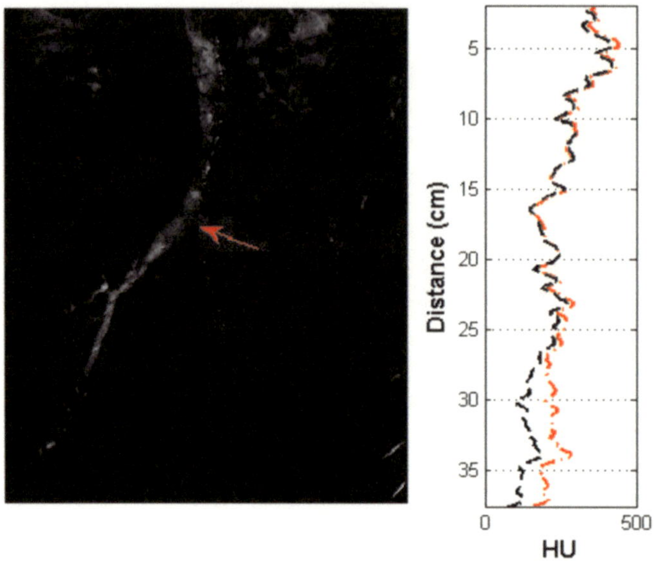

Fig. 2. The left plot is one of the DSA angiogram. It shows the occlusive vascular disease. The right plot shows the scan results of the adaptive-chasing method (dash-dot) and the constant-speed method (dashed).

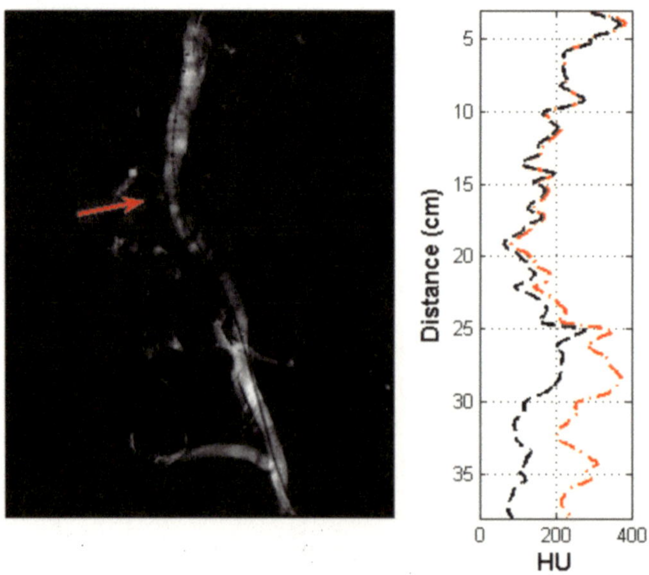

Fig. 3. The left plot is one of the DSA angiogram. It shows the occlusive vascular disease. The right plot shows the scan results of the adaptive-chasing method (dash-dot) and the constant-speed method (dashed).

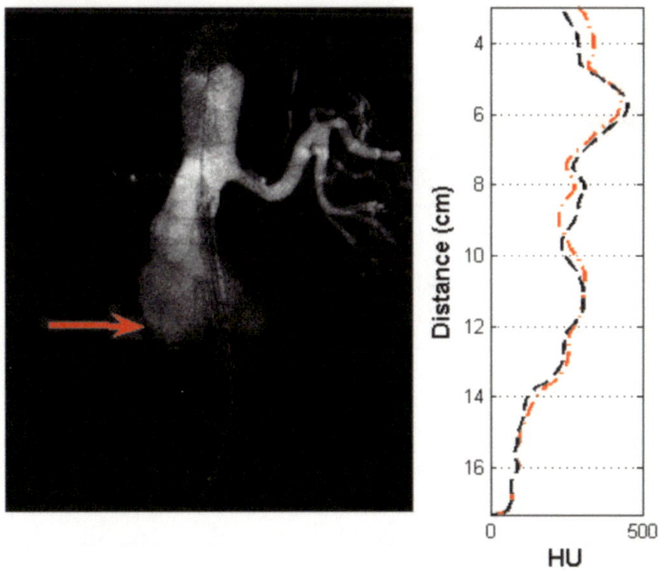

Fig. 4. The left plot is one of the DSA angiogram. It shows the abdominal aneurysm disease. The right plot shows the scan results of the adaptive-chasing method (dash-dot) and the constant-speed method (dashed).

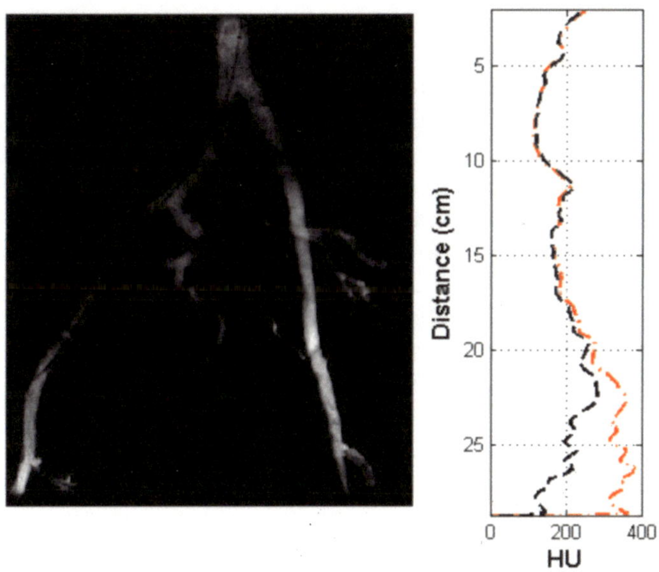

Fig. 5. The left plot is one of the DSA angiogram. No evident vascular disease is shown. The right plot shows the scan results of the adaptive-chasing method (dash-dot) and the constant-speed method (dashed).

Patient	Disease	Adaptive-Chasing method		Constant-Speed method	
		EED (msv)	PI	*EED* (msv)	PI
Patient 1	occlusive	4.95	0.97	10.73	0.84
Patient 2	occlusive	6.22	0.97	10.94	0.70
Patient 3	aneurysm	3.52	0.89	4.95	0.89
Patient 4	normal	6.57	0.96	8.25	0.79
Average		5.32	0.95	8.72	0.81

* *EED*: Estimated effective dose

Table 1. Estimated effective dose and PI for the adaptive-chasing method and constant-speed method, respectively.

4. Discussion and conclusions

The adaptive bolus chasing CTA with dose reduction is a new concept in dose reduction. It saves the radiation dose in two ways: 1) generally lowering the tube current, which is made possible through adaptive-chasing method. Though the adaptive-chasing method does not guarantee the scanned HU is greater than the expected, it generally has greater performance than the constant-speed method, which is validated in our simulations, and 2) tracking the bolus peak trajectory. The adaptive-chasing method allows the CT table to move fast when it is necessary under the condition to maintain the CNR for the scanned vasculature As we know, the faster the scan the lower radiation dose if all other parameters are kept the same.

Although the simulation is performed on a four-row detector CT scanner, this dose reduction approach could be easily extended to the 16- or 64-row detector CT scanners. Generally, 16 or 64 slice CT scanner has a wider field of view (in z direction) and moves faster. It provides much more information in a shorter time. On one hand, it is good to the control algorithm because more bolus information will make the chasing results better; on the other hand, it requires more computation capacity and challenges the real time control. This problem could be solved in following ways: 1) fast reconstruction algorithm with the advanced CPU techniques, 2) part reconstruction, which only reconstruct the images that around the region of interest. Those images are only used for real time control and the high quality CT images will be reconstructed after the scan.

The constant-speed method is not so bad for this short injection. This is because we choose a relatively good pre-set threshold to start the CT table. It is hard to set the right threshold, but a lot of contrast dose would be used to compensate for the deficit of the constant-speed method. On the other hand, adaptive-chasing method is not sensitive to the pre-set threshold. It can adjust optimal starting time by itself.

Patient 3 has an aneurysm in the abdominal aorta. When the contrast bolus flows there, it stays inside for a while until it fills the aneurysm. It is like the prolonged maximum geometry. Hence, the constant-speed method has almost the same PI as adaptive-chasing method does. However, the adaptive-chasing method saves the radiation dose by lowering the tube current while the constant-speed method does not.

We did not apply uniform slice thickness method in the simulation because it would not change the table increment, product of the tube current and collimator width, and dose savage. The only difference is the varying collimator width. We will try this method for the experiment on the CT scanner and evaluate the resultant CT image quality.

In a summary, we have proposed an adaptive-chasing method with dose reduction. The proposed approach ensures the vasculature to be scanned with higher bolus density and maintains a minimum CNR. The effective radiation dose is reduced through modulating the tube current and using the possible minimum time to track the contrast bolus. Simulation results show that the adaptive-chasing method has greater PI than the constant-speed method (0.95 vs. 0.81) and the effective radiation dose is reduced 39% on average. The proposed techniques also have great potential in optimization of contrast agent, which may save the exam cost and benefit patient who has kidney diseases. To that end, the future work will be focused on two areas: 1) the real experiment and evaluation on the resultant CT images, and 2) optimization of contrast agent.

5. References

Bai, E.W.; Cai, Z., MCcabe, R. & Wang, G. (2008). An Adaptive Optimal Control Design for a Bolus Chasing Computed Tomography Angiography. *IEEE Transactions on Control Systems Technology*, Vol. 16, pp. 60-69, ISSN: 1063-6536.

Bai, H.; Zeng, K., Bai, E. W. & Wang, G. (2008). Manual control of patient table for bolus-chasing CT angiography, *Journal of X-Ray Science and Technology*, Vol. 16, pp. 23-31, ISSN 0895-3996

Benítez, R.B.; Ning, R., Conover, D. & Liu, S. (2009). NPS characterization and evaluation of a cone beam CT breast imaging system, *Journal of X-Ray Science and Technology*, 17, pp. 17-40, ISSN 0895-3996

Brenner, D.J.; Elliston, C.D., Hall, E.J. & Berdon, W.E. (2001). Estimated risks of radiation-induced fatal cancer from pediatric CT. *American Journal of Roentgenology*, Vol. 176(2), pp. 289-296, ISSN 0361-803X

Cademartiri, F., van der Lugt, A., Luccichenti, G. & Krestin G.P. (2002). Parameters affecting bolus geometry in CTA: a review. *J Comput Assist Tomogr*, Vol. 26(4), pp. 598-607, ISSN: 0363-8715

Chow, L.C. & Rubin, G.D. (2002). CT angiography of the arterial system, *Radiol Clin North Am*, Vol. 40(4), pp. 729-49, ISSN 0033-8389

de Gonzalez, A. B. & Darby, S. (2004). Risk of cancer from diagnostic X-rays: estimates for the UK and 14 other countries. *Lancet*, Vol. 363(9406), pp. 345-351, ISSN 0140-6736

Fleischmann, D.; Hallett, R.L. & Rubin, G.D. (2006). CT angiography of peripheral arterial disease, *J Vasc Interv Radiol*, Vol. 17(1), pp. 3-26, ISSN 1051-0443

Fraioli, F.; Catalano, C., Napoli, A., Francone, M., Venditti, F., Danti, M., Pediconi, F. and Passariello, R. (2006). Low-dose multidetector-row CT angiography of the infra-renal aorta and lower extremity vessels: image quality and diagnostic accuracy in comparison with standard DSA, *Eur Radiol*, Vol. 16: 137–146, ISSN: 0938-7994

Kalender, Willi A. (2005) Computed Tomography, Fundamentals, system Technology, image quality applications, publicis MCD Verlag, ISBN: 978-3-89578-081-2

Liu, T. & Xu, J. (2009). Differential reconstruction for planar object in computed tomography, *Journal of X-Ray Science and Technology*, Vol. 17, pp. 101-114, ISSN 0895-3996

Mettler, F.A. Jr.; Wiest, P.W., Locken, J.A., & Kelsey, C.A. (2000). CT scanning: Patterns of use and dose. *Journal of Radiological Protection*, Vol. 20(4), pp. 353-359, ISSN 1361-6498

Rubin G.D. & Rofsky, N.M. (2008), CT and MR Angiography: Comprehensive Vascular Assessment, Lippinocott Williams & Wilkins, ISBN 978-0-7817-4524-3, Philadelphia

Rubin, G.D.; Schmidt, A.J., Logan, L. J., Sofilos, M. C. (2001). Multi-detector row CT angiography of lower extremity arterial inflow and runoff: initial experience, *Radiology*, Vol. 221(1), pp. 146-58, ISSN 0033-8419

Salmon, P.L.; Liu, X. & Sasov, A. (2009). A post-scan method for correcting artefacts of slow geometry changes during micro-tomographic scans, *Journal of X-Ray Science and Technology*, Vol. 17, pp. 161-174, ISSN 0895-3996

Sheafor, D.H.; Keogan, M. T., DeLong, D.M. & Nelson, R.C. (1998). Dynamic helical CT of the abdomen: prospective comparison of pre- and postprandial contrast enhancement. *Radiology*, Vol. 206(2), pp. 359-63, ISSN 0033-8419

Shrimpton P.C. (2009). Assessment of patient dose in CT: appendix C—European guidelines for multislice computed tomography. *European Commission project MSCT: CT safety & efficacy–a broad perspective Web site.* http://www.msct.eu/PDF_FILES/EC%20CA%20Report%20D5%20-%20Dosimetry.pdf. Published March 2004. Accessed May 28, ISSN 1527- 1315

Tublin, M.E.; Tessler, F.N., Cheng, S. L., Peters, T. L., & McGovern, P. C. (1999). Effect of injection rate of contrast medium on pancreatic and hepatic helical CT. *Radiology*, Vol. 210(1), pp. 97-101, ISSN 0033-8419

Wang, G. & Vannier, M.M. (1984). Logitudinal resolution in volumetric x-ray computerized tomography-Analytical comparison between conventional and helical computerized tomography, *Med. Phys.* Vol. 21(3), pp. 429-433, ISSN: 0094-2405

Wintersperger, B.; Jakobs, T., Herzog, P., Schaller, S., Nikolaou, K., Suess, C., Weber, C., Reiser, M. & Becker, C. (2005). Aorto-iliac multidetector-row CT angiography with low kV settings: improved vessel enhancement and simultaneous reduction of radiation dose, *Eur Radiol*, Vol. 15, pp. 334–341, ISSN: 0938-7994

Yan, G.; Tian, J., Zhu, S. Dai, Y. & Qin, C. (2008). Fast cone-beam CT image reconstruction using GPU hardware, *Journal of X-Ray Science and Technology*, Vol. 16, pp. 225-234, ISSN 0895-3996

Yang, L.; Cai, Z., Wang G., Zhao, J. & Bai, E. W. (2009). Preliminary experimental results on controlled cardiac computed tomography: A phantom study, *Journal of X-Ray Science and Technology*, Vol. 17, pp. 175-187, ISSN 0895-3996

Yin, Z.; Khare, K. & De Man, B. (2009). Parametric boundary reconstruction algorithm for industrial CT metrology application, *Journal of X-Ray Science and Technology*, Vol. 17, pp. 115-133, ISSN 0895-3996

Zeng, K.; Bai, E.W. & Wang, Ge (2007). A Fast CT Reconstruction Scheme for a General Multi-Core PC, *Int J Biomed Imaging*, Published online 2007 July 9. doi: 10.1155/2007/29160, ISSN 1687-4196

Zeng, K.; Fajardo, L.L.; Kao, S., Franken, E. A., Park, Jeong M., Jing, Z., Bai, E.W. & Wang, G. (2008). An in vitro evaluation of cone-beam breast CT methods , *Journal of X-Ray Science and Technology*, Vol. 16, pp. 171-187, ISSN 0895-3996

Zhang, Y. & Ruola N. (2008). Investigation of image noise in cone-beam CT imaging due to photon counting statistics with the Feldkamp algorithm by computer simulations, *Journal of X-Ray Science and Technology*, Vol. 16, pp. 143-158, ISSN 0895-3996